FIVE KEYS
TO *Successful*
Nursing
Management

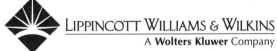

LIPPINCOTT WILLIAMS & WILKINS
A **Wolters Kluwer** Company

Philadelphia • Baltimore • New York • London
Buenos Aires • Hong Kong • Sydney • Tokyo

Staff

Publisher
Judith A. Schilling McCann, RN, MSN

Editorial Director
H. Nancy Holmes

Clinical Director
Joan M. Robinson, RN, MSN

Senior Art Director
Arlene Putterman

Clinical Editor
Kate McGovern, RN, MSN, CCRN
(project manager)

Editors
Jennifer P. Kowalak (senior associate editor), Stacey A. Follin

Copy Editors
Kimberly Bilotta, Heather Ditch, Amy Furman, Shana Harrington, Pamela Wingrod

Designers
Will Boehm (book designer), Donna S. Morris (project manager), Lynn Foulk, Elaine Kasmer

Cover Design
Larry Didona

Electronic Production Services
Diane Paluba (manager), Joyce Rossi Biletz (senior desktop assistant), Richard Eng

Manufacturing
Patricia K. Dorshaw (senior manager), Beth Janae Orr (book production coordinator)

Editorial Assistants
Danielle J. Barsky, Carol Caputo, Beverly Lane, Linda Ruhf

Librarian
Catherine M. Heslin

Indexer
Ellen S. Brennan

FKSNM – D N O S A
04 03 02   10 9 8 7 6 5 4 3 2 1

Library of Congress Cataloging-in-Publication Data
Five keys to successful nursing management.
    p. ; cm.
Includes index.
    1. Nursing services — Administration.
    [DNLM: 1. Nurse Administrators — organization & administration. 2. Leadership. 3. Nursing, Supervisory — organization & administration. WY 105 F565 2003] I. Lippincott Williams & Wilkins.
RT89 .F538 2003
362.1'73'068 — dc21
ISBN 1-58255-175-8 (pbk. : alk. paper)   2002008570

Contents

iii

PART THREE
Budgeting and finance skills

PART FOUR
Quality care skills

PART FIVE
Information technology skills

Contributors and consultants

Sally Austin, JD, ADN, BGS
Defense malpractice counsel
In-house legal counsel for several
 healthcare institutions
Marietta, Ga.

Marie Brewer, RN, LNC
Operations Manager
Georgia Pain Physicians/MD Pain
 Clinics of Georgia
Marietta

Gloria Ferraro Donnelly, RN, PhD,
 FAAN
Dean and Professor
College of Nursing & Health
 Professions
MCP Hahnemann University
Philadelphia

Melissa A. Fitzpatrick, RN, MSN,
 FAAN
Editor in Chief, *Nursing Management
 Journal*
Principal Healthcare Strategist, The
 Healthcare Division, SAS Institute
Cary, N.C.

George Harbeson, RN, MSN
President Elect American Nursing
 Informatics Association
Senior Systems Analyst
Texas Children's Hospital
Houston

Pamela S. Hunt, RN, MSN
Administrative Director of Surgical
 Services
Marion (Ind.) General Hospital

Martha Morris, RN, BSN, BC
Clinical Analyst, Project Manager
Borgess Hospital
Kalamazoo

Foreword

Over the years, I've had the privilege to work with so many of you — from the newest of nurse-managers to the most experienced in the profession. You've taught me about nursing management and all that it entails on a day-to-day basis. You've emphasized your firm standing in the health care system — right alongside the physicians. Most importantly, however, you've shared your common passion for safe, quality patient care.

Five Keys to Successful Nursing Management is for you because for nurse-managers — indeed, nurse *leaders* — quality patient care involves so much more than the best clinical bedside care. Whether you've been a nurse-manager for 2 or 20 years, this comprehensive text offers you hands-on practical advice for solving your day-to-day challenges. Its quick-reference style and clear guidelines will help you easily find new ways to succeed in today's evolving and varied care delivery settings. Hospital, emergency, subacute, outpatient, community, home health, and long-term care — you'll find unbeatable tips here to use anywhere you practice.

Individual chapters, written by some of the nation's top nurse-managers, cover what you need to know about nursing leadership, from managing and *inspiring* your staff, tracking finances, and planning budgets, to ensuring quality care, and applying the latest information technology. These chapters detail the characteristics and skills you need to meet patient care *and* budget demands, including objectivity, empowerment, flexibility, financial aptitude, attention to detail, business acumen, and time and resource management.

The book's accessible format promotes easy reading and quick retrieval of the information you need. In each chapter, graphic icons highlight *Manager's tips*—special insights into the manager role; *Coping with change*—suggestions to keep you from being overwhelmed by constant restructuring and reorganizing; *Case in point*—personal vignettes and real-life case studies to stimulate critical thinking; and *Questions and answers*—solutions to your everyday needs from seasoned nurse-managers.

I'm convinced that your passion for nursing is what keeps you whole and thriving as managers in the most complex of health care systems. Even during today's acute nursing shortage, your leadership opportunities and influence are obvious and invaluable.

Let *Five Keys to Successful Nursing Management* address your daily challenges and help you excel as a leader. And thank you for all that you do—nursing has never needed you more!

Theresa M. Steltzer
Editorial Director
Nursing Management *journal*
Planning Panel Member
Nursing Management Congress

PART ONE

*L*eadership skills

CHAPTER 1

Why leadership is important to nursing

Gloria Ferraro Donnelly, RN, PhD, FAAN

> "Let whoever is in charge keep this simple question in her head (not how can I always do this right thing myself, but) how can I provide for this right thing to always be done?" — Florence Nightingale, *Notes on Nursing*

This chapter offers both a broad and a specific understanding of *leadership*—what it is, how it works and acts, how it looks and feels, how it's different from and similar to management, and how it will shape the future of care delivery and the nursing profession.

Leadership is easy to recognize in action. However, many find it difficult to define. It occurs at every level of an organization. It's more a journey than a destination, with many detours along the way. It involves experimentation, failure, risk, and reward—and movement toward a specific vision and set of goals.

Dramatic changes in health care delivery over the past two decades are creating the demand for a new kind of nurse—one who easily deals with complexity, change, and uncertainty; one who is high tech and high touch; one who can work independently and interdependently; and one who holds quality care as the highest value. (See *Seizing the opportunity.*) Shrinking reimbursement, managed care, the need to do more with less, the graying of society, the increase in chronic illness, and staggering changes in technology are demanding that nurses assume leadership roles not only to respond to change but also to direct

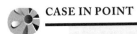

Seizing the opportunity

After working for 4 years as a staff nurse in a critical care unit, you apply for a nurse-manager position of a 40-bed medical surgical unit. This unit has had 3 nurse-managers in the past 5 years, at least 20% turnover per year among the 15 staff nurses, and a group of 6 licensed practical nurses who have worked an average of 10 years each on the unit. You've been restless for the past 6 months, and you need a new challenge. This position seems to be a good place to cut your teeth as a manager.

However, you have dreams of being more than just a manager: You want to be a leader — to dramatically improve care delivery and patient satisfaction, to help staff reach their potential, to contribute to the total organization, and to advance nursing practice.

Your nurse colleagues try to dissuade you. "Just because you're a great critical care nurse, doesn't mean you'll succeed on 4 South. They go through nurse-managers like paper clips," one colleague warns. "If you really need a challenge, wait until a position opens on a unit with fewer problems. You want to succeed, don't you?

Of course you want to achieve your goals, but it's really the experience of leading a staff that deeply interests you. During the series of interviews, you outline your vision for the unit, which includes developing a system of performance improvement, exploring problems and errors to find and correct root causes, focusing not only on achieving clinical excellence but on supporting families, upgrading staff through education and a focus on clinical learning projects, fostering an atmosphere of mutual respect, and considering the needs of other stakeholders in your unit, such as the physicians and other professionals involved in care delivery. You'll also need to focus on managing finances, given that the unit you'll be managing is the equivalent of a multimillion-dollar business.

Despite these challenges, you pursue the position. After the final interview with the Director of Nursing and a small group of staff nurses from 4 South, you're offered the position, and you accept.

Before you leave the critical care unit, your nurse-manager, one of the most respected in the hospital, wishes you well and offers the following: "You're going to a unit where resistance to change is the norm and where patient care and employee satisfaction have suffered. I think that on 4 South, you'll learn the difference between leadership and management and finally realize that leadership is what is so desperately needed there. Call me if you need an ear! I know that you can succeed if you're courageous and persistent." With a new challenge and a mentor in the wings, you're on the way to experiencing the realities of leadership in all of its dimensions.

changes for the benefit of patients, communities, and the nursing profession.

With these changes, the world is experiencing the most serious nursing shortage in the history of modern nursing. As a result, today's nurses are faced with two major challenges: to improve the quality of nursing care amid tumultuous change and to sustain and advance the nursing profession. Together, these challenges constitute the nursing leadership agenda for the twenty-first century.

Defining leadership

Every definition of *leadership* has four basic elements: relationship, context, purpose, and accountability.

Leadership and relationships

Leadership is a complex web of *relationships* that must be explored, understood, and fine-tuned. It is also a relationship with self. Effective leaders regularly explore their own motivations and reflect on successes and failures. They're especially adept at analyzing failures and extracting lessons that can help lead to success in the future.

When getting to know your staff — your direct reports, staff nurses, licensed practical nurses, clerks — consider the relationships among them as well as their work history. Although long-time staff members can provide useful clues about how a unit evolved, an individual's perspective and position on the unit will color those memories. Staff nurses are generally clinical contemporaries of the new nurse-manager, and most average 3 to 5 years on a unit. Your unit clerk may have been there for 15 years, whereas managers and staff have come and gone. Therefore, remember that each staff member can offer a different perspective and that there is never a definitive truth. As a leader, you must listen, keep an open mind, and sort information for its usefulness.

Getting to know your staff and how they relate to one another is key to building a team that will work with you and help you implement new goals, processes, and improvements. Although the nature of followership is as complex and difficult to grasp as the concept of leadership, it's key for all leaders to understand. Gardner[1] asserts that the need for a mission, a structure, and a hierarchy may be the very elements that bind "born leaders" and "born followers" together.

Some staff may choose not to become "followers" in the sense that they're inspired by you to reach the goal. It's reasonable to expect a few "mavericks" or "independents" among the staff, those who remain silent at meetings or are noncommittal when changes are introduced. However, you'll need to mobilize a coalition of trusted staff to plan with you, to implement, and to sustain the changes needed in the unit. A leader can't make improvements without staff support and "buy-in." Therefore, knowing your staff as individuals and discerning the relationship dynamics among them should be two of your first assessment priorities. (See *Your first steps to success,* page 6.)

Understanding staff relationships

Because negative groupings, such as factions and cliques, can interfere not only with change but also with the ordinary functioning of the unit, understanding the patterns of relationships among your staff is key. Your goal as a leader and manager is to form coalitions and to minimize the effect of factions and cliques. (See *Managing groups,* page 7, for the differences between factions, cliques, and coalitions, three types of groups that are commonly encountered among staff.)

Other relationships

Besides your staff, you must also cultivate relationships with other managers, the administration, consumers of the unit's services (sometimes called stakeholders), patients, families, doctors, and other professionals involved in patient care. Positive relationships are pivotal to your success as a leader. Poor or divisive relations with key individuals or groups can hinder your ability to achieve a leadership agenda. In fact, leading management theorists contend that the key to change in any facility lies in getting staff to participate, contribute ideas, do the work that leads to improvement, and have a stake in outcomes.

Leadership and context

The second element in any definition of *leadership* is *context.* Leadership never occurs in a vacuum. Rather, it's shaped by the context, or system level, in which it occurs. Different system

Your first steps to success

To begin a thorough assessment of your new situation, you should take the following practical actions in the first months of your new position.

➤ Review the personnel files of all staff members on every shift, paying particular attention to licenses and other credentials, past evaluations, commendations, and incident reports. If there are no files on the unit, ask the Director to give you access. A paper review gives you basic information not only about individual staff but also about unit management in the past.

➤ Schedule individual appointments with all staff members, and get their perspective on how the unit operates, how it's resourced, and how it might be managed differently. Ask not only about unit needs but also about individual needs — for example, need for education, development, goals, and aspirations. Take notes, and end by soliciting two or three recommendations from each staff member. Themes or commonalities will emerge from the recommendations that will give you important information about the directions you need to take.

➤ Request that the administration give you access to past incident reports, patient satisfaction data for your unit, or documented complaints from patients, families, and doctors.

➤ Give the staff progress reports on your meetings — the number of staff you have seen and the number and types of recommendations or themes you have received. Gather the information they've given you, particularly recommendations and perceived priorities. Keep in mind that the process of getting to know your staff is an ongoing one that should also include some informal social events.

➤ Take 5 minutes at the end of each day, and write a brief list of your successes and challenges for that day. (See the chart below.)

➤ Put your daily lists in a drawer, and take them out at the end of the month. Look for patterns among the successes and especially among the challenges so that you can begin a plan of corrective action.

Successes	Challenges
➤ Completed incident report summary by the deadline	➤ Avoided working on budget projections
➤ Explained and reassured the Smith family about their son's regimen	➤ Remained silent on an important issue at the nurse-manager meeting
➤ Convinced a pharmaceutical representative to provide tangible support for a unit grand rounds	➤ Put off talking with one of the staff about her "45-minute break"
➤ Worked through a problem with Dr. Jones and two staff members	➤ Didn't take time for lunch

levels include the patient unit, the facility, and the local health care system. Each system level has five basic components that need to be recognized:

➤ set of goals or a mission
➤ structure of groups

Managing groups

The chart below describes the nature of cliques, factions, and coalitions and provides tips for managing each type of group among your staff.

Type of group	Definition	Tips for managing
Clique	A social-emotionally oriented group bound together by need, negative emotion (such as a common enemy), or identification processes (such as racial or ethnic grouping or nursing education grouping). May operate out of such emotions as fear, hate, or anger.	The best means of dealing with clique behavior is gentle confrontation and getting issues on the table for discussion — for example, types of nursing education and culturally sensitive behaviors. Clique behavior often operates unconsciously and needs to be brought to the surface.
Faction	An ideologically oriented group that passionately believes in the truth of their position. Most are conceptually trapped and rigid in their views. They can't entertain other perspectives. They may passionately believe in "a right and only way to do things." They resist change mightily when ideologies are challenged.	Idealogues are difficult to deal with because their beliefs and opinions are fixed. Respecting yet differing with the beliefs of others is an important behavior for a leader. Bluntly confronting an ideology may result in the group digging in and growing more fixed in their perspective. Mutual respect can often lead to coalition building.
Coalition	A goal-oriented group focused on a mission or a problem. Its members may or may not share an ideology. However, ideologies don't stand in the way of accomplishing the goal or solving the problem. Coalitions are able to set aside social-emotional issues, and their members typically have well-developed interpersonal skills.	Coalition building is the goal of every leader, because this type of group will work through or set aside social-emotional and ideologic issues to reach the goal.

> ➤ structure of individuals
> ➤ set of tasks, roles, and responsibilities
> ➤ power system.

Some or all of these components may be present in the unit that you'll be leading and the facility in which it resides.

Context also includes the values and traditions of the unit or facility and the usual ways of getting the work done. One of the most important issues for you to consider as a new manager is whether you're a good fit for the position and the new setting.

Assessing your staff

You'll have many contextual elements to assess in your unit in the first months of your new role. Given that the unit is technologically modern and in good physical condition, some of the most important initial points of assessment are:

➤ Does the staff solve problems head on, passively, or as a team, or do problems tend to fall through the cracks until management intervenes? Does the staff, even the more senior staff, turn constantly to the manager for decisions that should reside at the clinical level?

➤ Are task assignments clear? Are the staff committed to completing the work and being accountable for it?

➤ Does the staff abide by hospital procedures and standards of care? Are the staff patient and family oriented — that is, do they go out of their way to meet patient and family needs above all else?

➤ What is the blend of cooperation, conflict, confrontation, and avoidance among the staff? When conflict arises, is it overt and solved relatively quickly, or is it covert and long-lasting?

➤ Are the staff supportive of one another, especially during high-census and high-acuity periods? Do they celebrate one another's successes?

➤ Does the staff work with management, or have they assumed a "we-they" stance?

➤ Is there a team spirit, or is there a high value placed on individuality?

➤ How does the staff deal with rumors — that is, do they check them out or spread anxiety?

➤ Are the atmosphere and the physical look of the unit orderly and routine or chaotic and disruptive?

For example, having succeeded for 4 years as a critical care nurse, will the move to a surgical unit — with a different staff, pace, values, and modes of operating — be a good fit for you? Will you, as the new manager, have the confidence, clarity of purpose, and persistence to set and achieve goals with the participation of a strong coalition of the staff? You'll need to effectively assess your new staff in order to successfully lead them. (See *Assessing your staff*.)

The ability to "get a feel" or "a read" of what is happening in your unit is a managerial competency that you must constantly hone as health care continues to change. You'll be called on not only to deal with the day-to-day routines and problems of operating a unit but also to be an agent of change, a politician, an innovator, a strategist, and a culture broker. Roaming the unit, being visible to staff and patients, and participating as much as possible in caregiving activities sends the message that you're deeply invested in the unit. Paying attention to context is like sending your antennae out frequently to sense the pulse of the unit: Is it strong and steady, weak and thready, or erratic? "Pulse" is a key indicator.

Leadership and purpose

The third element implied in the definition of *leadership* is *purpose*. The most obvious purposes of leadership in nursing are to provide the highest quality care to patients and families, to prevent disease, and to maintain health, even through periods of illness. Other purposes might be to create an environment in which staff can learn, do their best work, and fulfill their potential and to manage the unit as efficiently as possible, without compromising quality care.

Purposeful leadership unleashes leadership potential in others. Leadership isn't a destination; it's a journey and a process toward a set of goals. Therefore the overriding purpose of leadership is to fulfill goals — and when the goals are met, new ones are set.

Everyone defines *leadership* differently. Choose a definition that guides and inspires you; then take steps to incorporate its characteristics into your leadership role. (See *Definitions of leadership*, page 10.)

The role of influence

At the center of this web of relationships is the ability of the leader to influence — that is, to excite at least some of the staff with a vision of what the unit could be and to work with the staff to build a plan of action. The ability to influence implies positive, effective relationships among leaders and followers, clear communication and expectations, and a willingness on the part of the leader to ride out any resistance to change. Barking orders and giving ultimatums aren't strategies of influence. Rather, respecting those who resist, fully exploring and understanding resistance, negotiating for change, setting reasonable timetables for change, and persistently and humanely prodding the resisters are effective strategies for influencing staff. (See *Implementing a new system*, page 11, for an illustration of staff resistance to a small technologic change that could greatly enhance communication among the staff.)

Zuker[2] defines *influence* as the ability to affect others without exerting force or formal authority. This influence is evident only by its effect or result, which underscores the subtlety of the

Definitions of leadership

Select one or two of the following definitions to guide or inspire you. Type them in large bold print, and hang them in a prominent place so that you can begin to incorporate these definitions into your own leadership role.

Definition of *leadership*	Source
Leadership is "liberating people to do what is required of them in the most effective and humane way possible."	De Pree, M. *Leadership Is an Art*. New York: Doubleday Publishing, 1989, p. 1.
"Master Fushan Yuan said, 'There are three essentials to leadership: humanity, clarity, and courage.'"	Cleary, T. trans. *Zen Lessons: The Art of Leadership*. New York: Barnes and Noble Books, 1989, p. 8.
"Leadership is about a sense of direction. The word *lead* comes from an Anglo-Saxon word that means 'a road, a way, the path of a ship at sea.' It's knowing what the next step is."	Adair, J. *Effective Leadership*. Aldershot, England: Gower, 1983.
"Leadership is the capacity to create a compelling vision and translate it into action and sustain it."	Bennis, W. *On Becoming a Leader*. Reading, Mass.: Addison-Wesley, 1989.
"A leader is someone who has the capacity to create a compelling vision that takes people to a new place and to translate that vision into action. Leaders draw other people to them by enrolling them in their vision. What leaders do is inspire people, empower them. They pull rather than push."	Bennis, W., and Goldsmith, J. *Learning to Lead: A Workbook on Becoming a Leader*. Reading, Mass.: Addison-Wesley, 1997, p. 4.
"Leadership is the art of getting someone else to do something that you want done because he wants to do it."	Dwight D. Eisenhower, former President of the United States.
"The simplest definition of a leader is one who goes ahead to guide the way. ... The essential abilities required to lead — values, goals, competence and spirit — are expressed in two sets of requirements: the ability to set and articulate goals and reach them through the efforts of other people and the ability to satisfy the people whose judgment must be respected even under stress."	Greenleaf, R.K. *On Becoming a Servant Leader*. San Francisco, Calif.: Jossey-Bass Publishers, 1996, pp. 294-95.
"Leadership is a mindset and set of behaviors that often produces extremely useful change, often to a dynamic degree."	Kotter, J.P. *Leading Change*. Boston: Harvard Business School Press, 1996, pp. 25-26.
"Star leadership includes eight social skills: influence, communication, conflict management, the ability to initiate and manage change, the ability to build bonds, collaboration, cooperation, and team building."	Goleman, D. *Working with Emotional Intelligence*. New York: Bantam Books, 1998.

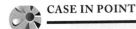
CASE IN POINT

Implementing a new system

A new e-mail system is to be implemented at your facility. This change seems insignificant and routine to you because you've been using e-mail at home for years — and you assume that most of your staff have had the same experience. Nevertheless, you believe that all staff will fully embrace the change because this way of communicating is so quick and efficient.

At the meeting where you're giving directions on how to get e-mail accounts, several staff ask why the change is necessary and whether communication by e-mail will be "mandatory." You're taken aback at this question, but you conceal your surprise. How could the staff not embrace e-mail?

After the meeting, a few staff members reveal their technophobia to you. "I don't have a computer at home," one staff member says. "Do I have to buy one?" Two other staff members confess that they've never used a computer other than the ordering system at your facility. They don't want to appear "stupid." You realize that you can't make light of their resistance. You learn that two staff members can't type, so constructing an e-mail message may take up to three times longer than jotting down a note.

How can you successfully implement a new e-mail system for staff members? Begin by relating matter-of-factly that everyone will be expected to use e-mail and that you will help get everyone fully oriented. Work individually with those staff members who are most resistant to the change. Make a pact with the two staff members who can't type that they can read and confirm receipt of e-mail with a simple OK and that if they need to respond at length they can call you, write a note, or come speak with you. Most important, treat the dissenters with respect, and ease them into using this technology with small, simple steps. Have a time goal to reevaluate the situation, and readjust the implementation plan as necessary.

process. Using positive communication, working with staff resistance, leading by example, and compromising with dissenters help to accomplish the goal. Listening to staff without judging them is crucial where influence is concerned. Determining what influences you also helps develop your own strategies of influence.

Leadership and accountability

The fourth element implicit in any definition of *leadership* is *accountability*. Nurse leaders are accountable to a complex web of constituents. You the nurse-manager are accountable to the health care organization in which you work, to managers to whom you directly report, to the state who grants your license to practice, to the staff on your unit who count on you to manage and lead effectively, and to patients, families, and in some cases communities. R.K. Greenleaf[3] wrote, the term *responsibility* is used to capture the essence of accountability:

> Responsibility...requires that a person think, speak and act as if personally accountable to all who may be affected by his or her thoughts, words and deeds. People are affected by neglect as well as by assertive actions. Therefore, responsibility is affirmative and imposes obligations that one might not choose. It is also negative in that it restrains or modifies what one might chose to think say or do.

Implied in this view of accountability and responsibility is the necessity of the leader to make careful judgments and decisions, to develop priorities for action, and to evaluate results through feedback.

Accountability and stewardship

Stewardship adds a necessary dimension to the concept of accountability. Block[4] defines *stewardship* as "the willingness to be accountable for the well-being of the larger organization by operating in service, rather than in control, of those around us." It gives all staff, regardless of their position, choices over how to serve the patient, the families, other stakeholders, and the organization. (See *Elements of stewardship.*)

Basic practices

Accountability requires continuous effort; thus, accountability practices should be integrated into every aspect of leadership and management. The following list includes practices that you can integrate into your day-to-day management to foster accountability to your staff, the administration, the patients and families, and yourself.

➤ Share your annual goals for the unit. Get feedback from your manager and staff, and revise if necessary. Then distribute the revised goals to management and staff, and display them in a prominent place for everyone to see.

Elements of stewardship

The following six elements of stewardship reinforce the idea of a partnership between the leader and the staff in the attainment of goals.

➤ Stewardship involves an affirmation of the spirit, of the notion that every staff member is truly central to the primary task at hand — the delivery of quality nursing care.

➤ Stewardship emphasizes a partnership between leader and staff that balances power and accountability in seeing day-to-day operations through and in initiating change.

➤ Stewardship gives value to staff empowerment, which means that everyone is responsible for creating the culture of the unit and for producing positive outcomes for patients, families, stakeholders, and themselves.

➤ Stewardship removes the lines between managing the work and doing the work. A general commitment to service by all is the focus of stewardship.

➤ Stewardship views change as a natural outcome of the service orientation, the partnership among leader and staff, and staff empowerment.

➤ Stewardship infuses the staff with ownership and responsibility, which simultaneously removes the barriers to quality and service.

➤ Keep the staff informed on fiscal matters, especially the development of the budget. Encourage participation in the budget's development so that the staff become more aware of fiscal realities. A budget is a quantitative expression of a manager's goals and strategies. Review your budget in light of your goals.

➤ Publish a calendar of staff meetings well in advance so that the staff can anticipate and plan to attend. Have a written agenda, and encourage the staff to submit agenda items beforehand. Track progress and issues by keeping minutes for all meetings.

➤ Keep management informed of incidents, potential problems, and conflicts. Your facility may have resources available to help you.

➤ Conduct annual reviews according to institutional policy and use real data to illustrate performance — that is, specific examples of excellent or problematic performance that illustrates patterns or trends.

➤ Celebrate and publicize the staff's success. For example, send a general e-mail or post a notice if a staff member returns to school, completes a degree or certification, publishes an article, gives a presentation, or designs a care or management innovation.

➤ Write and distribute an annual report, even if it isn't required. Include progress both on the goals you established for the unit and on staff successes. Establish some unit benchmarks concurrent with institutional priorities, and compare them from year to year—for example, number of admissions, staff turnover rates, patient satisfaction data, staff satisfaction data, number of students educated on your unit, and other benchmarks that might help you to track progress toward a goal.

➤ Participate assertively in your own evaluation process, and determine areas for your own improvement that can be incorporated into annual goals.

➤ If you're going to be away, at a meeting or conference for example, let the staff know where you'll be and how you can be reached. Leave someone in charge to ensure accountability.

➤ Expect the staff to update their knowledge and skills, and set an example in this area.

Accountability can become a pervasive value on your unit if you promote what De Pree calls "roving leadership," encouraging staff to participate and giving them a say in day-to-day operations. For example, you might permit one of the staff leaders to identify and work through a problem—while supporting her from the sidelines. What's critical is that you're open to sharing the ownership of issues and problems while at the same time being accountable for results. De Pree says, "Leadership is never handled carelessly—we share it, but we don't give it away."[5] (See *Sharing leadership.*)

Pitfalls to career progression

Since accepting the nurse-manager position and beginning your work with staff, you feel more confident and more assured of success in the role. You possess many characteristics of a good manager and leader. For example, you're organized, dedicated, rational, even-tempered, and responsible, and you have strong interpersonal skills. The day-to-day operations—such as assigning and evaluating care, staffing, delegating, budgeting, managing the physical environment, writing reports, and maintaining positive relationships with and among the staff—are functions that you confidently perform. Success in your new position, however, may

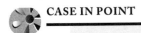

CASE IN POINT

Sharing leadership

At a staff meeting, several nurses raise the issue of the increased burden that having students on the unit creates. Several staff members want to severely restrict the number of students rotating through the unit. On the other hand, there's a nursing shortage, and you realize the inherent opportunities of giving students positive experiences and possibly recruiting them to the staff.

As you struggle to steer the discussion in a more positive direction, one staff nurse who is particularly interested in education volunteers to develop a plan that might improve student experiences and ease the burden on staff. The plan involves developing a short brochure with answers to the most frequently asked questions (FAQs). The brochure would be given to all new faculty members and students and would help orient them to the unit.

In the best example of roving (or shared) leadership, you approve the plan and stand by the sidelines as this staff nurse gathers the FAQs and the best answers. You give her clerical and design support as well as time to meet with each faculty member to obtain their input and to conduct a focus group with students on the brochure's design.

After staff review, the brochure is printed in its first draft in a pocket format and quickly becomes a model for other units in the hospital. In this case, roving leadership considerably reduced the pressure on staff by more thoroughly orienting students to the workings of the unit.

depend on how well you avoid those behaviors that interfere with career progression.

Based on behavioral research, the Benchmark System, a tool that evaluates an individual's management and leadership characteristics, enumerates six pitfalls to leadership effectiveness and, ultimately, to career progression.[6] (See *Strategies for avoiding pitfalls,* pages 16 and 17.)

Leadership and self-assessment

Self-assessment of behaviors and attitudes that underpin leadership is one of the most important activities of the leader. Gallwey[7] believes that continuous nonjudgmental observation of self can bring us to new levels of excellence and personal effectiveness. "Holding up a mirror," as he calls it, helps us to focus not only on our competencies and strengths but also on how we can get in our

MANAGER'S TIP

Strategies for avoiding pitfalls

Every leadership role has its difficulties. The key is to work through those difficulties and emerge a better leader. Some of the most common problem areas are described in the chart below, along with some strategies for improvement.

Problem areas	Strategies for improvement
Problems with interpersonal relationships	
➤ Behaviors include avoidance and passivity, anger, sarcasm, abrasiveness, lack of compassion, lack of sensitivity to others, lack of clarity concerning expectations, holding grudges, devaluation of the contributions of others, vindictiveness, emotionally explosive behavior, inability to use the lessons of your own and the staff's failures, paranoia, and obsessive checking up on staff.	➤ Participate in assertiveness training. Review the rights and responsibilities of your role and your scope of decision making with your supervisor. Keep a daily leadership journal to determine negative patterns.
Difficulty in molding a staff, including team building	
➤ Behaviors include lack of knowledge of group process, inability to deal with dominant or passive staff, inability to elicit participation, difficulty building and sticking to an agenda, and recruitment of staff who have difficulty fitting in or who are unprepared for the role.	➤ Obtain training in the following areas: group leadership, interviewing to select the best staff, and agenda building. Feel confident about delegating responsibility, exercising the rights of your role, giving both positive and negative feedback, and developing plans for corrective action. Be willing to accept both positive and negative feedback on your initiatives.
Difficulty making strategic transitions, including handling pressure well	
➤ Behaviors include inflexibility, unwillingness to make decisions or changes necessary to improve the unit's functioning or to get it through hard financial times, failure to transition mentally from a staff member to a manager, and withdrawal or overreaction when under pressure.	➤ Reflect daily on successes and challenges. Examine emotional responses that are counterproductive. Use centering or deep breathing to handle intense pressure. Consciously delaying emotional, verbal responses in highly charged situations.

Strategies for avoiding pitfalls *(continued)*

Lack of follow-through

> ➤ Behaviors include chronic lateness; failure to meet deadlines; failure to implement plans discussed with and agreed upon by the staff; procrastination on issues of staff conflict; failure to attend meetings where the manager's presence is needed; failure to meet deadlines for reports, budgets, or staff evaluations; failure to return phone calls; failure to answer e-mails or requests for assistance by staff, management, or patients; failure to attend important ceremonies; inattention to detail; and failure to complete work.

> ➤ Keep an up-to-date appointment book, and check it frequently. Schedule staff meetings months in advance, and keep to the often.
> ➤ Construct to-do lists, and check off items when they're completed.
> ➤ If you tend to procrastinate, take a time management course.
> ➤ If you're pressing a deadline, ask for a reasonable extension, instead of letting the deadline pass without a response.
> ➤ Return phone calls, and answer e-mails and letters.

Overdependence, burnout, and negativity

> ➤ Behaviors include feeling unappreciated, suffering in silence then becoming overemotional at the slightest provocation, whining, complaining to staff about the administration's lack of support (even if it's true), running out of steam quickly, and lacking persistence when situations are difficult.

> ➤ Proactively manage your morale. Communicate your beliefs, ideas, concerns, and dissent assertively.
> ➤ Know when to give up and move on to a new issue or initiative.
> ➤ Deal with the fear of delegating.
> ➤ Substitute the desire to be loved with the need to be respected.
> ➤ Engage in self-care activities outside of work — for example, exercise, hobbies, and social activities.

Strategic differences with management

> ➤ Behaviors include having irreconcilable differences with management that create unresolved conflict and work disruption and undermining management's initiatives.

> ➤ If you can't support management's initiatives, argue your case for change. Choose your battles with administration carefully, making sure that any contention pertains to substantive issues, not trivial ones.
> ➤ If you can't reconcile your differences with management, either lie low or move on.

own way. Lack of self-knowledge can hamper individual growth and development particularly in the leader role.

There are many routes to self-knowledge and many methods of self-assessment. Bennis and Goldsmith[8] identify four simple approaches: self-reflection, interacting with others, openness to others, and evaluating the internal and external consistency of our beliefs and actions.

Self-reflection

Self-reflection occurs when we purposely think about our experiences in a critical way. It may involve sitting quietly at the end of each day to review actions, experiences, conflicts, demands, successes, failures, and lessons learned. (See *Working toward self-awareness.*)

Using the ten characteristics of Greenleaf's[9] servant-leader concept, your periodic self-assessment should include the following questions.

➤ How well do I *listen* to the staff, to peer leaders, to administrators, and to patients, families, and other professional colleagues?

➤ Can I understand and *empathize* with coworkers and colleagues and at the same time give direct and accurate feedback on what might be unacceptable behaviors?

➤ Do I have the ability, skill, and intention to *heal* fractured relationships?

➤ What is my general level of *awareness*, including self-awareness, in situations?

➤ Are my powers of *persuasion* more developed than my tendencies for coercion? How successful am I at persuading the staff on conflicting issues?

➤ How well do I *conceptualize* problems and issues? Can I view issues and problems from a variety of organizational or theoretical perspectives?

➤ How well do I anticipate; how well honed are my *foresight* skills? Can I project multiple future scenarios and problem-solve each one?

➤ How strong are my tendencies toward *stewardship?* Do I view my role as holding the unit in trust for staff, patients, and families?

➤ Am I committed to the personal and professional *growth* of the staff? How do I operationalize this commitment?

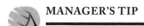

MANAGER'S TIP

Working toward self-awareness

Journal keeping is an activity that increases self-awareness. Before leaving your unit at the end of the day, find a quiet spot, take out your notepad, and ask yourself two questions:
1. What was the high point of my day?
2. What was my greatest challenge today?
   Briefly answer the questions as quickly as you can; then close the notepad. Do this exercise every day, and at the end of 1 month review the high points and challenges. Look for patterns and themes, progressions, and regressions. This simple exercise will help to familiarize you with your ways of thinking, perceiving, and operating.

➤ Do I strive to *build community* among the unit staff so that they feel ownership of the work and the goals?

Interacting with others

Bennis and Goldsmith's second approach to self-knowledge is interacting with others who will give us honest feedback. A trusted friend or colleague who can accurately and honestly describe our behaviors to us in the most humane way possible can provide points of contrast with self-perceptions. We usually don't see ourselves as others do, particularly in a leadership role. The contrast can help us eventually close the gap between our own and others' perceptions of our actions.

Openness to learning

Openness to learning is the third approach to self-knowledge. Lifelong learning is second nature to nurses, particularly for updating clinical knowledge and skills. A leader, however, needs to continually hone a second knowledge and skill that involves planning, operations management, evaluation of clinical care results and staff performance, and fiscal management. Openness to learning also involves periodic assessment of how the staff perceive your managerial performance so that you can make adjustments and improve the work environment. (See *Evaluating your leadership ability,* page 20.)

Evaluating your leadership ability

Once or twice a year, give the staff an opportunity to evaluate your managerial and leadership functions. Provided below is a simple tool that you can adapt or use in its current form to begin collecting data for the purpose of improvement. Give the staff time to think about the items and complete the form. Have someone collate the results. Summarize them for staff, and include in your summary how you intend to make improvements based on the data.

Use the following scale to rate the functioning of the unit manager (such as services provided to the staff over the past year). Please note that the scale ranges from 0 to 4. If you have no basis on which to evaluate an item, circle "0." Otherwise, use the scale from 1 to 4, with 1 being "ineffective" and 4 being "commendably effective."

Recommendations for improvement (use this section to offer recommendations for improvement in any area not addressed by the above items)

1. Communicates relevant information to staff in a timely manner.   0 1 2 3 4

2. Responds to issues and complaints in an appropriate fashion.   0 1 2 3 4

3. Oversees management of unit facilities (equipment, environment).   0 1 2 3 4

4. Treats staff, patients, and families with respect.   0 1 2 3 4

5. Provides effective liaison with hospital administration.   0 1 2 3 4

6. Advocates for staff when necessary.   0 1 2 3 4

7. Attends to administrative detail (meetings, agendas, reports, budget).   0 1 2 3 4

8. Acts as a mentor and an educator to staff.   0 1 2 3 4

9. Recognizes staff achievements appropriately.   0 1 2 3 4

10. Promotes a collegial, inclusive work atmosphere.   0 1 2 3 4

Add or replace items that match your own leadership situation. Most importantly, focus on the results and the level of participation of the staff working with you to improve the quality of care delivery and general operations. Getting the staff accustomed to providing regular feedback to which you respond will promote a sense of ownership in the unit's success.

Evaluating the consistency of beliefs and actions

Evaluating the internal and external consistency of our beliefs and actions is the fourth route to self-knowledge. A continuous assessment of the congruency between what we say and what we do is necessary not only to developing leadership but also to earning the respect of the staff. Leaders should be a living example of how the staff should conduct their work. You will command respect if you give respect. Carol Bartz, CEO of a billion-dollar technology company, asserts, "You have to show by example what is important. I tell my VPs that if their 10 year old has a concert that is only going to happen one time, the concert takes precedence over an executive meeting."[10] Bartz demonstrates the values that she espouses through action. Modeling behavior is the responsibility of those who aspire to leadership.

Case for analysis

You've been the director of a nurse-managed inner-city clinic for several years. Your mission is to offer primary care and disease prevention programs to residents of the community. The clinic staff is diverse, to match the population served, and is made up of five white, two Latino, and five black members. It's been your perception that staff work well together and are committed to the mission of the clinic.

It's one of those busy days: The phone hasn't stopped ringing, and you've had several walk-ins. The appointment book is full, and every client has been seen, except for one who didn't show up or call. You've been working on "no shows" with various reminders and incentives, but this client hasn't responded. As one of the black staff members is returning to her office, she overhears a conversation between two white staff members who disparagingly suggest that the client's lateness is somehow connected to their racial status. Upset and hurt, she repeats the statement to another staff member who is also black.

On the following day, you learn what happened and begin evaluating whether or not to have an open discussion of the incident. Hoping that the tensions will dissipate, you delay taking action. Although there were two call-outs this morning, the staff who are in appear to be working well. One of the call-outs is from the female staff member who overheard the conversation yesterday.

On the third day after the incident, the same staff member calls out. Of the staff present, one complains of a headache and another complains of stomach problems. You notice that the staff members are unusually quiet. You're the leader of the unit, and it's your responsibility to see that staff members work as a team to best serve clients. ●

(Case contributed by Brenda Lyons, RN, MSN.)

Critical questions

➤ How do you discover what's at the root of this situation? What is stereotyping, and how does it work?
➤ How culturally competent are you and your staff? Are you sensitive to the values and beliefs of other cultures?
➤ Should you, as leader, have immediately addressed the overheard statement made by the white staff members? How do you approach the situation now that time has passed?
➤ How will you verify your hunch that the staff who called out did so because of the incident that transpired 3 days ago?
➤ What strategies might you use to better evaluate the tension you perceive among your staff?
➤ If tension is present among the staff, how would you go about assessing and dealing with it?
➤ What opportunities are present in the above scenario?
➤ What strategies might you develop to explore values and perceptions of other cultural groups by you and your staff?

Points to remember

The following points summarize the importance of leadership in nursing management:

➤ Leadership is crucial to the nursing profession because of the unprecedented and tumultuous changes in health care and the demand on nurses to improve care delivery.
➤ Leadership is a process in which relationships, context, purpose, and accountability all come together.
➤ Stewardship is a form of accountability that emphasizes the empowerment and involvement of the staff working with the leader to accomplish goals. Leader accountability to the staff, stakeholders, and administrators is important in the stewardship model.
➤ The six pitfalls to leader career progression include problems with interpersonal relationships; difficulty molding a staff, including team building; difficulty making strategic transitions, including handling pressure well; lack of follow-through; overdependence, including burnout and negativity; and strategic differences with management.

References

1. Gardner, H. *Leading Minds: An Anatomy of Leadership.* New York: Basic Books, 1995.
2. Zuker, E. *The Seven Secrets of Influence.* New York: McGraw-Hill Book Co., 1991.
3. Greenleaf, R.K., et al. *On Becoming a Servant Leader.* San Francisco: Jossey-Bass Publishers, 1993.
4. Block, P. *Stewardship: Choosing Service over Self Interest.* San Francisco: Berrett-Koehler Publishers, 1993.
5. De Pree, M. *Leadership is an Art.* New York: Doubleday Publishing, 1989.
6. Center for Creative Leadership. *Benchmarks: Assessing Leadership Skills and Enhancing the Development Process.* Greensboro, N.C.: Center for Creative Leadership, 2002. *www.ccl.org/products/benchmarks/bmkover.html.*
7. Flower, J. "The Inner Game: An Interview with Tim Gallwey," *Health Forum Journal* 44(2):16-20, March-April 2001.
8. Bennis, W., and Goldsmith, J. *Learning to Lead: A Workbook on Becoming a Leader.* Rev. ed. Reading, Mass.: Addison-Wesley, 1997.
9. Spears, L.C. "On Character and Servant Leadership: Ten Characteristics of Effective, Caring Leaders." Greenleaf Center for Servant Leadership. *www.greenleaf.org/leadership/read-about-it/Servant-Leadership-Articles-Book-Reviews.html.*
10. Neff, T.J., and Citrin, J.M. *Lessons from the Top: The 50 Most Successful Business Leaders in America and What You Can Learn from Them.* New York: Currency Doubleday, 2001.

Recommended resources

Books on leadership topics

The Art of the Warrior: Leadership and Strategy from the Chinese Military Classics. Translated, compiled, and introduced by Ralph D. Sawyer, with the collaboration of Mei-chün Lee Sawyer. Boston: Shambhala Press, 1996.

This collection of writings from ancient Chinese generals and other military leaders offers many passages on leadership, the character of the leader, and leader-follower relationships.

Bennis, W., and Goldsmith, J. *Learning to Lead: A Workbook on Becoming a Leader.* Rev. ed. Reading, Mass.: Addison-Wesley, 1997.
  A valuable workbook that takes you on a journey of self-assessment pertinent to leadership. Warren Bennis is one of the leading experts in the world on leadership and how it works.

Block, P. *Stewardship: Choosing Service over Self Interest.* San Francisco: Berrett-Koehler Publishers, 1993.
  This book offers a very different view of how leadership can work. Stewardship emphasizes accountability to the organization and to staff as well as a dispersion of power and influence throughout the organization.

Cleary, T., trans. *Zen Lessons: The Art of Leadership.* Boston: Shambhala Publications; [New York]: Distributed by Random House, 1993.
  A group of lessons and quotations from ancient Zen masters on the nature of leadership. The lessons are brief but powerful and examine leadership from the viewpoint of self, followers, and community.

Collins, J.C., and Porras, J.I. *Built To Last: Successful Habits of Visionary Companies.* New York: Harper Business, 1994.
  This work explores the reasons underpinning long-term success in 18 visionary corporations. It's based on a 6-year research project at the Stanford University Graduate School of Business. It attempts to answer the question, What makes truly exceptional companies different from other companies?

De Pree, M. *Leadership is an Art.* New York: Doubleday Publishing, 1989.
  One of my favorite books on leadership. It's a personal, human yet practical account of leadership and followership. This author is passionate about leadership and what it takes to create an environment in which all can do their best work.

Gardner, H. *Leading Minds: An Anatomy of Leadership.* New York: Basic Books, 1995.
 This work explores the concept of leadership from the developmental point of view. Gardner examines the lives of different types of leaders and through them offers insights on how leadership works and leaders develop.

Greenleaf, R.K., et al. *On Becoming a Servant Leader.* San Francisco: Jossey-Bass Publishers, 1993.
 Robert Greenleaf is known as the father of the empowerment movement in business leadership. His concept of the servant leader is a humanistic approach to leadership. His explication of the ethics of leadership is clear and profound.

Hammer, M., and Champy, J. *Reengineering the Corporation,* 2nd ed. New York: HarperCollins Publisher, 2001.
 This already-classic work, now in its second edition, had a huge impact on how business introduced change and innovation in the 1990s. Many hospitals and health care organizations reengineered according to the principles of the reengineering process. If you worked in an environment that was "reengineered," this book will give you insight on why it worked or why it failed.

Hendricks, G., and Ludeman, K. *The Corporate Mystic.* New York: Bantam Books, 1996.
 This leadership book is for those with a spiritual bent, filled with what the authors refer to as "just in time wisdom." It focuses on how to improve commitment, communication, and honest feedback.

Hesselbein, F., et al., eds. *The Leader of the Future: New Visions, Strategies and Practices for the Next Era.* San Francisco: Jossey-Bass Publishers, 1996.
 This collection of essays on the challenges of modern leadership offers strategies to successfully lead in business and other arenas. Leaders in the business world and experts on the leadership and management author the essays.

Kotter, J.P. *Leading Change.* Boston: Harvard Business School Press, 1996.

Kotter clearly differentiates leadership from management by suggesting that leadership is about change and management is about dealing with daily complexities. This work offers specific strategies for introducing and sustaining substantive change in organizations.

Low, A. *Zen and Creative Management.* Garden City, L.I.: Anchor Press, 1976.

This little-known management book should be a classic. It explores the complexities and dualities of management. It also promotes Zen, or living in the present, and presence as a discipline for managers.

Morgan, G. *Organization,* 2nd ed. Thousand Oaks, Calif.: Sage Publications, 1997.

This work analyzes organizational cultures from several metaphorical lenses, such as organizations as machines, brains, cultures, political systems, psychic prisons, and organisms. It also validates the power of metaphor in thinking about and operating in organizations.

Musashi, M. *A Book of Five Rings: The Classic Guide to Strategy.* Woodstock, N.Y.: Overlook Press, 1974. (Originally published in 17th-century Japan. Translated by Victor Harris; London: Allison & Busby, 1974.)

This work is an ancient oriental military classic that succinctly describes the most effective strategies for winning at war. This work has become a powerful metaphor for leadership strategy in all venues.

Neff, T.J., and Citrin, J.M. *Lessons from the Top: The 50 Most Successful Business Leaders in America and What You Can Learn from Them.* New York: Currency Doubleday, 2001.

This work includes profiles of 50 of the most successful business leaders in the United States, summarizes the qualities that they share, and identifies six essential principles of business leadership.

Nightingale F. *Notes on Nursing: What It Is and What It Is Not.* Commemorative Edition. Philadelphia: Lippincott Williams & Wilkins, 1992 (original printing, 1859).
This is simply the greatest nursing book ever written.

Schwartz, P. *The Art of the Long View.* New York: Doubleday Books, 1991.
The prime work by the originator of scenario planning as a way of being ready for the future — and perhaps creating a bit of it.

Senge, P.M. *The Fifth Discipline: The Art and Practice of the Learning Organization.* New York: Doubleday, 1990.
This work revolutionized the concept of leadership and organizations and advanced the notion that organizations learn along with individuals. Learning about the four core disciplines — personal mastery, mental models, shared vision, and team learning — will be especially useful for managers and leaders.

Senge, P., et al. *The Fifth Discipline Fieldbook: Strategies and Tools for Building a Learning Organization.* New York: Doubleday, 1994.
If you liked Peter Senge's *The Fifth Discipline,* which introduced the concept of *learning organizations,* you'll love this book, which expands on the principles of building a learning organization and offers cases, exercises, and strategies for the modern manager or leader.

Sennett, R. *Authority.* New York: Knopf, 1980.
Understanding the idea of authority is important to successful leadership, and Sennett explores the concept in both theoretical and practical terms. This work demonstrates how the need for and the resistance to authority have been shaped by history, culture, and individual psychological factors.

Smith, P.B., and Peterson, M.F. *Leadership, Organizations and Culture: An Event Management Model.* Newbury Park, Calif.: Sage Publications, 1988.

A research-based work that looks at how leadership works in specific contexts. Contains a well-documented review of leadership research from the 1500s, when Machiavelli wrote *The Prince,* to the present.

Ulrich, B.T. *Leadership and Management According to Florence Nightingale.* Norwalk, Conn.: Appleton & Lange, 1992.
A clever excerpting of Nightingale passages on leadership and management. Given Nightingale's global effect on health care delivery, her thoughts on leadership and management are important. The book is well organized and well referenced.

Welles, J.F. *The Story of Stupidity: A History of Western Idiocy from the Days of Greece to the Present.* Orient, N.Y.: Mount Pleasant Press, 1998.
This work is an unusual look at the concept of stupidity, which has nothing to do with intelligence. *Stupidity* is defined as a person's inability to adjust internal schemas to the changing contingencies of reality. Examples of stupidity from ancient to modern times are explored.

Wills, G. *Certain Trumpets: The Nature of Leadership.* New York: Simon and Schuster, 1994.
This thought-provoking book explores the lives of individuals who exerted leadership in varying domains of life, including in diplomacy, the military, the church, sports, the arts, and business. Wills puts particular emphasis on the importance of followers in determining the success of leaders. He also describes types of leaders, including radical, charismatic, intellectual, traditional, and saintly.

Websites on leadership topics

The Center for Creative Leadership
This site features programs, products, and research reports on leadership. It also offers leadership evaluation tools, which are helpful for both experienced and novice leaders seeking to improve, and an e-newsletter to which you can subscribe.
Web site: *www.ccl.org*

The Change Project

This site features the work and insights of Joe Flowers on how change works, particularly in health care. The site includes models of change and practical advice on how to be a change master. Pay particular attention to the Change Codes and Change Processes. This site is rich with tools and insights for leaders.

Web site: *www.well.com/user/bbear*

Health Futures, Inc.

The site features the works of Jeff Goldsmith, a leading health care futurist who founded Health Futures, Inc., a company specializing in forecasting future health care trends. Leaders and managers who work in any corner of the health care industry should visit this site regularly. Goldsmith summarizes and synthesizes trends and recommends strategies for change.

Web site: *www.healthfutures.net/*

Leadership in Organizations

This site is a rich resource for the study of the nitty-gritty of leadership in organizations. "Overview of Leadership in Organizations," written by Carter McNamara, MBA, PhD, applies to nonprofits and for-profits unless otherwise noted. It presents models and theories of leadership, core competencies, and a section on basic skills as well as links to other leadership sites.

Web site: *www.mapnp.org/library/ldrship/ldrship.htm*

Florence Nightingale Museum

This site contains Nightingale's story, works about her innovations in health care, and some of her original works. When you visit, be certain to read "The Passionate Statistician," by Alex Attewell, a short essay that describes Nightingale's use of statistics to demonstrate efficacy of nursing care. You can find this article by clicking on "Resource Centre and Articles." Nightingale was one of the first health care professionals to use statistics as a tool to demonstrate the worth of nursing intervention.

Web site: *www.florence-nightingale.co.uk*

Plunkett Research, Ltd.

This site offers cutting edge, accurate, and timely information on various subjects, including health care. Overviews of the health care, biotech, and genetics industries clearly identify trends that will directly affect nurses in the future. The site also includes the 13 major trends affecting health care today.

Web site: *www.plunkettresearch.com*

Queendom

This site offers more than 100 self-assessment tools, many related to career and leadership. Click on "Personality Tests" and then on "Career." After you complete an assessment, the site will generate a brief report for you. Remember, the report is only a summary of what you said in your assessment. *Note:* Many of the tests require a fee.

Web site*: www.queendom.com*

CHAPTER 2

How leadership works: Myths and theories

Gloria Ferraro Donnelly, RN, PhD, FAAN

> "When I was young, I observed that nine out of ten things I did were failures. So I did ten times more work." — George Bernard Shaw

Perception and cognition undoubtedly shape our views of leadership. What follows is an exploration of familiar myths, early models, modern theories, and research findings on how leadership works and how such information may be practically applied in the leadership role.

Myths of leadership

A myth is a belief or story about some aspect of reality for which we have no explanation. Before the tools of science were available, the ancients created many myths about natural phenomena — for example, thunder and lightning occurred when the gods were angry, and people fell in love when Cupid's arrow struck.

Just as myths of natural phenomena exist, myths of leadership exist. Most persist because it's difficult to explain the complex conditions and factors that result in leadership. It's also difficult to reconcile the disparate theories about this behavioral phenomenon. Common myths include:

Myth 1: Leaders are born.
Myth 2: Leadership can be taught.
Myth 3: Leaders never fail.

Myth 4: Leaders promote change.

Myth 5: Leaders must possess charisma.

Myth 6: Leaders must be served.

Myth 7: Gender differences in leadership favor males.

Each myth is a sweeping generalization about some aspect of leadership. What they all have in common is their simplistic view of leadership. As you explore these myths, note the ones that have affected your professional practice, your dealings with "nurse leaders," and the development of your own leadership path. Use the romantic simplicity of the myths to appreciate more fully the complexity, practicality, and richness of leadership behavior.

Myth 1: Leaders are born

The myth that leaders are born is based on the notion that certain people have personality traits that facilitate leadership behavior. Associated with the trait theory of leadership, this simplistic myth discounts the interaction that occurs between leaders and their environment and the role that crisis and situational factors play in the emergence of leadership. Furthermore, the myth advances the idea that an inheritable trait or set of traits underpins the development of leadership — which is to say, some people have it and some don't. Think about the leaders you've known in your practice. Did they seem to be "born to the role," or did they become leaders through education, application, inspiration, and hard work?

Lavinia Dock was an early leader in nursing education and public health. She wrote the first textbook in nursing and was a leader in the fight for women's right to vote. She describes how the inspiration of Lillian Wald, the founder of public health nursing at the Henry Street Settlement in New York, awakened her own leadership potential when she was well into her thirties. A great mentor and societal need, rather than inheritable traits, were most influential in determining Dock's path to leadership.

"I continued to be too easily satisfied — not keenly observant — hazy, rather dreary — not sufficiently vigilant — too optimistic — I continued to wish only to do things I liked — my feelings for patients were compassion, or commiseration, or sympathy, rather than a warm personal care. I never began *to think* until I went to Henry Street and lived with Miss Wald. I was then about 38-years-old."[1]

To date, no research findings suggest that leaders have a specific set of inheritable traits. On the other hand, some personality characteristics may enhance leadership efforts, such as extraversion, a positive outlook, or even physical attractiveness. In a study of how nurses become leaders, Allen[2] identified five factors that influenced leadership development among 12 nurses who held formal leadership roles. Of those factors, two were related to personality characteristics, self-confidence, and innate leader qualities described by subjects as the tendency to lead since childhood. The other three factors were progression of experiences, successes, and influence of significant people and personal life factors that affected the seeking of leadership roles. Although leaders themselves may cite personality tendencies as predispositions to leadership, little direct evidence exists to support the notion that "leaders are born." Leaders evolve out of complex combinations of determination, inspiration, situational demand, and hard work.

Myth 2: Leadership can be taught

Leadership is both science and art. The science of leadership includes certain skill sets and behaviors that those aspiring to the role can learn. For example, one can learn how to communicate more assertively, how to plan an agenda and conduct a meeting, how to develop a strategic plan, how to develop a project plan and lead a group to complete the project, how to secure and manage resources both human and financial, and how to delegate and establish systems of accountability that ensure positive results.

Some aspects of leadership, however, seem nearly impossible to teach, because they're associated with more subtle behaviors — such as attitude, judgment, and timing — rather than with specific skill sets. Attitude is our personal orientation to aspects of experience. Senge and colleagues[3] describe three common orientations or attitudes toward experience:

> ➤ *reactive orientation* — the sense that you live in a world where forces outside of your control constantly affect you. This attitude may leave you feeling helpless, defensive, and negative,

and the organization may be fueling your reactive attitude by discouraging input, participation, and initiative.

➤ *creative orientation* — the sense that you can make things happen, change the organization, and motivate people to go along. Organizations that value this attitude expect that leaders will do what it takes to reach goals. Competition and rewards in this type or organization are often great.

➤ *interdependent orientation* — the sense that you are part of a system, of a greater whole, and that you're working with others in the organization to make a difference. This attitude may come naturally to you, and if the organization values responsibility and stewardship, this attitude will bring great personal satisfaction. What's more, some organizations consider a positive, interdependent attitude the primary characteristic when seeking out new employees. Kelleher, the CEO of Southwest Airlines, asserts the importance of attitude to the success of his organization: "We really focus on attitude. It's wonderful to have somebody with a good education, don't misunderstand me. And it's wonderful to have someone who has experience and ... expertise, but if they have a lousy attitude, we don't want them."[4]

Attitudes aren't easily changed through formal education. Rather, they change through openness to others and to the lessons of life experience.

Bell[5] describes leadership as "a sense of judgment — that is, judgment as to what is relevant and how to do things." Imagine that your unit is closing or that it's merging with another. Would you discuss the possibilities with your staff, or would you avoid raising their anxieties? Would you question your manager on this possibility, or would you wait until you're told? Could you effectively prepare data to make a case for the survivability of your unit? The strategies you develop to deal with this situation aren't easily learned. They involve risk, judgment, timing, keen observation, and well-honed communication skills. Even after a thorough assessment, your strategy may work, especially if the environment is rapidly changing or if there were contingencies beyond the range of your assessment. However, it's better to calculate the risks before fully disclosing what might happen.

Timing is another aspect of leadership that isn't easily taught. Yet, knowing when to act and when to delay can be crucial to

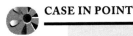

CASE IN POINT

Standing in the middle

You're preparing to fill a staff nurse vacancy when the Nursing Director hands you a résumé and strongly suggests that you "put it at the top of the pile." You and a group of senior staff have already determined what you're looking for in this next staff hire, and the suggested candidate falls short in more than one area.

Because it's summer and the census is running low, you decide to delay the interviews for a few weeks. You're counting on the delay to dampen the sense of urgency concerning the recommended candidate, who isn't among the four finalists to be interviewed. You know that the Nursing Director is going on vacation, and you ask, as is customary, whether she wants to interview the two finalists before you make your recommendation to human resources. She says, "No, that won't be necessary, since I'm leaving in 2 days and the census is on the rise again."

You complete the interviews, make your recommendation to human resources, and complete the hire. You decide not to mention the new hire unless you're questioned. And then, you'll say that all candidates were given careful consideration.

Depending on the circumstances, delays, imposing deadlines, early action, and surprise can be effective timing strategies.[6]

success in the leadership role. Without a specific deadline, taking early action may rob you of the opportunity to learn more about the situation and may expose you as a potential target for others. Conversely, being first provides the opportunity to set a standard or to take someone by surprise. A thorough assessment of the possible consequences of your actions should help in determining your timing. (See *Standing in the middle.*)

Bornstein and Smith[7] describe leadership as an ongoing process in which followers engage in conscious and unconscious evaluations of their leaders' credibility and subsequently make choices about buying into their vision and plan. (See *Six Cs of leadership credibility,* page 36.)

Myth 3: Leaders never fail

Failure isn't a welcome concept in clinical practice. Nurses learn early to take every precaution to avoid failures that may result in harm to patients. This fear of failure generalizes to other areas of professional practice. We're careful in our documentation and communication. We rely on written policy, procedure, and proto-

Six Cs of leadership credibility

Leadership credibility, as defined by Bornstein and Smith, has six criteria. They're listed below, with their positive and negative characteristics, to help you determine whether you're a credible leader.

Criteria of leadership credibility	Positive aspects	Negative aspects
Conviction	A strong, passionate belief in your goals and your ability to reach them; an unwavering commitment to pursuing the goals	Conviction can sometimes blind you to changing environment conditions and turn to rigidity.
Character	Ethical behavior that involves integrity, respect, and trust of self and others	Fine ethical behavior has no downside; however, a leader can be too trusting in some situations.
Care	Feelings and expressions of concern for the well-being of others, both personally and professionally	A leader can't be a psychotherapist or parent surrogate. Concern can turn into rescuing behavior and encourage staff dependency.
Courage	Willingness to take calculated risks, to confront others, to admit mistakes, and to change the course of action — or even the goal — in light of changing environmental conditions	A leader must carefully choose battles and keep negativity appropriately in check.
Composure	Display of grace and appropriate emotional responses, especially under pressure	Composure can sometimes turn to emotional numbness if the pressure is great. Leaders need appropriate outlets for stress.
Competence	Possession of the knowledge and skill set necessary to deliver and manage nursing care, including technical, communication, and organizational skills	Knowledge doubles at least every 10 years and perhaps more rapidly. Both clinical and managerial competencies need continual updating.

col to minimize the risk to patients and ourselves. We file incident reports when failures occur and take remedial action by counseling or reeducating the staff member who erred.

In analyzing past military failures, Cohen and Gooch[8] found that failures can be categorized as simple, complex, or catastrophic. *Simple failures* can further be broken down into one of three basic types:

COPING WITH CHANGE

Working toward change

When you wish to make a change that affects a number of people, such as staff members, the following actions can save time, reduce stress, and help avoid failure.

➤ Poll a few staff members to determine some of the realistic problems with the proposed change; gather feedback.

➤ Respect staff feedback by negotiating changes before initiating them.

All leaders experience failures — specifically, small and large tactical blunders in communication and organization. The important thing is to expect and face failure, analyze the situation that produced failure, and correct the course of action as often as possible. True leaders will build resolve from the experience.

To help keep yourself in check, constantly ask yourself, "Am I learning? Am I adapting? Am I anticipating?" If you answer no to any of those questions, take steps to change your leadership style so that when you ask yourself again you can answer each with a resounding yes.

➤ *failure to learn,* which involves missing cues, not seeing issues from the perspective of others, and not analyzing past experiences

➤ *failure to adapt* when new or unexpected circumstances arise in the course of everyday events

➤ *failure to anticipate* situations, in which cues may have been plentiful but the leader failed to predict the aversive action.

Complex failures occur when two of the three simple failures have taken place. Although difficult, recovery or repair is possible after a complex failure. *Catastrophic failures* occur when all three simple failures are operational. In catastrophic failures, it's nearly impossible to correct or recover without outside help. In the military and commonly in business, defeat and collapse are likely consequences of catastrophic failure.

In the exercise of leadership, failure is a great teacher. Because leadership involves risk and experimentation, failures are inevitable. What is key, however, is that the leader analyze these failures, learn from them, and apply those lessons to the next venture to reduce the possibility of failure. (See *Working toward change.*)

Tuchman, a leading historian who recorded the curious and recurring tendency of governments to pursue policies contrary to their own interests, describes a process of self-deception often engaged in by those in charge: "Wooden-headedness...consists in assessing a situation in terms of preconceived fixed notions while ignoring or rejecting any contrary signs. It's acting according to wish while not allowing oneself to be deflected by the facts."[9] It's also failing to benefit from experience that results in repetition of error. The overbearing need to be right or to exert power is often at the root of the problem. An effective leader is open to those who question the rationality of policies and changes rather than feel threatened by them.

Myth 4: Leaders promote change

Florence Nightingale's introduction of hygiene and management into the war hospitals of the Crimea is a study in change. Encountering resistance from doctors, military administrators, and occasionally her own staff, she persisted until the goals of lowering mortality rates and providing comfort and care to the foot soldier were completed.

Promoting change, however, isn't the leader's only role. Understanding change processes and appropriately timing change that leads to improvement are also leadership functions. The health care system has been changing at an unprecedented rate over the past 20 years. Managed care, the rise of for-profit health care systems, technology, and a more chronically ill population are just a few major societal changes bearing down on complex delivery systems. Leadership in today's health care environment involves not only introducing change where it's needed but also managing the rapid pace of change.

Change processes become more difficult to understand, predict, and control as health care delivery becomes more complex — that is, in the face of new knowledge, new diseases, new interventions and drugs, and new technologies. What's more, simplistic views of how change works can hamper the work of leadership. (See *Assessing your views on change.*)

Assessing your views on change

Review the following views on change to help identify where you lean in your own understanding of change and how to manage and promote it.

Traditional views of planned change	Contemporary views of systemic change
Change is more likely if persons affected by it have had a part in shaping it.	Change is the rule; it occurs constantly.
If proposed changes are understood, their acceptance is more likely.	Change is process, not content.
Change that's systematically planned is more acceptable and successful than serendipitous change.	Change begets change.
Change that doesn't threaten the security of any one group is more acceptable.	Every change has its price.
Change is more likely when it's linked to a group's value system and beliefs.	Change involves thinking, not merely rearranging prejudices.
Change is acceptable if it follows a previously successful change rather than a change that failed.	Change occurs according to a pattern or structure that may be unique to the system.
Gradual change is more acceptable than sweeping change.	Change tends to accelerate systems.
If people share in the benefits of change, acceptance is more likely.	Change doesn't guarantee success.

Myth 5: Leaders must possess charisma

Charisma is a set of personal qualities or gifts that enable a leader to reach and inspire followers. Striking physical appearance, unusual personality features, rhetoric abilities, and the capacity to formulate dramatic, symbolic, and highly understandable messages that spark the imagination of others are components of charisma.[10]

However, charisma isn't a prerequisite to leadership. Although it may help get broad, symbolic messages across to stir the spirit of the masses, it isn't necessary to help lead a group of clinicians down the path of improving care delivery. Expert knowledge — that is, knowledge of what care is and how it should be delivered in expert ways — is more necessary to the nursing leader than charisma. The culture of nursing demands that leaders or managers know the terrain and have the expertise to deliver what they're managing. Leaders do, however, need a sense of authority, "the strength and ability to guide others through disciplining them, changing how they act by reference to a higher standard."[11] Self-assurance, good judgment, and the ability to inspire respect, impose discipline on others, and have them respond positively are the essence of authority.

Myth 6: Leaders must be served

The most contemporary notions of leadership involve service to others. Greenleaf[12] describes servant leaders as those who are servant first to those they're aspiring to lead. Servant leaders also contribute to the growth of others — and encourage and guide them to be leaders themselves. According to Greenleaf, servant leaders have five constant concerns:

➤ a sense of responsibility
➤ openness to knowledge
➤ living and acting now as if the future is present
➤ personal growth
➤ purpose and laughter.

A servant leader isn't only someone who creates a sense of community and respect for staff but is also someone who pays attention to basic needs, such as the physical environment of the unit, the resources the staff need to perform their duties, and the need for celebration of achievements.

De Pree[13] echoes the view of servant leadership by focusing on its results — that is, followers who reach their potential, who learn, who serve others, who achieve required results, who change with grace, and who manage conflict. Servant leaders leave their units or organization in good financial health and with good reputations in the community. They're responsible for a sense of quality and for openness to influence, change, and dissent, which breed organizational renewal. They owe those served rationality, space, freedom to explore, and momentum to keep

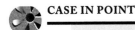

A case of sarcasm

It has been a harrowing day, with six admissions and two codes. With no time for breaks and the workload mounting, nerves are beginning to fray. One of your staff nurses doesn't respond well in such situations. She's prone to anger and sarcasm when under pressure. At a crowded nurses station, a student nurse approaches the staff nurse and asks her to check on one of her patients.

The staff nurse asks, "What specifically is wrong?"

The student nurse replies, "He seems very uncomfortable. ...I don't know..." as she gropes for words to describe the condition.

The staff nurse retorts, "Most people in here are uncomfortable. This is a hospital! I'll be down in a minute to check."

You're horrified at this interchange, especially in an environment where nurse recruitment is on everyone's minds. You follow the nurse to the patient's room and wait outside while she checks the situation. When the staff nurse emerges, you get a brief report on the patient to make certain that there's no impending emergency.

At the end of shift, you invite the nurse to your office and say, "I know that today was very pressured, but you can't continue to take your frustrations out on students or anyone else for that matter. If you need a break or help, ask."

The staff nurse is surprised at this feedback. She defends herself by saying, "Students need to learn. That's how I learned — from staff who tell it like it is."

You and she discuss the difference between appropriate feedback and sarcasm. You also give other examples of her tendency to flare up under pressure. The staff nurse apologizes to the student and turns the incident into a learning experience. You commit to giving her rapid feedback in anticipation of a similar event.

Over the next few months, the nurse shows marked improvement. Respect for others becomes a guiding principle of your unit.

pace with the vision for the future. Servant leaders are responsible for effectiveness and for maintaining civility and values in times of stress and change. Civility in the form of good manners and respect for others is especially needed in health care institutions. (See *A case of sarcasm.*)

As the nursing profession strove for decades to achieve equal status among health professional groups, the word *service* disappeared from the profession's vocabulary. Nursing service, for example, was changed to nursing administration. The concept of service is now back in vogue, particularly with respect to leadership. From the elevated position in the hierarchy, leaders serve to promote organizational strength and effectiveness. De Pree captures the essence of leadership as service: "The first responsibility of leader is to define *reality*. The last is to say thank you. In between, the leader is a servant."

Myth 7: Gender differences in leadership favor males

Gender differences in leadership are complicated by a tradition of cultural norms that promote men as natural leaders and women as followers or facilitators. Perceptions of leaders may be highly influenced by gender stereotypes. For example, in the 1970s, Broverman et al.[14] conducted extensive studies on gender stereotypes. They concluded that in American culture, masculinity and its associated behaviors — aggression, high self-confidence, ambition, independence, and so on — was more highly valued than femininity and its associated behaviors — dependence, emotionality, subjectivity, and submissiveness. Also in the 1970s, Bem[15] challenged the notion of traditional gender stereotypes. Instead she identified behaviors more highly valued by men and those more highly valued by women and developed a way to measure an individual's sex role identity. Some women possessed masculine behaviors; some men, feminine behaviors. The concept of androgyny, or possessing the best of both masculine and feminine behaviors, grew out of this work.

Powell[16] asserts that until the 1980s, most theories of management were based on the direct observations of male managers. However, no evidence exists to support the notion that men are better managers. Most theories of management describe behaviors that fit both masculine and feminine stereotypes. Stereotypes are resistant to change, even in the face of strong evidence. Powell further asserts that neither women nor men should bear the burden of living up to masculine stereotypes in leadership roles. Successful leaders in any organization usually exhibit high degrees of behavioral flexibility, depending on situational demands. Rosner[17] points out that women executives with an interactive style are successful in fast-growing, rapidly changing companies. Successful women in traditional companies typically used command-and-control styles. As more women rise to the tops of organizations, the question becomes whether they'll change the organizations or whether their experiences in the organizations will change them. We'll simply have to wait and see.

Models of leadership

From the time of Machiavelli, author of perhaps the first leadership manual, to the present, theories of what makes a good leader have abounded.

Machiavelli: Early concepts of leadership

In 1535, Nicolo Machiavelli, a minor Italian bureaucrat, wrote *The Prince,* the first book of its kind to explain the human relationship aspects of leadership and the role of politics in governance.[18] In it, he emphasized the role of human nature and relationships in leadership and diminished the importance of positional authority. Leaders weren't necessarily good or effective because they had risen to a position of authority. Nor could they lead by virtue amid corruption and intrigue. In fact, Machiavelli asserted that leaders must seek to understand self, others, and the goals of the organization for leadership to succeed.

Listed below are quotes from *The Prince* that demonstrate not only the wisdom of Machiavelli but also the timelessness of his recommendations for leaders.

➤ *"Only those defenses are good, certain and durable which depend on yourself alone and your ability."*

Nothing serves a leader more effectively than knowledge and experience in the field. Self-reliance is necessary in steering a course of action. Failure is a great teacher for the willing student. It's best not to blame others for failed plans. Instead, it's better to learn from mistakes and improve your behavioral repertoire. In the end, you have only yourself, your knowledge, and your integrity.

➤ *"He who becomes prince by help of the nobility has greater difficulty in maintaining his power than he who is raised by the populace."*

Connections are great in securing leadership positions; however, if the leader doesn't have the knowledge and skill to deliver, failure is inevitable. In most instances, the staff don't have the final say in choosing their managers. However, it's wise to seek input from the staff before appointing a manager. There is nothing more helpful to a leader than a powerful group of followers who will give open, honest feedback and who will own and participate in decision making.

➤ *"The first impression one gets of a ruler and of his brains is from seeing the men he has around him."*

Hiring or appointing only friends, those unwilling to question or challenge, or those with lesser credentials, knowledge, and experience is a sign of the leader's lack of self-confidence. A well-educated, articulate, questioning staff is always a reflection of the leader's competence and confidence.

➤ *"A prince must also show himself a lover of merit, give preferment to the able, and honor those who excel in every art."*

Even if a staff member is your worst personal enemy, if she performs well she should be publicly honored. Recognizing and honoring accomplishment publicly and privately reflects the leader's value of excellence.

➤ *"A man who wishes to make a profession of goodness in everything must necessarily come to grief among so many who are not good. Therefore it is necessary for a prince ... to learn how not to be good, and to use this knowledge and not use it, according to the necessity of the case."*

Every leader must be able to acknowledge her dark side. *"Being good"* is a subjective, relative phrase, and every leader should carefully examine its meaning. Florence Nightingale knew how and when "not to be good" to make accomplishing her goal more likely. Woodham-Smith's[19] and Cook's[20] biographies of Nightingale offers insight into her relentless battles with resistance and corruption. Her constant confrontations and behind-the-scenes strategies to defeat Dr. John Hall, the doctor who resisted the introduction of nursing to the war hospitals, are prime examples of Nightingale's mastery of how "not to be good."

➤ *"Is it better to be loved more than feared, or feared more than loved? One ought to be both feared and loved, but as it is difficult for the two to go together, is it much safer to be feared than loved."*

A need to be loved by all in one's professional life may be a signal of unmet dependency needs. Leaders should seek love in the personal arena and the respect and confidence of others in the professional arena. A solid foundation of self-esteem and self-knowledge will lessen the need and the demand for the staff's love and adulation. Respect for a leader is what fuels movement toward the goal.

Leadership and the cult of personality

It wasn't until the 1800s that more critical analyses of leadership were developed. Carlyle[21] advanced the concept of "heroic leadership" in his book *Heroes and Hero Worship*, published in 1841. With an interest in inheritable traits, Galton[22] asserted that those personality traits that result in leadership are inherited.

In the early 1900s, Weber[23] used the term *charisma* to describe the extraordinary "gifts" that some individuals possess in influencing others. Weber asserted that the historic bearers of charisma were the antitraditional oracles, prophets, warlords, and other leaders who created new world orders through the sheer power of their personalities. Charismatic leaders appear to create magic, miracles or victories, and dramatic successes single-handedly. The followers of such leaders are, however, partners in change driven by charisma. In fact, one of Weber's most important insights about leadership is the relationship between the personality of the leader and the social and organizational context in which the leader operates. Charismatic leadership depends on the willingness and inclination of followers to accept the vision. Although charisma may move staff to action in crises or times of unpredictability, it isn't a guarantee of success and could at times be risky. Charismatic leaders could encourage dependency rather than initiative.

Trait theories

Interest in the relationship between leadership and personality traits continued through out the early part of the 20th century. Stodgill[24] devoted his life to the study of the personal factors that contributed to leadership. He identified six categories of personal factors:

> ➤ capacity
> ➤ achievement
> ➤ responsibility
> ➤ participation
> ➤ status
> ➤ situation.

His research, however, concluded that "a person doesn't become a leader by virtue of the possession of some combination of traits."

McClelland[25] believed in the correlation between a high need for power and fulfillment of the managerial role. He also examined such motives as affiliation and achievement and their relationship to a manager's power. Although such trait and motive research is useful in describing a leader's personal dispositions and motives, it doesn't emphasize what actions and tasks leaders actually performed in their daily experiences. The focus on leaders acting in real-life situations became the next focus of leadership research.

Modern theories of leadership

Trait theories of leadership served as the springboard to behavioral and contingency models of leadership that attempted to account for the multiple factors interacting to produce leadership. The *Modern theories of leadership and management* chart summarizes the leading theories of leadership from the past 50 years. (See *Modern theories of leadership and management.*)

Identify the descriptions that make the most sense to you and ask yourself *why* they make sense. Choice of theory typically reveals more about the person choosing than about the phenomenon of explanation. The chart includes the name and author of each theory, the theory's unique view of leadership, and basic principles of the theory.

(Text continues on page 53.)

Modern theories of leadership and management

Theory name	Theory author	View of leadership process	Basic theory principles
Behavioral theories			
Managerial Grid Model	Blake, R.R., and Mouton, J. *The Managerial Grid: Key Orientations for Achieving Production through People.* Houston: Gulf Publishing, 1964.	Managers and leaders exhibit five basic leadership styles that integrate two variables: concern for people and concern for task accomplishment.	Five leadership styles: ➤ *Team Style* — integrates a high concern for both people and productivity. ➤ *Middle of the Road Style* — a balanced though not high concern for both people and productivity. ➤ *Produce or Perish Style* — high concern for productivity and low concern for people. ➤ *Country Club Style* — high concern for people and low concern for production. ➤ *Impoverished Style* — low concern for both people and productivity.
Theory X	McGregor, D. *The Human Side of Enterprise.* New York: McGraw-Hill Book Co., 1960.	People have an inherent dislike for work and are externally motivated by reward and punishment.	➤ The average worker must be controlled, directed, and motivated by reward and punishment to ensure the achievement of goals. ➤ Workers avoid responsibility, are not to be trusted, and seek security. ➤ Managers/leaders can be trained to control, direct, and administer rewards and punishment.
Theory Y	McGregor, D. *The Human Side of Enterprise.* New York: McGraw-Hill Book Co., 1960.	People intrinsically value work and are motivated not only by rewards but also by meeting goals and making a contribution.	➤ The goals of the individual worker and the organization can be integrated. ➤ Workers' commitment to objectives is inherently rewarding in itself. ➤ Workers can exercise initiative, imagination, and creativity in solving work-related problems.

(continued)

Modern theories of leadership and management *(continued)*

Theory name	Theory author	View of leadership process	Basic theory principles
Behavioral theories (continued)			
Theory Y *(continued)*			➤ Managers/leaders learn to focus on creating environments in which workers can commit to organization objectives through self-direction.
Cognitive/developmental theory			
Cognitive View of Leadership	Gardner, H. *Leading Minds: An Anatomy of Leadership.* New York: Basic Books, 1995.	Leadership is a process in which the leader "affects thoughts, feelings, and behaviors of a significant number of individuals." It's a cognitive process occurring and recurring within and between the minds of leaders and those led.	➤ Leadership can be direct or indirect. *Indirect* leaders influence others through their symbolic creations, such as writings, scientific discoveries, or art. *Direct* leaders, such as politicians or statespersons, deliver their stories directly to their audience. ➤ Leaders possess "personal intelligence" — that is, they know how to reach and affect followers, and they often possess "linguistic intelligence," the ability to convey their story. ➤ Theory values the uniqueness of the individual leader. It favors the "great person" concept because at the center of great social and economic change were important individuals driving or guiding the process.

Modern theories of leadership and management *(continued)*

Theory name	Theory author	View of leadership process	Basic theory principles
Contingency theory			
Contingency Theory of Leadership	Fiedler, F.E. *A Theory of Leadership Effectiveness*. New York: McGraw-Hill Book Co., 1967.	Leadership is a function of the interactions between the leader's behavioral style and "situations" that include leader-staff relationships, the formal position of the leader in the organization, and the nature of the task.	➤ Staff effectiveness is the result of the interaction of the leader's style (motivational system) and the favorability of the situation. ➤ An important measure of leader personality is the determination of the Least Preferred Coworker, such as the staff person with whom the leader has the greatest difficulty working. ➤ Levels of stress can also affect situational favorability in the leadership process. ➤ Training and levels of intelligence also interact with situational variables in the leadership process
Decision theory			
Vroom, Yetton, Jago Leader Participation Model	Vroom, V.H., and Yetton, P.W. *Leadership and Decision Making*. Pittsburgh: University of Pittsburgh Press, 1973.	Leadership is a function of applying one of a variety of leadership styles to the type of environmental contingencies at hand. Leaders who consciously determine their style according to environmental characteristics make the most effective decisions.	➤ Leadership styles are broadly categorized as autocratic, consultative, or participative (based on group decision making). ➤ The decision environment is broadly categorized into one in which obtaining the highest possible quality decision is most important and another in which getting others to accept the decision once it's made is most important. The model provides a series of step-type questions so that managers can arrive at the best approach. ➤ The model has high validity, as demonstrated by research on its use.

(continued)

Modern theories of leadership and management *(continued)*

Theory name	Theory author	View of leadership process	Basic theory principles
Interactional theories			
Theory Z	Ouchi, W.G. *Theory Z: How American Business Can Meet the Japanese Challenge.* Reading, Mass.: Addison-Wesley-Longman Publishing Co., 1981.	Building on MacGregor's Theory Y, leadership is democratic and rooted in holistic concern and respect for workers reflective of the Japanese culture.	➤ Leadership style is democratic, consensus-building, with shared responsibility among workers and managers. ➤ Leaders seek to match employee strengths to the work at hand. ➤ Using quality circles, employees and managers review approaches to work. ➤ Leaders support long-term investment in employees with job security and slow movement up the ladder. ➤ Leaders evaluate management decisions for their long-term effects.
Transformational Leadership	Burns, J.M. *Leadership.* New York: Harper and Row, 1978.	There are two types of leaders: *transactional leaders,* who maintain day-to-day operations using incentives to motivate subordinates, and *transformational leaders,* who inspire and empower others with their vision of what is possible.	➤ Leaders identify common values that capture the imagination and trust of subordinates. ➤ They inspire subordinates with a long-term vision that involves commitment from both the leader and the followers. ➤ Leaders constantly examine the effects of actions and make adjustments as needed. ➤ Leaders demonstrate a work ethic that inspires others to do the same so that goals will be achieved. ➤ The transformational leader is the definer of reality and the keeper of the dream.

Modern theories of leadership and management *(continued)*

Theory name	Theory author	View of leadership process	Basic theory principles
Motivational and style theory			
Path Goal Theory	House, R.J., and Mitchell, T.R. "Path-Goal Theory of Leadership," *Journal of Contemporary Business* 3:81-97, 1974.	Leadership involves coaching, guiding, and rewarding staff in choosing the best paths to reach organizational goals.	Leaders are flexible, using any of four leadership styles as the situation demands: ➤ Leaders use *achievement-oriented* style to set challenging goals and expectations for competent followers able to respond to challenges. ➤ Leaders use *directive* style to set expectations and methods of operation for followers. ➤ Leaders who need to consult and ask for follower's suggestions use *participative* style. ➤ Leaders who need to be friendly, approachable, and nonthreatening to followers use *supportive* style, especially useful in building followers' trust and confidence.
Quantum theory			
Quantum Leadership	Porter-O'Grady, T. "Quantum Mechanics and the Future of Healthcare Leadership," *Journal of Nursing Administration* 27(1):15-20, January 1997.	Leadership in an age of change is a function of the application of systems thinking, which is holistic, relational, integrated, and fluidly adaptive.	➤ Leaders must expect, embrace, and adapt to changes in services, structure, technology, and outcomes. ➤ Leaders should "read signposts" and "potentials" in order to manage change, instead of predicting the future, which is a gamble at best. ➤ Leaders are translators of information that should be used to support the users.

(continued)

Modern theories of leadership and management *(continued)*

Theory name	Theory author	View of leadership process	Basic theory principles
Quantum theory (continued)			
Quantum Leadership *(continued)*			➤ Leaders encourage staff to self-manage, engage in teamwork, and embrace the power of technology to transform work in the service of patients and providers.
Situational theory			
Hersey Blanchard Situational Leadership Theory	Hersey, P., et al. *Management of Organizational Behavior: Leading Human Resources,* 8th ed. Upper Saddle River, N.J.: Prentice Hall, 2001.	Four interrelated factors determine leadership style: the amount of direction given, the degree of social support, situational components, and the maturity of the staff and followers.	Leaders assess the maturity of the staff in order to select the most appropriate of four leadership styles: ➤ *Telling* is a high task/low relationship situation with low follower readiness. It's best applied in command-and-control situations. ➤ *Selling* is a high task/high relationship situation in which the leader is in primary control but is assisting the follower to build confidence. ➤ *Participating* is a high relationship/low task behavior in which leaders and followers share in decision making. ➤ *Delegating* is a low relationship/low task behavior in which followers are competent to perform and can assume full responsibility.

Leadership and management: The differences

The terms *leadership* and *management* are often used inter-changeably, as demonstrated in the *Modern theories of leadership and management* chart. However, distinct differences do exist as well as overlap in the two functions. For example, you may be able to articulate a vision of a highly functioning unit in which patient care is exemplary and the staff is performing to their highest potential. Yet, you can't expect staff to be inspired by your vision and work toward the goal if you don't effectively assume responsibility for day-to-day operations.

Managers who aspire to leadership must deliver as managers first, in the short term. Staff will watch you in your first months on the job. They'll assess whether you keep your promises, re-spond to their questions and problems, set limits, apply standards and expectations evenly among the staff, and perform instead of delegating your managerial duties. They'll assess how well you coordinate the work, keep them informed, and operate the unit with a minimum of chaos and turbulence. Staff respect for the manager's work ethic and integrity is the fuel that propels the group toward buying into the vision and working toward the long-term goals.

Managers with a leadership agenda create a level of predict-ability and excitement for the staff. They create a sense of order, confidence, and expertise in dealing with the complexities of care delivery while engaging in those disruptive activities necessary to move toward the vision or the goal.

Nursing offers relatively few opportunities to engage exclu-sively in leadership on the grand scale; however, opportunities abound for combining leadership and management functions. For nurses, managerial components are usually associated with leadership roles. In fact, leadership without basic management can result in chaos. (See *Comparing managers and leaders*, page 54.)

In your own role as a unit manager, you might think of leader-ship and management occurring on a time continuum. Ordinary and routine times will require that you manage operations with mastery and skill; however, extraordinary times involving a criti-

Comparing managers and leaders

The following chart draws on the theories of Zalesnik,[26] Kotter,[27] and Donnelly[28] to differentiate leaders from managers.

Function	Managers	Leaders
Purpose and aim	➤ Manage the complexities of everyday operations, including problem solving, decision making, planning, organizing, communicating, and evaluating	➤ Produce change, often dramatic, through the creation of a vision and the enactment of innovative strategies to attain the goals
Needed traits	➤ Persistent, tough-minded, intelligent, instinct for survival, ability to tolerate the mundane and routine, effective communicator	➤ Persistent, tough-minded, intelligent, inspirational communicator, ability to create and manage positive tension, ability to seek out and capitalize on risk
Creates	➤ Order and predictability	➤ Disorder before a New Order
Attitudes toward goals	➤ Goals relate to smooth operations and rise out of necessity; most often short-term and deeply rooted in the culture and history of the organization	➤ Goals often personal, active, and leading to substantive change; arise out of visions for the future, for fundamental change, and for setting new directions
Conceptions of work	➤ Work an enabling process involving a combination of people, processes, and actions that interact to complete a prescribed set of short-term goals	➤ Work a creative process involving a combination of people, processes, and actions that interact to create innovation and change in the long run
Relationship patterns	➤ Prefer working with and collaborating with others ➤ Maintain a low level of emotional involvement in working relationships and may not intuitively sense the thoughts and feelings of others ➤ Relate to staff according to the role they play in a sequence of events or a decision-making process ➤ Are concerned with roles in the process and the way to get things done ➤ Often play for time so that compromises will emerge that take the sting out of win-lose situations ➤ Usually strongly invested in and identified with the organization	➤ Work with others in a more emotional or connected way ➤ Concerned with ideas in a more intuitive and empathetic way ➤ Concerned with the meaning of events and decisions to staff ➤ Often involved in relationships that are intense and turbulent, especially if the goal is sidetracked ➤ May appear disorganized at times, especially if the path to the goal is unclear

(continued)

Comparing managers and leaders *(continued)*

Function	Managers	Leaders
Sense of self	➤ Are usually in harmony with the environment; protect and regulate the existing order with which they identify ➤ Self-worth enhanced by perpetuating and strengthening the existing organization, holding the ideals of duty and responsibility high, and participating in and conforming with organizational ideals	➤ Often experience a sense of separateness from the environment, including from other people ➤ May work in and value an organization but never belong to it or fully identify with its ideals ➤ Don't depend on memberships or work roles to determine their sense of self
Dealing with change	➤ Often view and approach change as incremental and as a planned activity ➤ May have difficulty with broad changes that require new rules or ways of operating; change is planned and managed	➤ Change often viewed in the gestalt, as a vision of what could be, as a new order with new rules and processes ➤ Change first led and then managed ➤ Change often precipitous
As described by subordinates	➤ Often described as inscrutable, detached, rational, and focused on maintaining control and equanimity	➤ Often evoke descriptions rich in emotional content, such as strong feelings of identification, loyalty, love, or hate; often described as inspirational

cal need for change precipitated by external factors or a crisis will demand that you lead.

Using theory in leadership

Theories and models are like lenses. They bring either clarity or confusion to the phenomenon at hand. Theories of leadership and management usually arise from the observation of patterns and relationships in the work setting.

Theory choice depends on your own world-view. For example, your attraction to command-and-control theories as opposed to transformational theories indicates your preferences for control or participation. If you prefer to control but your staff have

And the survey says...

Organizational changes and redesign undoubtedly affect nursing leadership. Researchers Gelinas and Manthey[29] surveyed more than 5,000 nurse executives and managers in 1993 and again in 1995 to determine just how much impact such changes have.

The 1995 survey data revealed that nurse leaders increasingly need to use tools to measure and manage outcomes, understand managed care, develop team-building skills, and change their management expertise. These skills are related to the demand for fiscal discipline, quality care, and leading change in health care delivery systems that are constantly evolving in structure and process.

strong needs to participate as stakeholders, the application of a command-and-control theory might not succeed.

No best theory of leadership exists. In fact, the complexities of the work and the environment may require you to apply more than one theory of management.

The most useful theories are those that can be validated through research. Leadership is such a complex phenomena, occurring in such rapidly changing environments, that meaningful experimental research is difficult to conduct. However, survey findings and descriptive research concerning nurses in leadership roles may contribute to the development of nursing leadership theory or to the refinement of existing leadership theories. (See *And the survey says....*)

Applying nursing theory to actual nursing leadership situations can also help clarify nursing approaches to leadership. Laurent[30] reminds us that although nursing theory has focused primarily on the management of patient care, it can provide a framework for leadership behavior. For example, using Orlando's model for nurse–patient negotiation, Laurent proposed a participative form of leadership, in which leader and staff members explore and agree on working arrangements. Nursing theories and models remain untapped as sources for leadership theory development.

Case for analysis

How exciting — the Director of Intensive Care Units (ICUs), your good friend and colleague for many years, has invited you to join an ICU that has been without strong leadership for 3 years. The director confided to you that the leadership position is yours for the asking. The possibilities are endless in making this a great unit, even though it will take much time and effort. You accept the position of senior clinical coordinator, in which capacity you'll be working with three clinical coordinators, all of whom have worked on the unit an average of 4 years.

As soon as you join the staff, rumors begin circulating that your joining the staff is a signal of bigger changes to come, including the elimination of one or two existing clinical coordinators. During a staff meeting, the director is confronted with some of these rumors. She responds cryptically that each clinical coordinator, including you, will be evaluated, and thus confirms the rumor's likelihood. You're now between a rock and a hard place. The staff and the other clinical coordinators begin to isolate you, making it difficult for you to learn the ways of the unit. You have so many questions, but no one answers them, including the director who recommended you for the position. How have patient assignments been made in the past, and how can you improve the system? When are schedule requests due? Should you take patient assignments?

You begin to feel overwhelmed. During a staff meeting, a nursing assistant remarks, "I don't know who you think you are. You don't know how things work around here. You can't come up here and think you're going to change our ways!" Before you can reply, the director intervenes and goes quickly to the next agenda item. You feel hurt and compromised. Your director advises you to "figure it out" and adds, "You're being too hard on yourself, and you can't do everything perfectly immediately." However, she offers no specific strategies to get you through this situation. You're determined to succeed, but you need to regroup. Where do you go from here?

What is resistance? Why does it manifest itself so often in response to change? What theories of change help in dealing with resistance? ●
(Case contributed by Christine Rapacchiano-Kimber, RN, BSN.)

Critical questions

➤ What are the best strategies for integrating oneself into a new work unit?
➤ Is there a timing to the introduction of new ideas? Considering this case, what might be the best times to introduce your ideas to the staff and clinical coordinators?

➤ When you seek information from other staff members and they don't respond, how might you interpret this, and what can you do to get a different response?

➤ How do you deal with the anger and hurt you're feeling, while still maintaining a positive attitude about your new position and its potential?

➤ What is your assessment of the director's role in creating this situation? For example, how does the staff perceive the director's intervening in your behalf?

➤ What is your estimate on how long the staff will test you? How will you know that you have been integrated into the work unit? What will be your signs?

➤ What are the most important lessons for leadership development in this case?

Points to remember

The following points summarize the myths and theories about nursing leadership:

➤ A myth is a constructed view of reality that explains phenomena in the absence of direct evidence. Seven common myths of leadership are that leaders are born, leadership can be taught, leaders never fail, leaders promote change, leaders must possess charisma, leaders must be served, and gender differences in leadership favor males. By exploring myths of leadership, we can better understand leadership phenomena, and guiding principles or theories can be developed and tested.

➤ Machiavelli was one of the earliest leadership theorists. His principles for leadership and governance, written in 1535, emphasized the importance of human nature and self-awareness in the exercise of leadership. Machiavelli was the first to describe leadership as practice rather than as prescribed.

➤ The relationship between leadership and personality was used as a framework for some of the earliest theories of leadership, particularly Weber's concept of charisma and the later trait theories of leadership.

➤ Modern theories of leadership attempt to account for the complex interactions of views of work, interpersonal interaction, task roles, and environmental factors. Theories of leadership have become more complex and have moved their emphasis to leader-staff participation and creating environments where leadership can shift and each staff member can fulfill her potential.

➤ Research on the challenges and strategies of nurse leaders and executives can provide useful data on how nurses can apply leadership in the service of improved care delivery.

References

1. "Lavinia Dock: Self-Portrait," *Nursing Outlook* 25(1):22-26, January 1977.
2. Allen, D.W. "How Nurses Become Leaders: Perceptions and Beliefs about Leadership Development," *Journal of Nursing Administration* 28(9):15-20, September 1998.
3. Senge, P., et al. *The Fifth Discipline Fieldbook: Strategies and Tools for Building a Learning Organization.* New York: Currency Doubleday, 1994.
4. Neff, T.J., and Citrin, J.M., eds. *Lessons from the Top: The 50 Most Successful Business Leaders in America and What You Can Learn from Them.* New York: Currency Doubleday, 2001.
5. Bell, D. "A Conversation with Daniel Bell," *Harvard Gazette* pages 5-6, October 1992.
6. Pfeffer, J. *Managing with Power: Politics and Influence in Organization.* Boston, Mass: Harvard Business School Press, 1992.
7. Bornstein, S.M., and Smith, A.F. "The Puzzle of Leadership," in Hesselbein F., et al. *The Leader of the Future: New Visions, Strategies, and Practices.* San Francisco: Jossey-Bass Publishers, 1996, pp. 281-292.
8. Cohen, E.A., and Gooch, J. *Military Misfortunes: The Anatomy of Failure in War.* New York: Vintage Books, 1991.
9. Tuchman, B. *The March of Folly from Troy to Vietnam.* New York: Alfred A. Knopf, 1984.
10. Gardner, H. *Leading Minds: An Anatomy of Leadership.* New York: Basic Books, 1995.
11. Sennett, R. *Authority.* New York: Knopf, 1980.
12. Greenleaf, R.K., et al., ed. *On Becoming a Servant Leader.* San Francisco: Jossey-Bass Publishers, 1996.
13. De Pree, M. *Leadership is an Art.* New York: Doubleday, 1989.
14. Broverman K., et al. "Sex Role Stereotypes: A Current Appraisal," *Journal of Social Issues* 28(2):59-78, spring 1972.
15. Bem, S.L. "Gender Schema Theory: A Cognitive Account of Sex Typing," *Psychological Review* 88(4):354-64, July 1981.
16. Powell, G.N. *Women and Men in Management,* 2nd ed. Newbury Park, Calif.: Sage Publications, 1993.

17. Rosener, J.B. "Differences Make a Difference." *Healthcare Forum Journal* 35(5):62-67, September-October 1992.

18. Machiavelli, N. *The Prince*. New York: Bantam Classics, 1981 (first published 1513).

19. Woodam-Smith, C. *Florence Nightingale 1820-1910*. London: Constable, 1950.

20. Cook, E. *The Life of Florence Nightingale*. New York: Macmillan Publishing Co., 1913.

21. Carlyle, T. *Heroes and Hero Worship*. Boston: Adams, 1907 (first published 1841).

22. Galton, F. *Hereditary Genius*. New York: Appleton, 1870.

23. Weber, M. *The Theory of Social and Economic Organization*. New York: Oxford University Press, 1947 (first published 1921).

24. Stodgill, R.M. "Personal Factors Associated with Leadership: A Survey of the Literature," *Journal of Psychology* 25:35-71, 1948.

25. McClelland, D.C. *Power: The Inner Experience*. New York: Irvington, 1975.

26. Zalesnik, A. "Managers and Leaders: Are They Different?" *Harvard Business Review* 55(3):67-79, 1977.

27. Kotter, J.P. *Leading Change*. Boston: Harvard Business School Press, 1996.

28. Donnelly, G, et al. *The Nursing System: Issues, Ethics and Politics*. New York: John Wiley & Sons, 1980.

29. Gelinas, L.S., and Manthey M. "The Impact of Organizational Redesign on Nurse Executive Leadership," *Journal of Nursing Administration* 27(10):35-42, October 1997.

30. Laurent, C.L. "A Nursing Theory for Nursing Leadership," *Journal of Nursing Management* 8(2):83-87, March 2000.

CHAPTER 3

Leadership, change, and the future

Gloria Ferraro Donnelly, RN, PhD, FAAN

> "Not everything that is faced can be changed, but nothing can be changed until it is faced." —James Baldwin

Nurses in all segments and at all levels of the profession are facing massive change. The ability to read the signals and to initiate, respond to, manage, and cope with change are key predictors of a leader's and staff's success.

Drivers of change in the health care system

The pace of change in health care delivery continues at unprecedented rates. It's propelled primarily by advances in technology, the aging of the population, the high cost of health care, the growing number of uninsured patients, the corporatization of health care, and critical workforce shortages, particularly in nursing.

Technology and health care

Advances in information and other technologies continue to play a primary role in the health care system's rapid evolution. The most revolutionary and rapidly evolving power source of this century is information processing. To illustrate, the power of the warehouse-size computer of 1945 is comparable to the silicon chip, small as a baby's fingernail, in today's digital watch. Further,

Techno-toolkit for leaders

Information technology skills are basic tools for every nurse manager, given the role that technology plays in the evolving health care system. Mindful of that fact, every nurse should embrace technology.

Ask yourself the following questions to assess your basic knowledge about information technology. If your goal is to be a truly effective nursing leader, you should be able to answer yes to every question.

Basic information technology skills assessment

➤ I own and regularly use a personal computer.	Yes No
➤ My employer gives me access to the Internet and to e-mail.	Yes No
➤ I regularly explore the World Wide Web for information that will enhance my clinical practice and leadership-management knowledge.	Yes No
➤ I regularly use e-mail in my work and personal life.	Yes No
➤ I regularly use a standard word processing program.	Yes No
➤ I can develop a budget or simple financial analysis on a computerized spreadsheet.	Yes No
➤ I can prepare a computerized slide presentation and use the computer to present it	Yes No

a modern supercomputer can execute 1 trillion multiplications in the time it takes you to read one page of text.[1]

These developments have facilitated the mapping of the human genome, which in turn will provide a growing number of sophisticated therapies. Among these are new pharmaceuticals, gene-based diagnostic tests, and customized gene therapies for diseases and conditions once thought to be incurable. The use of advanced computer technologies is increasing the speed of laboratory research techniques and the development of new interventions. Huge databases are now available to researchers interested in specific diseases, health care behaviors, use of prescription drugs or health care services, and medical records, to name a few.

Hospitals and other health care organizations are moving rapidly to link health care providers and consumers on the web, and use of the Internet continues to offer health care professionals more sophisticated ways to extract, analyze, aggregate, and evaluate data and information used in clinical decision making. (See *Techno-toolkit for leaders* to assess your basic information technology savvy.)

With respect to consumers, the Internet is creating a shift in access to health care knowledge from the provider to the patient. Of the 275 million residents of the United States, more than 100 million have access to the Internet and 52 million regularly seek health information on the web and will continue to demand the latest drugs, treatments, and higher-quality care.[2] It's likely that some patients and their family members are checking the latest diagnostic and intervention information on a website devoted to research and practice issues. They may also have visited your facility's' website before admission. Patients can also join virtual communities of individuals with similar conditions where care comparisons are shared and recommendations made. Goldsmith[3] asserts that the Internet is "often the first destination of a patient newly diagnosed with a serious, chronic health problem." Consumers not only get advice, support, and information but also can purchase medicine and products and explore alternative interventions.

More than any new technology in the past 50 years, the Internet has the potential to unalterably change the structure and processes of health care.[4] A leader who is resistant to its use will severely compromise her ability to quickly assess trends and access information, in the service of patients and staff.

The aging population

Demographics are also quickly changing the landscape of health care delivery, and life expectancy is extending. By 2030, 19.6% of the population will be older than age 65, compared to 9.5% in 1970, and 2.4% of the population is expected to be disabled.[5]

Related to the growth in population of elderly people, the incidence of illness is shifting from acute to chronic. In 1995, for the first time in the 20th century, more people died of chronic than acute illness. This shift has dramatic implications for facilities attempting to adjust their services to meet the changing demands.

Further, expenditures in nursing home care increased from $4.2 billion in 1970 to a projected $117.6 billion in 2004.[6] The Balanced Budget Act was the government's attempt to slow Medicare spending. (See *Balanced Budget Act of 1997*, page 64.)

Balanced Budget Act of 1997

The Balanced Budget Act (BBA) was signed into law by President Clinton in 1997. It was proposed with the intention to decrease federal spending by restructuring the program rules of Medicaid and Medicare. The BBA was projected to save the government $130 billion over 5 years. For more information about the BBA, visit *www.hcfa.gov/regs/bbaupdat. htm.*

However, prescription drug benefits in demand by so many elderly people may reverse this trend.

The growing population of elderly people, the rise of chronic disease, and end-of-life care will increase the demand for all levels of nursing services.

The cost of health care and the uninsured

Over the past 3 decades, U.S. health care costs have risen at an astounding rate. Projections are that U.S. health care expenditures will rise from $1.31 trillion in 2000 to $2.17 trillion in 2008. Managed care was moderately successful in slowing health care costs in the late 1980s and early 1990s; however, this trend has reversed. Health care premiums rose 2% to 4% annually from 1994 to 1997 and continued to rise from 9% to 12% at the turn of the twenty-first century.

Despite the fact that the United States spends more of its gross national product on health care than any other country, 15.5% of Americans, or more than 40 million individuals, are without health care coverage.[7] In 1989, Goldsmith[8] predicted that the successful hospital of the future would focus more acutely on early diagnosis and management of chronic illness as well as on reaching out to homes and residential communities, including electronic outreach. Although profits may slowly improve for some facilities, many facilities are still in danger of closing. Documenting quality care through outcomes measurement and improving outcomes by reducing errors will continue to challenge nurse-managers, making identifying trends and interpreting data very important. (See *Tracking trends.*)

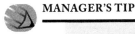

Tracking trends

You've worked at your facility for more than 5 years, and now you're in a management/leadership position. But how much do you know about trends in care and cost at your facility? How much of the big picture do you have?

You should know the following about your facility so that you can plan for the future of your unit and possibly foresee changes that will affect patient mix, staffing, workload, and care delivery.

Identifying hospital trends

➤ What is the average age and length of stay of patients in my facility, on my unit? How has this changed, if any, over the past 5 years?
➤ How is acuity measured in my facility, and what are the 5-year trends?
➤ What is the ratio of staff to beds, and how does this compare with national benchmarks?
➤ What is the trend in number of beds and services over the past 5 years?
➤ What community or geographic area does my facility serve, and what are the changing demographics of that community?
➤ What is the cost per day for an average patient on my unit, and how has this cost changed over the past 5 years?
➤ What is my facility's ratio of insured to uninsured patients?
➤ Does my facility have for-profit or nonprofit status? Is it part of a larger system? Have I visited the facility or corporate website lately? If my facility is a for-profit, how has the price of its stock fared over the past 5 years?
➤ What is the turnover rate for nurses at my facility and on my unit? Has it changed dramatically over the past 5 years? How does it compare internally, regionally, and nationally?

The corporatization of health care

Since the 1970s, hospitals and other health care organizations across the country have been at the business of integration. Of the 4,915 community hospitals in the United States, 3,544 belong to a system or a network. The American Hospital Association defines a *system* as either a multihospital system, which can include two or more hospitals under the umbrella of a central organization, or a diversified single hospital system, which includes three or more owned or leased nonhospital, preacute, or postacute health care organizations. A network may include groups of doctors, hospitals, other providers, and community agencies that collaborate in delivering a broad range of services.[9]

Over the past 3 decades, the for-profit sector of the health care industry has grown. For example, of the 4,915 community hospitals in the United States, 749, or 15%, are investor owned, for profit.[10] The health care industry is big business, which can put the clinician at a disadvantage because clinical education hasn't always stressed knowledge of the business side of health care. Nurses commonly focus on care and cure, assessment, diagnosis, intervention, and the quality and continuum of care, which includes not only the principal patient but also the family.

The health care industry at the macro level is focusing on market segmentation, financial outlooks, continuous quality improvement, benchmarking and outcomes, branding, and cost-quality trade-offs. The language and the focus between clinicians and those who manage health care systems are very different, which is precisely why nurse-managers and leaders need to better understand the business of health care.

Byers[11] stressed that marketing is an important part of the leadership equation. Because consumers are becoming more sophisticated, competition for market share among hospitals, health systems, and other provider organizations has increased. Nursing leaders, with their deep understanding of patient needs and knowledge about quality clinical care and outcomes, can play an important role in designing and implementing marketing plans that target both patients and potential staff. Retaining staff and attracting new staff to the facility also involve marketing efforts. (See *Marketing your workplace.*)

Nursing workforce shortages

According to an American Hospital Association bulletin in June 2001, 75% of vacancies in hospital staff positions are for nurses and 126,000 nurse positions are open.[12] The National Council of State Boards of Nursing reported a 26% decline overall from 1995 to 2001 in graduates sitting for NCLEX, the licensing examination for nurses.[13]

In addition, the average age of the working registered nurse is climbing. The U.S. Government Accounting Office reports that by 2010, 40% of all registered nurses will be older than age 50.[14] The convergence of a tight labor market in general and the aging of the nurse workforce will worsen the nurse workforce shortage

Marketing your workplace

Question: *How can I market my facility as the best place to work?*
Answer: The following approaches can be used to market messages about your facility or your unit to various audiences.

Marketing strategy	Purpose	Audience
Publication of clinical outcomes	To give the staff a sense of pride in clinical care and a desire to improve outcomes	Staff, patients and families, and potential patient markets
Patient testimonials	To recognize the staff and to promote the facility's excellence in clinical care	Staff, potential patient markets, and current patients
Patient satisfaction results	To give the staff a sense of pride in clinical care and a desire to improve outcomes	Staff, potential patient markets, and current patients
Accreditation results	To promote the facility's compliance with standards and level of excellence	Staff, potential patient markets, and current patients
Awards received by the facility or staff	To recognize the staff and to promote the facility's excellence in clinical care	Staff, potential patient markets, and current patients
New or improved programs, technologies, or services, such as cutting-edge therapies, patient education programs, community service programs, and disease management programs	To promote the facility's commitment to meeting the needs of patients and communities and to improving the lives and health of patients and communities	Current and potential patient markets and potential staff
Human interest stories involving patients, staff, and quality outcomes	To recognize the staff and to promote the facility's excellence in clinical care	Current and potential patient markets and potential staff
Snapshots of noteworthy clinicians and staff	To recognize and retain staff, to recruit new staff, and to interest young people in a career in health care	Current and potential patient markets, potential staff, and individuals who might be considering a career in health care

and affect access to care. Burnout and dissatisfaction among nursing staff are on the rise, and the American Hospital Association's FutureScan reports that union activity among health care professionals, both doctors and nurses, is on the rise.[15]

Retention is also an issue because there are now many more employment opportunities for nurses in organizations other than hospitals. These include managed care, the insurance industry, long-term care, and pharmaceutical companies and clinical research organizations conducting clinical trials. In previous nurse shortages, employers put resources into recruitment. The current and worsening shortage is demanding an infusion of resources into both recruitment and retention, with the emphasis on retention, given the shrinking pool. The retention issue implies that employers need to design and implement career trajectories for nurses so they have paths for advancement in the system and increased compensation. The twenty-first century has presented an even greater challenge to the nursing profession — to learn to market nursing careers aggressively and competitively in an environment where all career paths are open to both sexes.

Competition to attract individuals into the nursing profession and qualified nurses to the workforce will be fierce over the next 10 to 15 years. Nurse leaders will be challenged to create positive and safe work environments where staff can grow personally and professionally and where turnover rates are relatively low. At the same time, nurse leaders will be challenged not only to respond to change but also to initiate strategies that position both the unit and the total organization for success.

Challenges and change

Advances in technology, the aging population, the high cost of health care, the growing number of uninsured, the corporatization of health care, and critical workforce shortages aren't the only external trends that impinge on your leadership. The changes in your own facility and unit — including new systems, programs, policies, staffing challenges, and restructuring, to name just a few — also affect it.

Change is a function of perspective. You might not be able to control the internal and external forces creating change in health

How do I think about change?

To assess how you perceive and grapple with change, think about and answer the following questions.

➤ When I sense that change is needed, do I concentrate more on defining the problem or on projecting the outcome of change?

➤ Do I believe that rapid change is deleterious?

➤ Do I value stability and status quo rather than experimentation and change?

➤ Am I willing to entertain ideas contradictory to my own?

➤ Is there a pattern or pace to change in my work environment, and am I comfortable with it?

➤ Can I view a proposed change from another person's or system's point of view?

➤ How many changes have occurred recently in my life, particularly in my work?

➤ Can I change a premise from positive to negative and examine both critically?

➤ Can I arrange my plan for change in sequential order, change the sequence, and examine potential effects?

➤ Do I isolate critical factors in my change problem?

➤ Do I examine a change problem from a historical perspective, knowing that many of those who don't know history are doomed to repeat it?

➤ Do I project various effects or scenarios that result from change, and can I examine them critically ?

care delivery, but you can change the way you think about change. Even in the best of circumstances, managing change can be challenging. The natural tendency is to resist change, because of the need to understand and adjust to change on the operational level. A brief assessment of how you think about change might prepare you to flex your perspective and develop more agility where change is required. (See *How do I think about change?*)

Change is never a panacea. In fact, the most beneficial changes will always create a new set of issues and problems. Even a positive global change such as "world peace" can have both positive and negative effects far beyond our imagination. Models and theories of how change works are important conceptual tools for the nurse leader.

Models of change

Think about your unit and your leadership perspective in four dimensions: being, or identity; behaving; becoming, or developing; and believing.

Being

The first dimension is *being*, or *identity*. The unit on which you work is made up of staff, patients, a physical environment, a structure, properties, and boundaries that distinguish it from other units in the organization. These elements interacting together result in the unit's identity, which can be either very distinct or amorphous in the total organization.

With respect to being, ask yourself:

➤ What distinguishes my unit, staff, and leadership from others in the organization?

➤ How do we want to be? How do we want patients, staff, administration, and other stakeholders to perceive us? What is our vision of the unit's potential?

➤ What are the values that drive how we want to be? Clinical nursing excellence, a healing milieu, a place of comfort for patients and families, a rich environment for staff growth?

Behaving

The second dimension of your unit is *behaving*, which consists of all transient, reversible, and repetitive changes over time. Stability or change within limits is a pattern of behaving. Your unit exhibits patterns of behaving that your leadership as well as multiple other factors can influence day to day.

With respect to behaving, ask yourself:

➤ Does the unit operate according to a rhythm or pattern? Is the atmosphere one of "smooth operations" or "crisis-oriented management"? Is it "serious and high pitched," "calm and deliberate," or "chaotic"? Work with your staff to chose a phrase that characterizes your unit's operational style, and then decide whether you need to make adjustments.

➤ Do staff members have a sense of their place and responsibilities in the operations of the unit? Do normal processes—for example, admissions, care delivery, equipment monitoring, clerical tasks, and interdepartmental communication—go smoothly?

Becoming

Becoming, or *developing*, is the third dimension of your unit. Unlike behaving, becoming consists of enduring and irreversible changes that bring the unit to a different state. This dimension involves and demands leadership functions more than any other.

With respect to becoming, ask yourself:

> ➤ How do you and the staff create and respond to change? Is there a spirit of experimentation, a tolerance for failure, or an untidiness when change is occurring?
> ➤ Is there strong resistance to most changes proposed — a tendency to be the last holdout? What are your strategies for leading change? Are they effective?

Believing

The final or fourth dimension of your unit is *believing*, which is about viewpoint and perspective. Our views of the world, the lenses through which we observe, have great influence on defining reality.

With respect to believing, ask yourself:

> ➤ Do you view compromise as loss? Do you tend to be an optimist or a pessimist? Does an issue need always to be framed along dimensions of right or wrong, or can you live with ambiguity? Identity, behaving, and becoming are all influenced by our world-view.
> ➤ When a staff member questions your directive, do you view this as insubordination, challenge, or an opportunity to further explore the issue?
> ➤ When an administrator doesn't approve your request, do you view this as rejection, or do you resubmit plan B and then C?

Believing greatly influences being, behaving, and becoming because perspective and world-view are frameworks for observation and action.

A classic model of change

In an era of rapid change, classic change models can be helpful in understanding change processes. One such model is the theory of

Defining first- and second-order change

Type of change	Definition	Example
First-order change	Change that occurs within a system, with the system itself remaining essentially unchanged — that is, there's no change in the basic rules or structure of the system, merely a rearrangement or manipulation of a part or parts of the system. First-order changes: ➤ appear to be based on common sense ➤ address the cause of problems or issues — that is, are origin or cause oriented ➤ are usually based on precedent or a "more of the same" approach.	After encountering problems or documenting need, a decision is made to introduce a new piece of equipment, a new ordering system, new staff, or a new evaluation system.
Second-order change	Change that provides a way out of the original system and changes the rules and internal order of the structure, thus changing the system itself. Second-order changes: ➤ sometimes appear weird, illogical, unexpected, puzzling or disruptive. ➤ are action- or results-oriented, instead of origin- or cause-oriented; change techniques deal with effects, not causes. ➤ are usually based on a solution-oriented approach that abandons precedent.	The organization implements a two-way information system by which patients can communicate with staff of the unit they'll be admitted to, before admission and after discharge. This empowers patients and families and nurtures the staff–patient relationship.

first- and second-order change. (See *Defining first- and second-order change.*)

First- and second-order change

Watzlawick et al.[16] have advanced a theory for understanding change processes within systems. Rooted in mathematic logic, the theory is concerned with the interdependence of change and stability and with changes across system boundaries and among hierarchic levels.

Think about your organization: A major change at one level trickles down or fans out like a pebble in a pond. If you initiate successful changes on your unit, the administration might mandate such changes on other units. If your facility becomes part of a larger system, changes are likely at all levels.

Change in Watzlawick's theory is a constant that's similar to an idea of the Greek philosopher Heraclitus, who believed reality to be a "continuous process of change and becoming, a world of dynamic stresses, of creative tensions between opposites."[17]

At the heart of Watzlawick's theory are two types of change: first-order change and second-order change. First-order change is most common in organizations. They're the ordinary changes brought about by new demands on the system, by efforts at continuous improvement, or by problems that need to be solved.

First-order changes are sometimes ineffective because they don't address the level at which change needs to occur. For example, one problem might be that the organization's evaluation system is ineffective in promoting staff improvement. To address this problem, new evaluation forms are adopted (a first-order change), but the problem continues. In this case, change should have been introduced with the level of management that has the power to create an environment with a higher level of accountability and a greater range of responsibility and authority. Such an environment would change the rules and the relationship between management and staff. With such changes, most of the nursing staff functions at a higher level — and the issue of the evaluation form becomes moot.

Occasionally, first-order changes are all that are needed to support staff or to make things more efficient. For example, staffing has been very lean and lateness and absenteeism are up. You know that adding an LPN to the staff to perform certain functions would greatly improve staff productivity and reduce absenteeism. You calculate what you have spent in agency nurses to fill gaps during the past 8 months. Based solely on the numbers, you easily make your case for the additional staff member.

However, management instead brings in a high-powered consultant to examine and then propose new work processes. You and the staff are so stretched that you have no time to learn a new system. The consultant is frustrated and is getting in the way of the staff. Sick time increases by another 10% over the next month. At the end of 6 weeks, the consultant recommends the addition of an LPN to your unit and the maintenance of current work processes with some tweaking, all first-order changes. The rules didn't need to be changed; the system merely needed additional support to function at maximum. Attempting second-order change where only first-order change is necessary can push systems into chaos.

Neither first-order change nor second-order change can be said to have a greater value. Either may be effective, depending on the nature of the problem. Therefore, it's the leader's responsibility to assess the situation and determine what level of change is needed.

Leading change: Kotter's model

With external and internal forces driving enormous change in health care, leaders need action-oriented models that offer specific strategies for promoting successful change. Kotter,[18] an expert on business leadership, asserts that change will continue at the same rate and that competition in most industries will accelerate. Health care is no exception. After studying the patterns of restructuring, reengineering, downsizing, quality improvement, acquisitions, and other organizational transformations for 15 years, he offers not only some powerful insights on why change often fails but also a road map for "leading change."

The need to reduce costs, improve quality, find opportunities for growth, and increase productivity demands leadership rather than management skills to effect change in the health care system. Kotter defines *management* as planning and budgeting, organizing and staffing, and controlling and problem solving. He differentiates leadership as establishing direction and aligning, motivating, and inspiring people. Effective management produces predictability, order, and the possibility of positive short-term results. Leadership, on the other hand, produces change that's often dramatic and extremely useful. Effective management is needed once new directions are set so that change doesn't turn into chaos. As Kotter asserts, "All highly successful transformation efforts combine good leadership with good management."[19]

Kotter recommends an eight-stage process for implementing successful change. We'll examine each one in light of the vision for the unit in your new leadership role.

Stage 1: Create a sense of urgency

If the staff are comfortable in their ways and don't perceive a need for change, they'll resist it. Think about the staff on your unit. For example, say they aren't satisfied with the documentation system because it creates too much paperwork. They're whispering in your ear about two peers who aren't "pulling their weight." When you attempt to address productivity issues, no one speaks up. Staff meetings often evolve from the beginnings of problem solving to complaining about management or another department. You've been reluctant to give direct feedback because you're new and still feeling your way. And, although staff may complain to you about others or about systems, when you encourage putting their issues on the table, they don't respond.

Kotter identifies several sources of complacency that may fit the pattern of your unit. Senior management may not discuss real problems enough. A focus on "being positive" may overshadow real problems and issues, causing denial to become the pattern. Complacency prevails when giving direct feedback is viewed as hurting people's feelings, creating conflict, and lowering morale. However, it's the leader's responsibility to give direct feedback and to encourage the staff to do the same. Direct feedback can be given in a respectful manner, and once the leader has demonstrated that the intent of feedback is to foster improvement, the staff will learn to give and receive constructive feedback with one another and with the leader.

Even if your staff has no sense of urgency to change, it's your job to raise that level of urgency within them. Give them information about productivity and budget. Look at the numbers together, and when performance is low, discuss strategies for improving productivity or cutting costs. Share the pressures of leadership with the staff. If patients and families complain, have the staff confront their complainants. When a staff member whispers about problems with a colleague, insist that the person give feedback directly. Expect the staff to communicate freely, directly, and respectfully with you and with one another. Most important, keep staff fully informed about the goings-on of the organization, future opportunities, and organizational threats. Because the staff can easily slip back into complacency, you'll need to monitor the pitch of the urgency to ensure that it remains high enough to catalyze and moderate enough to permit the staff to function.

Stage 2: Create a guiding coalition

You alone can't drive unit transformation. Every leader needs help, a group of committed staff who will guide change at all levels. You might begin this process by forming an executive committee of the unit, a group of staff who represent the following characteristics and will work with you.

➤ *Expertise in nursing practice.* Choose a nurse to whom the staff go when they need practice advice.
➤ *Credibility.* Choose a nurse or support staff member whom the staff trusts and respects.
➤ *Leadership.* Choose staff members who show leadership tendencies and are problem solvers and team players.
➤ *Positional power.* Invite a trusted member of the administration to sit in on your meetings from time to time, to provide a check against the total organization's direction.

After the coalition is formed, have frequent contact in social environments and in work. Kotter points out two important features of coalitions: They tend to fall apart if the need for change isn't deeply felt, and a commitment to excellence and a desire to have the unit perform at the highest level are what keep successful coalitions together.

Stage 3: Create a vision and a strategy

Creating a vision implies that you can project a picture of what your unit will be in, for example, 5 years. Kotter identified six characteristics of an effective vision, which are embedded in the following assessment questions.

➤ Is the vision *imaginable?* Can the guiding coalition paint a realistic and appealing picture of what the unit can become?
➤ Is the vision *desirable?* Are the staff excited about it? Can they view it as in their best interests? Would it appeal to patients, doctors, and other stakeholders?
➤ Is the vision *feasible?* Can you really get there, and does it match the parent organization's direction?

A vision of the future

The following is a sample vision for a nursing unit: "Our vision is to become a unit that delivers the highest quality patient care, has positive clinical outcomes, and has the highest level of patient-family satisfaction in the organization. Our unit will become a magnet for staff who wish to achieve a high level of professional growth, excellence in practice, and service to the organization and to one another."

In two or three sentences, write a first draft of a vision statement for your own unit.

> ➤ Is the vision *focused?* Is it clear enough that obvious methods and approaches exist to help the staff attain that vision?
> ➤ Is the vision *flexible?* Can you change course in response to internal and external flux?
> ➤ Is the vision *communicable?* Can you describe it in less than 5 minutes?

Vision statements take time and patience to craft. Seemingly simple and elegant statements can take months to develop. When developing a vision statement, remember that you're creating the future. (See *A vision of the future.*)

Stage 4: Communicate the vision

When you and the staff have settled on a simple, jargon-free vision statement, communicate it widely and repeatedly in various forums, unit staff meetings, managers meetings, and administrative meetings. Print the vision statement on unit notepads, and display it on bulletin boards, remembering that repetition of ideas breeds comfort.

The vision will be undermined if it's too out of line with organizational structure. For example, excellence in clinical practice may be a goal, but the organization may be so focused on cost containment that the vision becomes unattainable. A high level of professional growth may be very desirable, but the organization may not put enough resources into formal or continuing education for staff.

Finally, the leadership must take every opportunity to live the vision by example. If excellence is the goal, then the leader must always strive for excellence. There can be no double standard when implementing a vision.

Step 5: Empower the staff to act

Empowerment is a controversial concept. A colleague who worked in a busy managed-care company described with disdain how her manager had latched onto the empowerment issue. He left the following message on his voicemail, "Good day. I'm unavailable to speak with you now; however, I am empowering you to leave a message, and I'll get back to you." Of course, we don't empower others to do simple things like leave messages. We can, however, create environments in which individuals believe they can act and make a difference.

Action is born of confidence and trust. Kotter identifies four barriers to empowerment:

> *structure* — Formal structures, such as reporting lines, documentation systems, and many layers of management, can create unwieldy bureaucracies that inhibit action. The staff will avoid acting if to act means a formal report in triplicate and a review by four levels of management before approval.
> *authority* — Controlling managers who wield authority, second-guess, and are hypercritical of staff are likely to inhibit action.
> *skill deficit* — Lack of knowledge and skill will certainly inhibit action. The organization or unit with a patient- and staff-focused vision of the future will need to invest in the lifelong learning of its staff. Education may be the most empowering strategy of all in the long run.
> *personnel systems* — A misalignment of personnel systems with the vision will inhibit action. For example, the vision pictures a highly functioning, professional staff, but support for staff to attend conferences and meetings and wide access to clinical information on the Internet or through other technologic devices are missing. The annual evaluation doesn't include items that directly relate to elements of the vision. A vision is an alignment tool. It will function to identify the gaps in the organization that impede progress toward the goal.

Stage 6: Produce short-term wins

Change is always difficult, which is why tangible wins and gains that the staff can celebrate are necessary. For example, after working only 6 months toward the vision, absenteeism is down

60% and incidents are down 40%. To help those around you see such short-term wins, you should review this information with the staff and disseminate it to administration and to key stakeholders. Kotter points out that short-term wins offer data that extra effort is worth it, recognize and reward change agents, validate the vision and strategies, undermine the naysayers and resisters, earn the extra support of management, and incite further momentum.

Short-term wins don't happen serendipitously, and they aren't about empty cheerleading. They're about data that reveal results. Leadership must plan the demonstration of such wins. Tracking important clinical issues — such as rates of infection, number of patients deceased, number of falls and other incidents, and improvement — gives staff a sense that their results aren't a function of luck, crisis, or other factors outside their control. Planning and achieving results are empowering. If the plan doesn't work, you can always revise your strategy. Short-term wins also create the impression that results could be better, so the staff maintains the urgency to continue changing.

Stage 7: Consolidate gains and create more change

With reasonable success in the first six stages, you've moved significantly closer to fulfilling your vision — but you aren't finished. How many times have you worked on a unit where the promise of change was great yet, in a year, you were back to the old systems and ways? (See *Another new system,* page 80.)

Resistance is always lurking at the underbelly of change. In fact, resistance never completely disappears. After all, the successes on your unit may be creating pressure for other units to comply, which may further undermine your efforts. Hospitals, home care systems, and long-term care agencies, to mention only a few, are complex, interdependent systems in which change in one part can interfere with operations in another. If the interdependency is unnecessary, it needs to be removed so that change can proceed.

To consolidate gains, you must frequently return to the vision and then initiate more change. Additional resources, including support from administration, are also needed. According to Kotter: "Systematically targeting objectives and budgeting for them, creating plans to achieve those objectives, organizing for imple-

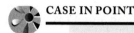

Another new system

Shortly after the new corporation acquired the facility, the first major change was announced: Patient-focused care, a popular model in the 1990s, would be introduced on all units. This model focused on increasing the registered nurse workforce, at a time when there were many licensed practical nurses (LPNs). New titles were developed, and LPNs were to be called patient care associates (PCAs). Three-month training periods were implemented to clarify the work redesign and multitasking that would now be expected. Training included team building, delegation, and management skills for nurse-managers.

For a while, things seemed to be working, although there was no real data to demonstrate that the new system was any better than the former one. Relationships among the nursing staff began to erode, particularly between the registered nurses and the PCAs. Each group believed that the other did not do enough, and managers used much of their time mediating battles. After a year, the new system was working on only a few units, where staff seemed to have the skills to implement the change. The project was abandoned after 18 months, and a new system was introduced.

mentation, and then controlling the process to keep it on track—this is the essence of management."[20] Expert management combined with leadership is the key to maintaining momentum and consolidating the unit's transformation.

Stage 8: Secure the transformation in the culture

It's been a long road since that first day you walked onto that new unit with high hopes of making significant change. After 3 years, your unit is humming along, productivity is up, clinical outcomes are outstanding, patient satisfaction is high, the staff is more educated, doctors request that their patients be sent to your unit, and you and the staff have successfully held down costs. Your unit is realizing its vision, but powerful cultural forces are at work that could create significant setbacks. This is why it's important to understand the concept of organizational culture. *Culture* is the shared values, ways, and norms for interpreting signs, symbols, and actions in a group. For example, in a community hospital, a crisp white uniform may be a sign of professionalism, but in a bustling university hospital green scrubs serve the same function. All change in an organization involves the context of culture. However, you can't wait for the culture to change before

Changing the culture of health care

Beginning in the 1850s and until her death in 1910, Florence Nightingale went about legitimizing nursing as work for women, creating an educational system to prepare nurses, designing health care facilities, and profoundly changing the delivery of health care worldwide. After she completed her work, the culture of health care was changed forever

you implement change, and you must monitor the culture's response to change to prevent regression. Kotter points out that culture will always be the last element of an organization to change, and cultural change is most dependent on results and a great deal of verbal instruction. Cultural change may also involve a great deal of turnover.

While transforming your unit, you'll need to heed the culture and its response to your efforts. Respect the culture through timing and underplaying what might be threatening, until you can demonstrate results. Transforming health care systems will always require a persistent, masterful blend of leadership and management. Change rates will continue to bear down on health care as a function of the five external driving forces: advances in technology, the aging of the population, the high cost of health care and the growing number of uninsured, the corporatization of health care, and critical workforce shortages, particularly in nursing. Hence, creating change for the future to strengthen the reach and quality of health care will require leaders with courage, commitment, and clarity of vision. (See *Changing the culture of health care.*)

Coping with change

For a leader, change is the constant. Some individuals and organizations seem to thrive on change, whereas others seem to wither into defensiveness. Flowers[21] identifies five attributes for flourishing through chaotic change:

➤ *husbanded resources* — A system, a unit, or an individual that conserves its energies, capital, and resources has more options and defenses when it's threatened. For example, if your unit is producing positive outcomes for patients and staff and is managing cost effectively, it's less likely to be a target for closing or merging when the organization needs to consolidate.

➤ *abundant relationships*—Relationships tend to be constrained and confined to subunits in large, complex organizations. Forming positive connections with the staff in other units and other departments, with other professional colleagues, and with administrators builds reputation and systems of support. Such connections can provide great advantage in periods of rapid change.

➤ *abundant information*—Information and knowledge connote power. Holding back information is a form of control. When the staff are well informed about not only the successes but also the problems and threats, anxiety in times of change can be held in check.

➤ *distributed power*—Many theories of leadership, as well as Kotter's model of change, emphasize that power distributed throughout the staff results in constructive action and in teamwork. If the leader is the sole source of power, information, and decision making, the unit will be severely compromised in times of threat and rapid change.

➤ *a common story*—A well-articulated, accepted vision can generate a common story about the direction and goals of the unit and the staff's commitment to them. Under pressing change, the common story will be a unifying factor for the staff.

Leaders sense the pulse and patterns of change. They not only have inborn capabilities but also gravitate to situations that test and shape their leadership qualities. Leaders are standard bearers. They raise the bar with their self-confidence and their quest for excellence. Leaders treat successes and failures as opportunities to grow and learn. A leader is a lifelong learner, building knowledge and skills and moving comfortably in highly competitive environments of ambiguity and change.

A Zen master identified the three essential elements of leadership:

➤ *humanity*—implies positive regard and respect for others
➤ *clarity*—suggests proper behavior, a sense of duty, and the ability to distinguish the safe from the dangerous, the wise from the foolish, and right from wrong

➤ *courage*—implies stepping forward and seeing things through.

"When all three of these are present, the community thrives. When one is lacking, the community deteriorates. When two are lacking the community is in peril, and when there is not one of the three, the way of leadership is in ruins."[22]

Case for analysis

The rumors are flying. After 3 years of fiscal ups and downs, your facility is merging with the dominant health system in town. The official announcement is made to all nursing managers with the codicil that changes, particularly consolidations, will be coming. At least two services will disappear or move to the parent institution, and other general care units will be reviewed for further consolidation.

You're the nurse-manager of one of the general medical-surgical units, and your staff is feeling particularly vulnerable. You have two brand-new staff nurses, who have been with you for 1 month and a group of seasoned veterans, two of whom have spent 12 years working on your unit. Given that your census has fluctuated wildly over the past 8 months, you don't know which way things will go. You've always encouraged rumor checking but are beginning to regret your openness, because each morning you're besieged. The flu season is ending, and you're experiencing another drop-off, so you believe that your unit might be a likely target. ●

Critical questions

➤ How much do you know about the health system into which your hospital has merged—for example, its vision, management philosophy, staffing patterns, and patient and employee satisfaction?

➤ How much do you know about the external environment in health care and the internal environment of your organization, with respect to possible impact on your operation?

➤ Do you have a clear picture of how your unit has functioned over the past 3 years in the areas of census, patient profile, staffing, budget performance, and so on?

➤ What do you know about your unit's productivity in relation to others?

➤ Should you be proactive for your unit, given your data? If you're proactive and some other unit closes, what adverse effects on your unit staff and you might you anticipate?

➤ What alternatives might you offer to the administration with respect to closing versus consolidation, based on the 3-year data?

➤ How do you interpret the ambiguity of the situation to your staff?

➤ What insights might you apply from the various theories and models of leadership that you have explored?

➤ What are the best strategies for preparing your staff for a closing or a merger with another unit? How might you do this without flaming the rumor mill?

➤ How much flexibility is there in your staff to move, retool, and so on?

➤ How flexible are you in the face of such changes?

➤ What strategies have you developed for yourself in the face of change?

➤ What alternatives might you offer to administration with respect to closing versus restructuring?

➤ What strategies might you develop to always have your staff ready to face, adapt to, and optimize rapid changes in the external environment?

➤ How will you assist your staff to put their potential anger, fear, and loss to the best possible use for themselves and one another?

➤ What opportunities are inherent in this change situation, and how can you take the most advantage of them?

Case for analysis

As director of the hospital-based Family Planning Center, it's your responsibility to recruit staff. There is a position open for a women's health nurse practitioner (NP) to replace the NP who had worked so well for the past 5 years. You know that she'll be a tough act to follow. In response to advertising, there are four promising applicants. You've put a small committee of the staff together to interview all four, and you all generally agree on the final selection.

This new NP had lost her former position in the downsizing of a large hospital in a booming metropolitan area where part of her role was to make home visits in depressed inner-city communities. She loved the work, the clients, and the big city. Also, she was very close to her family, especially her mother, with whom she had lived since her divorce.

Accepting the position at your center meant moving away from home and family in the city and relocating to a much smaller, rural town. You believed that the adjustment to your clinic pace would be an easy one for the new NP because of her experience in a busy urban clinic. However, you begin to have doubts. She isn't integrating with staff or into the workflow as you had expected. Other staff members complain of "never getting done on time." Patients complain of waiting too long to be seen. Two of the regular patients have requested not to be assigned to the new NP again. At the same time, there are patients who praise the NP for taking extra time with them.

You speak to your director about the problems. She wants you to "Make it work!" because so much time and money has gone into recruitment and orientation. The end of the NP's probation time is getting closer. ●
(Case contributed by Jean Hoover, RN, CRNP.)

Critical questions

> What are the salient issues in this situation? Who are the main players in resolving the issues?
> How strictly do you enforce the end-of-probation date to decide whether the NP can meet expectations?
> What qualities of leadership will you need to employ when talking with the NP about issues and problems? Will you focus more on task completion or consideration of the staff member?
> If you successfully negotiate with the NP for improvement, how will you measure success and in what time frame?
> What arguments and data will you use to convince your director of the best course of action?
> When and how might you involve the staff in improving the situation?
> If termination is the solution, what lessons learned might you apply in the next recruitment?

➤ If termination is the solution, how do you interpret this decision to the staff? How do you enlist their support and assistance through another transition period?
➤ What are the most important lessons for leadership development in this case?

Points to remember

The following points summarize how change affects leadership:

➤ The major external drivers of change in the health care system are advances in technology, the aging of the population, the high cost of health care and the growing number of uninsured, the corporatization of health care, and critical workforce shortages, particularly in nursing.
➤ Change is a function of perspective. Even under the best circumstances, managing change can be challenging. A natural tendency to resist change exists because of the need to understand and adjust to change on the operational level. You can't control all internal and external forces that drive change, but you can be aware of the way you think about and respond to change.
➤ There are four dimensions through which you can view your unit and leadership: being, or identity, which refers to the distinctive characteristics of the unit; behaving, which refers to transient, reversible, or repetitive changes over time; becoming, or developing, which consists of enduring and reversible changes that bring the unit to a different state; and believing, which is the lens through which we observe and influence reality.
➤ Watzlawick et al.'s theory of first- and second-order change is helpful in understanding change processes. First-order change occurs within a system, with the system itself remaining essentially unchanged. Second-order change provides a way out of the original system and changes the rules and internal order, thus changing the system itself.
➤ Kotter's model of change identifies an eight-stage process for leading change: Create a sense of urgency, create a guiding coalition, create a vision and a strategy, communicate the vi-

sion, empower the staff to act, produce short-term wins, consolidate gains and create more change, and secure the transformation in the culture.

➤ Flowers identified five attributes for flourishing through chaotic change: husbanded resources, abundant relationships, abundant information, distributed power, and a common story.

References

1. Davidow, W.H., and Malone, M.S. *The Virtual Corporation.* New York: HarperCollins, 1992.
2. Society for Health Care Strategy and Market Development. *Future Scan 2001 Millennium Outlook 2001-2005.* American Hospital Association. *www.aha.org/resource/Statistics/Statistics.asp.*
3. Goldsmith, J. "How Will the Internet Change Our Health System?" *Health Affairs.* 19(1):148-56, January-February 2000. *www.healthfutures.net.*
4. Goldsmith, J. Op. cit.
5. *The Aging of the U.S. Population, 1970-2030.* Social Security Administration. Office of the Actuary, 2001.
6. Plunkett Research, Ltd. "National Health Expenditure Amounts and Average Annual Percent Change by Type of Expenditure: 1970-2008." *www.plunkettresearch.com/health/health_statistics_5.htm.*
7. Plunkett Research, Ltd. "Overview of the Health Care Industry." *www.plunkettresearch.com/health/index.htm.*
8. Goldsmith, J. "A Radical Prescription for Hospitals." *Harvard Business Review* 67(3):104-11, May-June 1989. *www.healthfutures.net.*
9. American Hospital Association. "Fast Facts on U.S. Hospitals from Hospital Statistics." 2001. *www.aha.org/resource/newpage.asp.*
10. ibid. Op. cit.
11. Byers, J.F. "Marketing: A Nursing Leadership Imperative," *Nursing Economic$* 19(3):94-99, May-June 2001.
12. American Hospital Association. "Workforce Data Fact Sheet." June 5, 2001. *www.aha.org/workforce/resources/FactSheetB0605.asp.*
13. American Association of Colleges of Nursing. *"Nursing Shortage Fact Sheet."* August 2001. *www.aacn.nche.edu/media/backgrounders/shortagefacts.htm.*
14. U.S. General Accounting Office. Testimony Before the Subcommittee on Over-sight of Government Management, Restructuring, and the District of Columbia, Committee on Governmental Affairs, U.S. Senate. "Nursing Workforce: Multiple Factors Create Nurse Recruitment and Retention Problems." Statement of Janet Heinrich, Director, Health Care — Public Health Issues, June 29, 2001. *www.gao.gov.*

15. Society for Health Care Strategy and Market Development. *Future Scan 2001 Millennium Outlook 2001–2005.* Op. cit.

16. Watzlawick, P., et al. *Change: Principles of Problem Formation and Problem Resolution.* New York: Norton, 1974.

17. Koestler, A. *The Sleepwalkers: A History of Man's Changing Vision of the Universe.* London: Hutchinson, 1959.

18. Kotter, J.P. Op. cit.

19. Kotter, J.P. *Leading Change.* Boston: Harvard Business School Press, 1996.

20. Kotter, J.P. Op. cit.

21. Flowers, J. "The Change Project." 1999. *www.well.com/user/bbear.oindex. html.*

22. *Zen Lessons: The Art of Leadership.* Translated by Thomas Cleary. Boston: Shambhala Publications. [New York]: Distributed in the U.S. by Random House, 1993.

PART TWO

People skills

CHAPTER 4

The human capital component

Melissa A. Fitzpatrick, RN, MSN, FAAN

> "First study the science, and then practice the art which is born of that science." —Leonardo da Vinci

Leading and managing health care professionals and support staff requires exceptional "people" skills. It also requires that we connect with those we're leading and managing on a human level and that we understand their needs, fears, hopes, and dreams.

Leading in today's turbulent times is challenging: Where do we find answers to that never ending barrage of questions? How do we pave the road for others when we're just as anxious about where the road might lead? How do we balance the mandates of providing high-quality, cost-effective, innovative, and outcome-based care with the need to nurture and support our team members?

This chapter provides potential answers to these questions. However, in the final analysis, it all comes down to people skills.

People caring for people

Our goal as leaders is to bring out the best in our employees, to maximize their potential to achieve their goals, and to ensure that they have the tools and resources needed to practice effectively. Every employee has different capabilities. These include knowing what to do and how to do it as well as knowing whether the necessary resources are available for doing it. These capabilities are commonly referred to as competencies, knowledge and skills, resources and tools, processes, and organizational training. Our commitment to developing these capabilities in our employees helps ensure their ongoing growth and development and quest for continuous improvement.

Another part of the human capital equation is commitment. Nurses bring a true commitment to their patients and families, which when at its highest level, can expand their capabilities. A leader's role is to nurture the employee's commitment and make sure it doesn't wane over time. Such commitment requires that the employee wants to do what she's doing, knows why she's doing it, and perceives leadership's commitment to it as well. Usually, employee commitment is related to economic interdependence, an emotional reward, the feelings of fit and belonging, status and identity, and trust and reciprocity. These provide the basis for commitment on the employee's part and help ensure that the employee sees the activity, project, or new endeavor through to its fruition. When successful, the leader maximizes employee capabilities and employee commitment, thus maximizing human capital.

However, leaders must possess diligence and determination to find their way through the health care maze to make the vision of high-quality, cost-effective care, and competent, satisfied staff members come to life. Furthermore, because nurses are the strongest force advocating for patients and their families in the health care system, attention to all issues related to human capital is essential. These represent the very essence of nursing—the fundamental value of caring. No matter what role the nurse will play in the future, adherence to the fundamental value of caring will mean the most to the patient and his family, will provide the greatest satisfaction to us as nurses, and will in so many ways set us apart from others in our organizations. With patients needing more complex care as time passes, it's only logical to assume that their need for humanistic and holistic care will also grow exponentially. The same can be said for employees, who will need more compassionate and humanistic care from leadership and employers. It will be the role of the staff nurse leader to ensure that the patient isn't lost amid technologies and treatments and that the care that only nurses can provide shines through so that patients and families safely move through the health care system.

Norma Lang, former Dean of the School of Nursing at the University of Pennsylvania said it well: "The complexity of humanistic caring provided by nurses is also increasing dramatically and will require the most intelligent and humane men and women to become nurse-leaders of the 21st century."[1]

It's the leader's job to ensure staff support so that they can provide the kind of care that patients and families require. To do so requires unceasing attention to the employees and all that they bring to work each day. It's the leader's job to bring out the best in the staff, to help them feel whole as they provide care, and to nurture their growth and commitment so that they stay in this profession for the long haul. We may best fulfill our leadership role by helping our team members "take after a kid: believe in the impossible, dream and imagine, be passionate, be creative and innovative, don't worry or feel guilty, and learn enthusiastically."[2] These qualities will bring out the best in our team members, will enhance the effectiveness of the team, and will make the care environment a fun and innovative place to practice.

Interviewing skills: Finding the right fit

The old adage "people are your most important asset" is wrong: The right people are your most important asset.[3] Finding the right fit is an essential part of leadership today and one that requires honesty and a keen awareness of the realities of the work environment and its requirements. Not every candidate is a good fit for your leadership style or your team. Not every candidate fits within the organizational culture that's in place or shares the vision of those determining the future direction of the organization. Finding good fits involves assessing candidates to find those who share the team's goals, those who bring new and diverse skills to the team, those who have different ways of thinking and approaching situations, and those who want to help the team achieve its vision. These qualities will make the team more robust. (See *Who to hire.*)

Supervisors should be carefully selected because positive management practices and a high performance workforce all start with good supervisory selection and effective interviewing processes. A true leader and coach attracts the best and the brightest to the team, even if that means hiring those who have

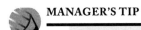

Who to hire

Effective nurse leaders openly show passion and vision to prospective hires, inspiring them to join — and remain with — their team. They show care-givers their commitment and willingness to teach and support their development. This is paramount, and doing so up front will save resources, time, and energy down the road. The best leaders get it right from the start by investing in the hiring process and hiring selectively. They seek not just to fill a position but to fill it with the candidate who's the best fit for the department and who will bring the broadest skill set to the team.

"Upright and licensed" doesn't work anymore. Nursing must attract the best and the brightest in order to sustain the profession through difficult times.

better credentials, more education, broader experience, or better skills than he has. Many leaders hire "clones" of themselves: those who don't challenge the status quo, those who don't "cause trouble," those who "do what they're told," and those who don't "show them up." Such teams lack innovation and creativity, are full of "yes" people, and never experience the most robust dialogue or decision making. They have members who go through the motions, passing time and breathing air, yet they never create an environment in which excellence is expected or achieved. These teams are ill prepared to meet the challenges that face health care leaders and to move our organizations forward.

Effective leaders know that frontline input and support to hiring and building a work culture are irreplaceable, which is why they afford all employees some decision-making authority. Team members are engaged in the hiring process, voice their opinions regarding candidates, and help to determine who will fit most effectively on the team. They tell the truth about workload, the care environment, the team members, the ability to balance personal and professional life, and the current status of the organization. Those at the frontlines of care delivery can provide the most realistic and vivid description of work life for prospective candidates and can help ensure that the candidate has the best information possible to make a good decision about employment. Such involvement in the hiring process also provides a greater commitment on the part of team members to ensure the success of the new hire that they recommended to the team.

Another key component of finding the right fit involves hiring the heart. Most leaders recognize that you can only teach so much technique and skill and that competence and technical prowess only take you so far. The rest involves what a candidate has in her heart and what she brings to the care delivery system beyond technical competence. You can't teach passion and personality, so it's essential to assess the candidate for these human qualities before making a hiring decision. Would you want this employee to care for your own loved one? Does the candidate have both the technical and the human capability to provide the level of care that you'd want for your family member? If the answer is "no," then the candidate wouldn't be a good fit on your team.

Involving staff in the hiring process, assessing all aspects of "a good fit," and hiring the heart are essential to the leader's success in recruiting candidates who will make the team more effective and robust. These issues are at the heart of the recruitment and retention challenge, and are critical to the success of health care organizations. If you do these things well, your individual leadership efforts, coupled with the efforts of your team, will result in an energized organization.

Knowing your employees

To be a servant leader, you must truly get to know your employees as people and understand the full array of issues that affect their performance, satisfaction, and commitment. Because the health care system has become depersonalized, a more personal, empathetic, and humane system must be established if workforce issues in nursing and health care are to be resolved. Leaders who become fully aware of the life issues that affect employees can better empathize with them and support their efforts to juggle the demands of their hectic lives. When employees feel the support and empathy of their nurse leaders, they're much more apt to be supportive and flexible in return.

In the past, nurses were taught "not to get attached" to their patients. They were told that they would lose objectivity and not be able to make good decisions if they were too personally in-

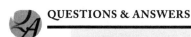

QUESTIONS & ANSWERS

Gaining new insight

Question: *How do you get your staff's attention?*
Answer: A key issue for nurse managers is finding ways to capture the attention and precious free time of their employees. The first step in doing so successfully is to know and understand the staff's many personal and professional demands and to support their ability to wear many hats in as healthy and balanced a manner as possible.

volved. Many nurse-managers were taught the same philosophy when it came to involvement with the staff. Many were encouraged to "rule with an iron hand" and to "let the employee know who was boss." They were discouraged from socializing with the staff and from "letting their guard down." This approach created distance and tension between frontline staff and the nurse leader, making communication one way only. As a result, staff members were reluctant to "pitch-in" when needed and had a "what has she done for me lately" attitude. Such barriers, whether real or perceived, have been in place much too long and have prevented many teams from achieving their goals and from creating true environments of care — for patients and for employees.

The demographics of the American population have changed dramatically, which is why it's more important than ever for nurse leaders to get to know their team members. Immigration into the United States is at an all-time high, and by 2013, those with a Spanish language heritage will be the largest minority group in the United States at over 42 million.[4] Households are becoming more diverse, with new patterns of marriage, cohabitation, and family structure. The domestic concerns of working parents, dual-worker families, and single parents are requiring greater flexibility in our organizations and a true commitment from nurse leaders to support the domestic and personal obligations of their employees. (See *Gaining new insight*.)

Staff nurses today are required to care for more patients who come from multicultural backgrounds. To meet this demand, they must be equipped with the understanding and knowledge of a multicultural community. Incorporating diversity into the staff nurse's caring practices refers not only to race but also to such issues as individuality, cultural differences, spiritual beliefs, gender, ethnicity, disability, family configuration, lifestyle, socioeconomic status, age, values, and alternative therapy preferences. Such attention to diversity helps ensure that patient and family needs are met in a way that's most meaningful to them.

However, the issue of cultural competence is as important for nurse managers as it is for staff nurses. A new function of nurse leaders is that of chief diversity officer. This role requires that nurse leaders be sensitive to diversity and recognize, appreciate, and incorporate differences into the management of care environments. Once the nurse leader is culturally competent, she must then put that knowledge to use and fully appreciate and support the cultural perspectives and demands of the workforce. The effective nurse leader is one who embraces and values diversity and inclusiveness and who builds diverse and robust teams. Are you prepared for this role?

In truly getting to know employees, nurse leaders must spend time with them, ask them questions, and build an interpersonal foundation with them that's based on respect, honesty, mutuality, and caring. How often do you ask employees how they are and actually take the time to listen to the answer? Are you aware which issues are at play in your employees' lives, and how those issues affect their performance at work? How much time do you dedicate to "being" with the staff and to truly understanding and appreciating what they do and the difference that they make every day? Today more than ever, our employees need values based on leadership, love, compassion, and healing. A key focus for nurse leaders must be on building consciousness, human awareness, and empowerment.[5] These are the attributes that will sustain nurse leaders and their teams through difficult times. Nurse leaders who understand this will win not only the heads and hands of their team members, but also their hearts.

The most effective nurse leaders get personal with their teams, aren't afraid to care deeply about the people they serve, and tap in to the heart and soul of all team members on a human level. Some say that by tapping into heart power, and capturing the heart, you capture the employee.[6] Effective nurse leaders capture the hearts of their team members with a compelling vision, a balance between work and family, and celebration and fun, inciting them to become more dedicated and to work harder. What's more, even though the focus in school and on the job is on im-

What's your staff thinking?

Are you fully aware of the most pressing issues and concerns of your team members? Have you taken the time to personally get to know them? How do the following results of the American Hospital Association's "Reality Check III: Searching for Trust" Report[7] reflect the feelings of your staff members?

➤ Nurses identify patient safety as their number one professional concern.

➤ Most nurses don't believe their hospitals are in financial difficulty.

➤ Nurses believe hospital leadership doesn't spend enough time at the frontline of patient care.

➤ Nurses are generally wary of the benefits of unionization.

➤ Nurses aren't positive about nursing as a career today or for the future.

plementing strategy, planning techniques, reading financials, and other important matters, nurse leaders recognize that leadership is fundamentally about understanding and motivating people.

Think about these recent quotes from *Hospitals and Health Networks*[8] regarding the nursing care environment: "It is a hostile environment. Nurses feel respected by their patients, but not by their employers." "Nurses rarely see top management until union contract negotiations begin. Then they suddenly begin acting as though they're our best friends. It's so transparent it's laughable." "The proliferation of union-organizing campaigns should be a wake-up call. If your hospital is facing an organizing drive, there's a reason for it. Industry-wide, there's a very large communication, credibility, and trust gap between registered nurses and upper administration. Nurses want a voice and priority attention paid to their issues."[9] At the base of many of these issues is the fact that nurse leaders and hospital administrators don't take the time to truly get to know their employees, or to understand the issues that are most important to them. Too often, hospital leaders "assume" what the issues are — and in many cases assume wrong. Decision making would be so much more effective and on target if nurse leaders went to the source for information, the one closest to the patient and to the issues: the staff nurse. (See *What's your staff thinking?*)

Learning what satisfies staff requires that leaders take the time to ask. Some health care organizations do an employee opinion survey every 10 years and think that keeps their finger on the pulse of their employees. That approach may have worked in some markets years ago, but it's equivalent to professional suicide

Employee response

Studies[10] have shown that employees respond most favorably to leaders who provide them with:
- a sense of mission
- support in developing their abilities
- recognition of performance
- an opportunity to share ideas
- an opportunity to grow.

today. Human resource leaders, working closely with operational leaders, must assess the needs and desires of their employees frequently enough so that issues can be identified and addressed. Health care leaders are finally realizing that the issues surrounding employee relations, employee satisfaction, and quality of work life have a dramatic and lasting effect on financial performance, patient satisfaction, and quality of care. They require ongoing and continuous attention.

Truly getting to know the staff and recognizing the link between leaders and team members can't be minimized. A study of 25,000 employees from a wide range of companies found that 69% of employee job satisfaction was derived from a manager's leadership skills.[11] In a time of personnel shortages and high turnover, it behooves all leaders to focus on their relationships with staff and to commit to responding to employee needs, both professional and personal. (See *Employee response.*)

Understanding the issues

For any initiative to be successful, the frontline management team must effectively understand, communicate, and advocate it. Failure to gain the understanding and support of the workforce has tangible consequences: You lose staff, quality suffers, and you lose the union campaign. Therefore, you must honestly assess the work environment and behaviors of the team members. Don't assume that you know the issues, although you can bet that the primary concerns usually have to do with work-life issues, such as overtime, scheduling, workload, acuity, assignments, and compensation and benefits.[12] Perform a management audit or assessment to understand the managers' and supervisors' perceptions and feelings, and assess the extent to which they're valid and reflective of employees' perceptions and feelings. Then provide supervisory training to secure the effective support of frontline managers—provide them with the skills, tools, and motivation necessary to respond to and address employee issues and concerns. Use a questionnaire to ascertain and measure employees' feelings toward their work environment. Measure employee alienation, which predicts behaviors and attitudes affecting employee relations, morale, and productivity. Use assessment findings to drive your strategy and to focus on key issues.

Once you know the key issues, you must be prepared to act swiftly to address them. This requires a strategic approach that's based on a core element and the essence of effective leadership: using exceptional interpersonal skills to connect with people and to gain their trust and commitment. Although this approach may seem basic—and a given for health care leadership—many organizations don't follow this approach. These organizations are paying a severe price for their lack of insight into what drives employees today and how to effectively connect with staff to obtain their support and creativity.

Tending to the human element of our nursing leadership roles can only have a positive impact on all involved. Building a strong foundation of people caring for people creates a true "us" environment and eliminates divisiveness. What's more, when we get to know the people in our organizations, there's no telling what we can achieve.

Points to remember

The following points summarize the importance of people skills in management:

➤ Leaders need to bring out the best in their employees. This includes assisting them in realizing their capabilities, providing tools for growth, and encouraging them to achieve their goals.
➤ Hiring the right fit of staff members is crucial to build a cohesive, strong work culture.

➤ A personal, empathetic, and humane system helps to resolve issues in the nursing and health care workforce. Employees who feel that they're valued as people are more apt to be supportive and flexible.

➤ Leaders must assess the work environment and behaviors of team members to better understand work-life issues and address them effectively.

References

1. Lang, N. University of Pennsylvania Alumni Newsletter, 1997, 4-5.
2. McGee-Cooper, A. *You Don't Have to Go Home from Work Exhausted! The Energy Engineering Approach.* Dallas: Bowen & Rogers, 1990.
3. Collins, J. "Turning Goals into Results: The Power of Catalytic Mechanisms," *Harvard Business Review* 77(4):71-82, July-August 1999.
4. Romano, G. "Including All," *Association Management* 52(6):30-37, June 2000.
5. Scott, C., and Jaffe, D. Managing Organizational Change: A Practical Guide for Managers. Menlo Park, Calif.: Crisp Publications, Inc., 1989.
6. Dow, R., and Cook, S. *Turned On: Eight Vital Insights to Energize Your People, Customers, and Profits.* New York: HarperBusiness, 1996.
7. American Hospital Association. *Reality Check III: Searching for Trust Report: America's Message to Hospitals and Health Systems.* Chicago: AHA, 2000.
8. Bilchik, G. "Norma Rae, RN," *Hospitals and Health Networks* 74(11):40-44, November 2000.
9. ibid.
10. ibid.
11. Anderson, M. *Companies Don't Succeed...People Do!* Aurora, Ill.: Successories, Inc. USA, 1998.
12. O'Grady, T. "Collective Bargaining: The Union as Partner," *Nursing Management* 32(6 Part I):30-32, June 2001.

CHAPTER 5

Getting your team together

Melissa A. Fitzpatrick, RN, MSN, FAAN

> "Vision without action is a daydream. Action
> without vision is a nightmare" —Japanese proverb

Nurse leaders must define the work and expectations of team
members so that everyone is singing from the same sheet of music from the beginning. Leaders must take the time to help employees understand which roles they play in the organization and
how their roles help to move the organization in a positive direction.

Organizational culture

An essential element of cultivating successful people and successful relationships in health care organizations is understanding organizational culture, the major influences on the culture, and the
role that each team member plays in either perpetuating that culture or changing it. Because health care organizations are highly
bureaucratic and political, nurse leaders must hone their political
skills and understand their place within the culture of the organization to achieve the greatest influence and effectiveness. By
mastering organizational dynamics and politics, nurse leaders become the most effective advocates for patients and families and
for employees.

In order to lead deep and fundamental organizational reengineering, nurse leaders must establish an organizational culture
that revolves around a new work contract that's based on people

The work contract

A work contract entails employees building a new type of relationship with the organization, one that involves:
➤ new expectations of what employees give and get from the organization
➤ a new understanding of the nature and scope of work
➤ a new willingness to do what it takes to achieve success.

principles, interpersonal skills, and mutuality. Long gone are the days in which employees stay at the same place of work for an entire career. No longer is it commonplace for employees to retire from the employers who gave them their first job. Today's work environment and the expectations of employers and employees must be re-articulated and new groundwork must be laid. (See *The work contract.*)

Nurse leaders must articulate their expectations in such a way that employees feel part of the greater organization and understand the role that they play in its success. They must help employees see the "big picture" and to embrace the vision and mission of the organization at large, including its strategic goals and objectives and the methods that will be used to achieve them.

Clear articulation of organizational culture, dynamics, and expectations provides clarity when challenging circumstances arise. Such clarity and articulation comes from presence and requires that nurse leaders and other organizational leaders are visible and have taken the time to establish credibility in the eyes of their employees. This also requires that nurse leaders are fully informed and involved in all aspects of strategic decision making so that they can fully inform and include their team members in supporting and nurturing the organizational culture in a positive way.

How decisions are made and how communication occurs are important components of organizational culture that affect many aspects of team satisfaction, inclusion, and commitment. Although health care organizations have been traditionally hierarchical and bureaucratic, many health care and nurse leaders are realizing that such bureaucracy can impede decision making, hamper empowerment, and limit resourcefulness. (See *Creating solutions.*)

QUESTIONS & ANSWERS

Creating solutions

Question: *Who is best prepared to create new systems and to brainstorm solutions to everyday issues?*

Answer: In a time of constant change, dwindling resources, and demands to do everything better, quicker, and cheaper, those closest to patients, families, and the teams that support them are the best ones to ensure that good decisions are made and that resources are allocated most effectively.

Leaders in successful organizations create cultures that focus on helping empowered employees define service standards and create a work environment and an organizational culture that are healthy for the people receiving care and for the ones giving it. Nurse leaders garner the support of team members and encourage them to channel creative dissatisfaction into better ways of delivering care. They take risks, extend themselves, and use their knowledge and skills in new ways to meet organizational needs.

In doing so, many leaders are creating flatter organizations and moving toward a culture of "adhocracy" rather than hierarchy and bureaucracy. They've realized that bureaucracy must be eliminated to be successful in today's changing work environment. They've moved beyond form, structure, and organizational charts to develop and lead cross-functional teams. They've moved from territorial to global in their perspective and in their approach to work, recognizing that interdependence is integral to successful organizations. These effective leaders are comfortable being on point on some projects and as team members on others. They're less interested in adhering to the boxes on the organizational chart and more interested in assembling the right people with the right skill sets to get the job done.

MANAGER'S TIP

Like it or not, effective nurse leaders learned a long time ago that to give up control and power yields far greater returns in the long run. Such nurse leaders have adapted their styles, roles, titles, structure, and power bases as needed to respond to the forces at play in the health care industry. ●

Two forces are leading many organizations into a more ad hoc, or temporary, environment. The first is a movement from an internal, management-driven focus to an external, customer-driven focus. The second is a movement from a stable, control-oriented mindset to a more flexible, adaptive mindset. These two forces together create adhocracy, which is the opposite of the hierarchy. Driving adhocracy is today's competitive environment, which requires speed, customer responsiveness, innovation, teamwork, and creative thinking.[1] Nurse leaders and their employees must see beyond their narrow, rote job descriptions and embrace the interconnectedness and interdependencies of all players on the health care leadership team. They must focus on the big picture, and the connections between functions. In strengthening the organizational culture, nurse leaders must create processes that work and close the inefficient gaps between functions that are common in traditional hierarchies, like hospitals. This requires that they create cultures in which team members want to understand and own the entire process, not have a "that isn't my job" mindset.

An organizational culture of adhocracy calls for spontaneity, innovation, and entrepreneurial spirit. Hierarchy calls for rules, regulations, and structure. Hierarchy emphasizes positions and functional titles; adhocracy emphasizes accountability and cross-functional teams. Hierarchy can work when managed effectively, but hierarchy should exist only to support the higher purpose or the mission. Nurse leaders who are comfortable with the ad hoc become customer-driven, not management- or hierarchy-driven. They're less generous with management direction and exert far less job structure from above. They arm their team members with a vision and ensure that resources and tools are available to them to succeed in achieving the vision. They tend to be more "hands-off" and encourage autonomy in their team members at all levels. These ad hoc leaders have created enough structure to support the team, but not enough to strangle them and to stifle creativity and autonomy. They're the antithesis of micromanagers and tend to be those that team members really like to work with and for. They're the vision keepers and the culture builders, but they leave the "how to" to those who know it best and to those who are closest to the issues.

Keeping their distance and not micromanaging their team members doesn't imply that these ad-hoc leaders are disinterest-

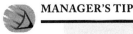

Setting the tone

At one time or another, you've likely found yourself at a meeting in which someone has delivered news in a negative, bitter, and angry way. Delivering information in this manner immediately set the tone for how that information was to be received.

The lesson? Leaders must use their influence to create positive energy, direction, and vision — and, in doing so, they'll capture the energy and commitment of their employees.

ed and don't care. They care deeply, but their focus on outcomes and team autonomy and development enables them to mentor and coach from afar, rather than having their hands in the day-to-day details of operations. These leaders get much more out of their team members, who know that support is there when they need it, but that they have the freedom to grow, to try new things, and to make mistakes.

More self-management and self-leadership with personal initiative is needed at all levels in organizations because time is precious. Priorities shift rapidly, with unceasing ambiguity and blur, therefore nurse leaders must be in charge of themselves and function as thinkers and independent problem solvers — they must build teams that can function in the same way. This underscores why a common sense of direction is essential. Empowerment, greater independence, and personal accountability define the new kind of following and the new kind of leadership needed in the ad hoc organization of the future.[2]

Nurse leaders play an integral role in establishing the successful organizational cultures of health care delivery systems. In leading the largest employee groups in these systems, nurse leaders have tremendous influence over the ways in which organizational dynamics play out and the ways in which they're interpreted and translated. It's essential today more than ever that such influence is positive, flexible, creative, and inclusive. (See *Setting the tone*.)

Organizational depression

Being negative, burned out, and entrenched in old thinking are symptoms of organizational depression and an extension of organizational cultures that are stale, inhibiting, and mediocre at best. Organizational depression is an indictment of leadership and is symptomatic of leaders who are present in title but not in action and vision. Organizations become depressed when they're led by a negative vision, risk avoidance, and downplaying threats. Such cultures require a movement toward transformational ways, rather than transactional ways, and they put employees, patients, and families at risk by sustaining negativity, blame, and lack of accountability.[3] Oftentimes, the basis for such negative organizational cultures is related to the rules of engagement that have been established, whether formally or informally.

Rules of engagement drive organizational culture and help set expectations of practice. In organizations with high morale and great teamwork, a common characteristic prevails: well-defined rules of engagement, with each team member being held accountable to them. There's zero tolerance of behaviors that derail or degrade, ongoing support to do the right thing, and tremendous role modeling at all levels. It becomes clear that those who don't follow the rules of engagement don't fit in and must either change or leave.

To assess your unit, department, and organization, ask yourself first what your rules of engagement are. Are they clear? Are they role modeled? Do you "leave wounded on the battlefield"? Is there an ethical framework in place that you're proud of? Do you stand together and support each team member, or are you divided? Is yours a learning environment in which failure is celebrated and improvement is continuous? Can you speak favorably to your family and friends about your organization and the practice environment and culture that you've created?

Clarity about professional and organizational rules of engagement goes a long way toward solving some issues. It helps to reinforce and replicate all that's good in nursing, and at the same time, it helps weed out that which is divisive and unhealthy. If this exercise works, all will undoubtedly benefit, including our patients.

Improving the culture

Establishing a healthy culture at all levels of the organization is paramount to leadership success. Such cultures endorse and nourish a healthy, creative dissatisfaction with the current state of affairs and encourage all parties to create solutions that work. The impact of organizational culture on quality, satisfaction, productivity, recruitment, and retention can't be underestimated, and nurse leaders must take the helm in ensuring that their cultures evolve in a way that best supports the people they serve.

Effective communication

Effective nurse leaders create meaning through communication. To have high levels of commitment, people must be aware of the overall and specific organizational mission, philosophy, and goals, and their relationship to them. Essential to creating a healthy organizational culture is establishing dialogue and communication that connects people throughout the organization. Effective teams are built on a foundation of inclusiveness, collaboration, communication, relationships, vision, and accountability—and communication is one of the most critical elements.

MANAGER'S TIP

Clear, open, honest, and concise communication is the best way to achieve awareness and consensus. Managers who are reluctant to share power are often reluctant to share information because they don't trust employees or other managers. ●

Organizations that emphasize management rather than leadership are frequently less willing to communicate openly. When in doubt, effective leaders communicate with their employees, talk to them in person, tell them the truth, and express their own feelings, using self-disclosure as a powerful strategy.[4]

Disclosing feelings and concerns about issues and sharing personal and professional experiences is an effective way to connect with team members and create a shared bond and empathy between them. Too often, leaders keep their feelings and worries to themselves, fearing that disclosure may make them appear weak or not in control. However, in most settings and circumstances,

What employees want

Employees want straight talk, communication, integrity, problems openly presented and discussed, and belief in the credibility and core values of their leadership. The more openly you share information, the less vulnerable your organization is to disagreement, apathy, alienation, and unionization. Openly sharing information includes the routine sharing of business plans, organizational goals and strategies, financial performance, and satisfaction results. It includes sharing the good news and the bad, admitting mistakes, and celebrating and rewarding innovation and commitment.

people usually respond favorably to those who use self-disclosure effectively and who share what they've learned and mistakes they've made. These connections lay the groundwork for trust, teamwork, and mutuality and help sustain us when times are tough. They also help break down the walls between frontline staff and formal leaders and close the gap between "us and them."

Communicating effectively is an essential element in our leadership repertoire. Leaders take information and strategies and translate them into understandable terms for patients and their families and for members of the health care team. By linking all care disciplines, nurse leaders keep things from falling through the cracks. Because you know your team members and your work so well, you're able to use examples and analogies that make sense to your audience, whether they're consumers or professionals. Communication becomes the vital link among all levels of the organization, therefore you must be able to communicate up and over, not just down.

A clear communication strategy is imperative to give and receive feedback and input effectively. This can hopefully evolve to the point at which employees become the messengers so managers aren't the only ones responsible for communicating. When employees feel their input is valued in the vision-building process, they feel included and are less likely to seek third-party representation. The goal is to move from information sharing to collaboration and consensus building. (See *What employees want.*)

Too many leaders want to be absent when difficult messages are conveyed. Leaders must be visible, clear, and direct, or people will assume the worst. Avoid sending double messages. One of the most common reasons for cynicism in a changing organiza-

Avoiding crisis mentality

One of the most commonly voiced complaints by team members is that leaders dilute team efforts with too many priorities. Every issue is treated like a crisis, and every request is accepted and made a top priority, detracting from the focus on the vision. This crisis mentality leads team members to disregard the leader's priority setting.

Use these suggestions for a better approach:

➤ Work with team members to establish priorities, recognizing that in the health care industry, priorities can change on a daily basis.

➤ Fully inform team members of all of the issues.

➤ Allow team members to participate in reprioritizing as needed.

By putting these suggestions into play, team members will be better able to support decisions and get the job done on time.

tion is the incongruity between what the change leaders say and what they do (like when they invite people to share ideas and become empowered, and then try to micromanage their behavior). People believe behavior more than words. The more you manage, the more you give others the message that their ideas aren't wanted. The more you lead, the more you send the message that you care what people think and want to work with them to create solutions.

Communicating vision

Nurse leaders create attention through vision by articulating what an organization or team can and should become or accomplish. Team cohesion results from a unified commitment to the goal and the relinquishing of self to the team that's in pursuit of that goal. (See *Avoiding crisis mentality*.)

Loss of focus on the vision or goal doesn't occur as the result of incompetence, lack of ethics or morality, character flaws, or any other simple explanation. Rather, it occurs because the problems are complex, the strategies for solving the problems are even more complex, and the degree of collaboration required involves intense and constant concentration in order for the vision to be attained.[5] The nurse leader must be able to focus, despite distractions in the environment. However, this is easier said than done. It requires the leader to have a strategic plan clearly defined and articulated to all key stakeholders and the ability to say no sometimes, even to superiors. If a request doesn't "fit" with the plan,

MANAGER'S TIP

I have a vision

You don't have to be the most experienced manager in the department to lead your staff toward a vision. When you hold your vision in clear view at all times and don't get distracted by daily demands, you can chip away at the broken systems and create ones that work. That's why communicating your vision should be at the top of your to-do list every day.

then it's easier for the leader to say no and to cite the strategic agenda and the focus on the vision as her rationale.

Nurse leaders have a vision of what excellent care is and of the knowledge, skills, and behaviors that every team member needs to make that vision a reality. Communicating this vision and articulating expectations of team members is essential to the attainment of the vision. It's up to the leaders to spell out this vision, to help unify the team, and to convince team members they *can* do something. In learning organizations, vision generates a creative tension between what is and what can be. In this kind of environment, leaders become designers, stewards, and mentors. Nurse leaders galvanize others around the vision and have the ability to lead by the power of their vision and not solely by their status or authority. (See *I have a vision.*)

Politics and personal agendas seem to be the greatest threats to vision attainment and goal clarity and, consequently, to effective leadership and teamwork. Did you ever wonder why teams work so well in crisis situations—such as traumas, floods, snowstorms, or hurricanes—yet they sometimes struggle to perform effectively when it's "business as usual"? Perhaps a big part of it is that in crisis situations, people generally tend to leave their egos, politics, and personal agendas at the door and focus completely on the issues at hand. There's no time for petty antics, rivalry, and competition. Such antics can make the difference between life and death, and no one tolerates them in a crisis situation. The focus is crystal clear, and everyone gets it. What a difference that focus makes in outcomes and in the way team members feel about the work they've accomplished. The nurse leader's ability to communicate a vision is paramount to creating a work environment in which the focus is clear on a daily basis, petty antics are never tolerated, and the team is successful in achieving organizational goals.

Communicating values

Communicating values is essential in the nurse leader role. The nurse leader is the guardian of the values, and values are the glue of successful teams and organizations. In the ever-changing health care environment, the effective work group operates not only by following tradition but also by employing vision and shared values. Team members must make more independent decisions, and the function of the nurse leader is to keep them enthused and directed toward the targets they have set.[6] The nurse leader's values are exemplified in guiding principles and are used to make every decision and in every relationship. The nurse leader demonstrates the organization's core values by consistently doing what she says she's going to do. Every opportunity is taken to tell stories that exemplify her values and to use such exemplars for discussion of opportunities for improvement. On all unit and department visits and in all meetings, the nurse leader reinforces her values and doesn't tolerate anything that threatens them. Adherence to these core values gives the nurse leader stability in the face of constant change and gives her employees the confidence to know that she'll stand by her values regardless of the obstacles, challenges, and threats that she faces.

When the nurse leader can clearly articulate her vision and values, it creates and environment in which employees are expected to do the same. This expectation establishes a forum for dialogue and communication that sets the framework for teamwork, cooperation, and collegiality. Common values that come out of discussions to create a sense of team and community include openness, localness, ownership, partnership, accountability, diversity, generosity, equity, respect, service, meaning, and lifelong learning. These values sustain the team through the tough times and promote an understanding of the key links needed to help everyone see the whole more clearly. The leader is responsible for conveying the issues clearly, for creating a setting for dialogue and design, and for keeping the rules of engagement. The team does the rest when empowered to do so and when it has a leader who is a positive role model of living her values and guiding principles every day.

Such a leadership focus on communicating vision and values has another positive outcome. When employees "practice" articulating values and establishing team norms and group expectations, they're better prepared to fulfill a core leadership competency that's required today more than ever before: ethical competence. Today, nurses report being confronted with ethical issues or problems on a routine basis. These issues — such as end-of-life decision making, informed consent, incompetent practice, breaches of patient confidentiality, and futile treatment — are prevalent today and will become increasingly so in the future. As team members coordinate the care of the patient, they need to play a more active role in addressing these ethical issues and need to possess the knowledge, skill, and diplomacy to best serve the patient as an advocate and moral agent. A team focus on values and expectations serves them well in this regard, and the role modeling of the nurse leader in preparing the staff to perform in an ethically competent and values-driven manner can't be underestimated.

Effective leaders communicate well — and often. Their key messages are precise and direct. They use inquiry and anticipate questions, problems, and concerns. They also know how to ask the right questions — questions that will give them greater understanding of a situation or help clarify ideas and evaluate the effectiveness of their communication. The best communicators believe in abundance, not scarcity, and can see endless possibilities. They continue to use inquiry and clarification skills until all possible ideas and solutions have been heard. An effective communication strategy is to follow the example of Mark Twain when he said, "I was gratified to be able to answer promptly, and I did. I said I didn't know."[7] Effective leaders and communicators are comfortable admitting what they don't know and which resources to tap to find the answer. Then they follow up with the team members and provide the newly obtained information in a timely manner. Above all, effective communicators never lie. They don't embellish the truth or tell half-truths. They tell it like it is, take the heat, and keep on moving. In doing so, they create trust and ensure that honesty and integrity are the cornerstones of team communication.

Communication is a two-way street, and effective nurse leaders are exceptional listeners. They listen attentively and with empathy. They tune in to team members' body language as well as their own. ●

Nurse leaders can effectively change their communication strategy in a split second to connect with the audience, because they know them so well and can read when they're losing them or talking over their heads. They truly listen to their team members, and they use clarifying statements to ensure that the messages and intent have been received. Such leaders make themselves available to the members of the team in order to hear issues and ideas and do so using various strategies, including open forums, staff meetings, brown bag lunches, off-shift rounding, and one-on-one dialogue, to name a few.

Communicating philosophy

Some of the most effective nurse leaders embrace the communication philosophy and style that the employees should know everything that they know. They share detailed financial information, strategic agenda discussions, and specific information regarding the organization's performance in order to ensure that employees understand issues that clearly affect their job security and their job satisfaction. When armed with information, employees can have a dramatic and long-lasting impact on quality, patient satisfaction, financial performance, and staff retention.

These leaders work every day to demystify information and to take secrecy out of the equation that's all too commonly found in health care organizations. There's nothing magical about financial reports. The data that they reveal can be understood by team members and should become part of daily communication and planning. The same holds true for quality data, satisfaction data, and human resource statistics. Of course, some information may be confidential or sensitive in nature and should be treated accordingly. But these data are more the exception to the rule, and most of the time information can and should be shared so that employees also get the full picture of the organization's performance. Nurse leaders who share information openly and who use this strategy with employees typically yield the best results and build the strongest teams.

Creating a culture of effective communication requires effort and time. Staff nurses, nurse managers, and nurse executives need to take time away to have a dialogue about leadership. Such a dialogue must be built upon the ground rules of safety, honesty, problem solving (not complaining), and ownership and accountability, rather than blaming. Such a dialogue allows all parties to share their experiences, frustrations, vision, and hopes and to come to consensus on the future direction of nursing within the organization. Time away also allows each team member to see the others in a different light, and hopefully bury the past and focus on the future. Such a dialogue provides fertile ground for setting expectations of all team members, including staff nurse expectations of the nurse leaders and vice versa. Once the preliminary values, vision, goals, and expectations are set, the team's energy can be put to establishing a priority list or action plan for how to get the work done, with consideration of the needs and opinions of all team members.

If out of this dialogue comes a discussion of shared governance or participative management, then the players are in the room to define the roles that all levels will play to make that a success. Another key topic must be to define leadership roles of staff nurses, nurse managers, and nurse executives and to establish methods of communication that work between and among the roles. Another discussion deals with the organizational structure and how each role can best relate to the others in order to optimize synergy. The key is to get as many stakeholders together as possible, to build consensus, and to take action. Everyone hates sitting in these "retreats" when nothing tangible comes about. Employees and nurse leaders alike want to see the fruits of these discussions and to see improvement in the environment of care, in team building, and in the interpersonal relationships among the team members. Taking time to develop the "people" side of the business can pay great dividends down the road. (See *Dealing with naysayers.*)

Oftentimes, issues of control are at the heart of communication, negotiation, and resistance to change. Forces that lead to employee dissatisfaction (and ultimately to collective bargaining) drain human capital. These include:

> ➤ a lack of employee input on hiring decisions
> ➤ not sharing financial information with employees

Dealing with naysayers

Every working environment has its naysayers — and you know exactly who they are. They're the same people who oppose every suggestion; who usually say,"we tried that before, and it didn't work"; and who have their heels dug in to resist change.

Here are some hints for dealing with these employees:

➤ Be direct with the nonsupporters and naysayers; establish ground rules.
➤ Demonstrate personal integrity: Say what you mean, and mean what you say.
➤ Be willing to talk openly about any issue.

Genuineness and authenticity in what you say are perceived as integrity, and build a culture of open communication and honesty. This strategy is an essential first step for laying the foundation for a team or work group that feels respected and valued and that feels that they matter to you. Personal purpose, vision, and passion energize leaders and encourage followers. Even the naysayers can join the bandwagon when they see daily evidence of leadership and when they receive adequate information. Helping team members understand that reinventing themselves is a lifelong and continuous learning process may help them see the positive and not just the negative.

➤ not terminating employees who perform unacceptably
➤ asking for staff input after the fact, rather than before you make decisions.

Such factors widen the communication divide between managers and employees, and exponentially increase staff alienation as well as union vulnerability. Nurse leaders who recognize that sharing information and communicating openly and truthfully strengthens their position and enhances their power base will cultivate teams that are empowered, that communicate well, and that also feel no need for third-party representation.

Too often, the middle managers are left out of the satisfaction assessment. Nurse leaders are so focused on retaining frontline caregivers that they forget about the vital managers who support them. To include managers in an assessment of overall satisfaction and to gain their perspectives on the effectiveness of communication strategies is essential and can lead to greater support from the middle-manager team. To enhance communication between administration and management team members, a survey may be helpful in assessing all levels of management — for example, their views about management training, information sharing, and span of control, and their ability to cooperate and communicate across department lines. The survey should also include an alienation index to indicate the degree of alienation the manager

Elements of a strategic plan

Most successful leaders and communicators consider these fundamentals as core elements of their strategic communication plan:

➤ They have a clear, compelling mission, and they communicate it to all parties in terms they can relate to, understand, and put into practice.

➤ They pinpoint the essence of the business by defining services and the philosophy of care.

➤ They know their customers and their needs, and they actively involve them in their treatment and in all decisions that affect their care.

➤ They organize their business around their customers and provide services, meals, procedures, and tests at times that meet customer needs.

➤ They focus on the basics and achieve excellence in providing them.

may be experiencing. Oftentimes, alienation in the manager group may be a sign of trouble in the staff group too.

Communicating strategic priorities

In a time when nurse leaders are bombarded with so much information on a daily basis, it may be difficult to sort out what information to communicate. Because information is power, some leaders hold on to too much of it, thinking that it increases their power base. However, the most effective leaders and communicators share information freely and in a style that makes the information understandable and easy for the audience to retain.

Even high-level strategic plans and agendas can be shared with frontline staff in a way that's meaningful to them and that co-opts them into the processes involved. Senior administrators have realized that communicating strategy to doctors and caregivers is more important today than ever. Such communication helps to ground the members of the team and provides a focus for all efforts and energy. (See *Elements of a strategic plan.*)

At a time when the focus in health care continues to be on cost reduction, efficiency, and productivity, it's more important than ever that leaders communicate in a way that connects people to the issues and strategies, and lets them know that the focus must continue to be on the quality of care delivery above all else. When employees hear the truth about all the imperatives facing their organization, they'll be more willing to bring their ideas forward and to participate in the solutions, rather than sitting on the sidelines and derailing progress.

Communicating data

Nurse leaders must be informationally competent as organizations build infrastructures that support the acquisition of data at any point of care. They must be able to speak the language of informatics, to prioritize the incredible amount of data that is at their fingertips, and to turn that data into useable information that better supports patient outcomes and organizational needs. They must be able to synthesize and interpret multiple, sometimes conflicting sources of data and use expert judgment to respond effectively in dynamic situations. Gone are the days when nurse leaders can rely exclusively on what worked before and on intuition. The information age requires that they be data driven and promote evidence-based practice and decision making. Building a compelling case using data is the surest way to accomplish the established goals.

As nurse leaders in health care delivery systems attempt to manage information and stay ahead of the game, they use comparative data to measure the cost of care, the clinical and functional outcomes that result from care, the satisfaction of those receiving care, and the impact that care has on the health of communities. Some might say, "That isn't my job," but think about it: Who better to look at the cost of care delivery than those entrenched in that care 24 hours a day? Who better to assess where there's waste in the system, what could be eliminated, and where the system needs to be fixed in order to support patient care delivery than those who deliver the care and support the care providers? When nurse leaders inform their teams about what supplies actually cost, team members can help make better purchasing, supply allocation, and utilization decisions — and ultimately help the team save money.

Nurse leaders can also help reduce length of stay by pulling together the appropriate team members to dissect the delivery of care into its component processes and parts. They lead the team in taking out work that doesn't matter, change medication prescriptions that prolong ventilator days and length of stay, and ensure that days in the hospital aren't wasted due to lack of early nutritional intervention or prolonged wait times for tests or procedures. Nurse leaders affect cost and quality in many ways. The key is that in each of the above examples, nurse leaders viewed that as part of their job, and were empowered to bring their vast knowledge and expertise to bear in order to make meaningful change. They role modeled collaboration, multidisciplinary teamwork, expert communication, and negotiation, and emphasized data and the best way to communicate it.

Becoming more evidence-based in leadership can help nurse leaders promote the use of data and arm them with the information they need to enhance care delivery and to achieve organizational outcomes.

Communicating with patients and families

It would be impossible to think about people and communication in health care without considering our patients and their families. The role of the nurse leader today interfaces directly and often with the consumers of care. Today's patients are less resilient, more vulnerable, less stable, more complex, and more unpredictable than yesterday's patients — and they need more resources. They are older, have numerous chronic conditions, and are better informed. Patients today clearly want to be partners in their care delivery, not passive recipients of that care. Patients and their families have access to comparative data now, to consumer "report cards," and they come asking what their predictive morbidity and mortality will be for open heart surgery. They want the new medication that they heard about on CNN prescribed for them, and many won't take no for an answer. Today's patients are members of large and powerful lobbying groups who put pressure on their legislators to ensure appropriate care. Just look at the impact that AARP and the Gray Panthers have on health care delivery.

Nurse leaders must develop and hone communication skills that are specific to and effective for the recipients of their care. It's increasingly challenging to communicate with informed consumers who want to play an active role in decision making regarding their treatment. It's challenging to ensure patient and family satisfaction when such informed consumers may know more about a specific treatment, experimental drug, or complementary therapy than the nurse leader. Effective communication with patients and families requires time, patience, humility, and empathy. They want information and data; they don't want to hear "do what I say" or "because the doctor said so." Nurse leaders must view this communication as a blessing, as we educate the public, heighten their awareness, and arm them with data so that they can be full participants in their care experience and not merely passive recipients as in the past.

This philosophy should extend to care providers, who communicate closely with care recipients. Taking time with patients and families, listening to their questions and worries, and teaching them is one of the most fulfilling aspects of nursing care delivery and can't be seen as a bother. Nurse leaders must cultivate a workforce that's knowledgeable, articulate, and able to answer the questions of these informed consumers — and, at the very least, a workforce that knows where to get the information the patient needs.

Effectively honing communication skills specific to care recipients and their loved ones has an important impact on the way patients and families perceive the quality of the care they receive. The caring touch, the tone of voice on the telephone, the flexibility in visiting hours, the competent caring that extended beyond the patient and to the family, the consideration of the patient's holistic needs — these are all factors that nurses have total control over and that can make a difference for patients.

How many times, despite the loss of a loved one, has a family member told you that your team made an unbearable situation bearable? That through your attention to their needs, your teaching, planning, and leadership, they had a positive experience that will live in their memories always, even though their loved one died? These examples occur every day and have a dramatic effect on the image of your organization in the community and on the choices patients and families make when considering where to receive their health care. It's essential that nurse leaders and their employees cultivate expert communication skills with patients and families. After all, our roles exist to support them.

Communicating across the continuum of care

The degree of interdependency and communication required by all parts of the organization has never been greater. Patients require a much greater level of care coordination than before, and it's your team members who provide that coordination. They must consider not only the patient's present condition, but what led up to it and what will happen to the patient once he leaves your unit. No longer is it appropriate to send the patient to the step-down unit and consider yourself done with him, using the out-of-sight-out-of-mind approach. Now, through the use of clinical paths and with the help of case managers, utilization reviewers, community health care providers, and insurers, the responsibility is on nurse leaders and team members to plan for the patient's care along the continuum and for the resources he'll need on the step-down unit, in the extended-care facility, and in the home or community. Some may say "that isn't my job"; however, leaders on the health care team are the ones best prepared to ensure that care is communicated and delivered with the full continuum of the patient's needs in mind.

Nurse leaders need to consider how to prepare the workforce to play a greater role in telehealth initiatives, bringing their knowledge and faces into patient's homes, physicians' offices, schools and other community settings, and health care organizations within their networks and beyond. Again, some might say "that isn't my job," but who better to prepare the patient for discharge; to interact with colleagues in community health; to provide education at health fairs, in schools, and in community centers; and to be the interface to patients once they've left the facility than nurse leaders and their team members?

In many communities, the staff nurse role has already started to transition across the continuum of care. Examples are numerous of inpatient staff nurses following their patients into the clinic setting, or seeing surgical patients preoperatively in their homes. Many staff nurses are seeing roles defined for them in transitional units, in day facilities, and in patients' homes, as the push continues to shorten inpatient lengths of stay and to curb the cost of inpatient care. Staff nurse expertise is being placed at the other end of the telephone, triaging patient calls and concerns, clarifying their questions, and in many cases eliminating the need for the patient to come to the emergency department or to be readmitted to the hospital—talk about improving cost, utilization, and quality!

Nurse leaders are also experiencing a broadening in the scope of their roles to include leading those in facilities across the continuum of care and facilitating teamwork and communication among a multitude of care providers in various care sites. These expanded roles — and mentoring employees as their roles expand — requires a new mindset for many nurse leaders, and one that's more flexible, less structured, and more inclusive. Cultivating a mindset that sees beyond walls and boundaries is imperative in nurse leaders and their team members and will be even more so in the future as the lines between facilities in integrated delivery systems blur.

Moving forward

The greatest obstacles to effective communication in nursing are found between the ears of staff nurses, nurse managers, and nurse executives. At all levels, you hear the obstacles verbalized every day. (See *Let's change our tune,* page 122.)

Thank goodness not all staff nurses, nurse managers, and nurse executives share negative viewpoints. Each negative comment, no matter who says it, is an effort somewhere along the line to be either a victim or a controller. Negative comments halt communication, place blame somewhere else, and strengthen the walls between "us and them." Unfortunately, in many cases, the "us and them" participants are nurses. (See *Expanding communication,* page 123.)

Nurse leaders can change the perceptions that they and others have of nursing by changing the way that they communicate who they are and what they do. You can start by following these guidelines:

➤ Introduce yourself as a professional nurse who has a tremendous impact on the health and well-being of your patients.
➤ Don't allow an employer to prevent you from wearing your nursing credentials with pride. Wear those credentials and educate your patients, families, and other team members about what they mean and why they matter.
➤ Actively contribute to your patients' care plans. Don't abdicate your role as a patient advocate because you're too busy.
➤ Keep key messages on the tip of your tongue that precisely and unequivocally articulate your role and your impact on outcomes.
➤ Enhance your work environment and your team's effectiveness by taking responsibility for the obstacles that exist.

Let's change our tune

The following statements show how views can differ according to level of employment.

Staff nurse	Nurse-manager (colleagues)	Nurse executives
➤ "It isn't my job."	➤ "I have to do it for it to be done right."	➤ "I'm all for empowerment as long as it's done my way."
➤ "He isn't my patient."	➤ "If I don't do it, it won't get done on time."	➤ "The staff isn't ready to take on this kind of responsibility."
➤ "That's the nurse manager's job."	➤ "I'm the one who is accountable, so I'm making the decisions."	➤ "With all of the sick calls, the staff doesn't have the commitment to make shared governance work."
➤ "I'm not paid to do that."	➤ "The staff don't want to own their practice; they want me to."	
➤ "I'm just a nurse."	➤ "I've tried to get the staff to participate, but they never follow through."	➤ "I'd be afraid of what the staff might say if they were put into some of these forums with all of the other players at the table."
➤ "I'm too busy."		
➤ "I'm not coming in on my day off."	➤ "The staff tried self-scheduling, but they only did the easy part. Then they gave the schedule to me full of holes to fix."	➤ "It's too expensive."
➤ "They don't do their jobs, so I can't do mine."		➤ "That isn't in the budget."
➤ "They don't understand what I do."	➤ "If I'm not empowered by my boss, how am I supposed to empower my staff?"	➤ "I tried this before, but never saw any outcomes from it."
➤ "Nothing's going to change, so I give up."	➤ "The staff want me here at their beck and call, yet when I need something done, no one comes forward."	➤ "I can't be accountable for the staff's morale; they have to own that."
➤ "We tried that with the previous consultants, and it didn't work."		
➤ "I had to learn the hard way, so you should, too.		

➤ Allow the pride that you take in your chosen profession to shine.

➤ Communicate optimism, and make positive strides each day to celebrate who you are and to communicate the difference that nurses make.

Just a nurse? Never.

Team building

In these times of extraordinary change, nurse leaders can only survive and thrive if they build strong teams, relationships, and coalitions. It has been said that leadership is collective and that leadership by one person is a contradiction in terms. Therefore nurse leaders must network well and look to those outside their own sphere for ideas, criticism, and support. Nothing exists in isolation and very little falls exclusively within one's individual

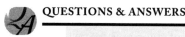

Expanding communication

Question: *How can I hope to communicate effectively outside my profession when I have so much work to do within it first?*

Answer: Too often, nurses focus on the differences between them and other nurses and don't move toward synergy and true professional unity. Only when you break down the communication barriers between you and other nurses and create a shared vision with common goals will you create a truly superior climate of care and tap the limitless potential on your team.

To communicate effectively, nurse leaders need to communicate positively with all team members, both within and outside of nursing. Through effective communication, you can create an environment of optimism and renewed pride in nursing. It may sound simple, but one way to start is to eradicate the expression "I'm just a nurse" from your vocabulary. This phrase is typically prefaced with a large sigh, usually some degree of hand wringing, and an "isn't it awful" facial expression — body language that screams oppression and victimization. Obviously, this isn't the countenance that assures patients, exudes competence to colleagues, or inspires others to enter the nursing profession. It's this phrase and others like it that keep nurses down and hold us back from truly reaching our professional potential and assuming our place of leadership in the health care industry.

domain. In the interdisciplinary world of health care, it's imperative that nurse leaders value and respect the contributions of others and that they find ways to use all talent and expertise in the most effective ways possible. The lines between professions may blur and activities that have been historically in the exclusive domain of nursing may become shared. Although this paradigm shift may be difficult or even painful to accept, nurse leaders can facilitate acceptance by changing their thinking to what the patient and family need and creating systems accordingly, rather than holding on to turf and titles at the expense of synergy and collaboration. Creating strong teams and cultivating the essence of teamwork is essential if nurse leaders are to effectively address the issues of dwindling resources, increased demand, and limited supply. These are all people issues that can be resolved only when nurse leaders use their human resources to their fullest advantage through effective teamwork.

FRONTLINE MANAGEMENT TEAM. One strategy that's effective in addressing the significant issues of the day is to create a sense of team and community in the workplace, beginning with frontline managers. Middle management is one of the most difficult and high-stress jobs in health care. Nurse managers are pulled from every direction, and oftentimes aren't given the resources they need for team building and development. This key interface between staff, executives, and patients represents the first line of defense against alienation, low morale, turnover, and unionization. Therefore, nurse leaders must ensure that these managers have the resources and tools they need to do their jobs. This includes allocating time and money to building and coaching teams so that outcomes are achieved.

For managers, taking on the goal of creating community in the workplace can give personal meaning and focus to what can feel like a thankless job[8] and can offer consistency in an ever-changing landscape. Instilling a proactive, team-oriented mindset in the management team will help them to anticipate issues and to focus on solutions. It will also help them shift toward the role of coach and facilitator.

There are many strategies for team building in the literature. All involve bringing team members together in a way that encourages communication and open sharing of ideas, and that directs the team toward a common goal or vision. In too many cases, though, the vision is handed down to the team from above, and never fully gains the support of those who are responsible for executing the strategies to achieve the vision. The most effective teams set targets and objectives together and clearly define each team member's role in achieving the vision. (See *Getting it together.*)

Creating a strategic approach builds the team from the start by having all team members help create the vision and articulate what is most important to them in determining the direction of the team. With key players fully participating, they'll provide the most realistic appraisal of the way things are now and will probably not mince words in describing what needs to improve. They're closest to the issues at hand, therefore their solutions will have the greatest probability of success. This is an iterative process, and the team members need to know that their ongoing input and feedback is required and welcomed. This approach re-

Getting it together

Consider this simple strategy[9] to gain buy-in of frontline managers and to minimize threats to morale, retention, and autonomy.
➤ Create a vision together.
➤ Conceptualize the vision to build a shared mental model.
➤ Look at the way things are now.
➤ Talk about ways to move from now to the vision.
➤ Pick priority actions from those ideas.
➤ Begin the action steps and schedule check-ups.
➤ Recognize problems, but spend most of the time celebrating the positive.
➤ Continue creating the vision together.
➤ Continuously freshen the process and repeat the steps.

flects a continuous improvement philosophy, in which frequent check-ups are completed to assess progress toward stated goals. It doesn't matter which approach you take to building a team, as long as it's inclusive, participative, and iterative.

COLLABORATION AS A TOOL. The most effective leaders are masters at combining talents into effective teams, like Herb Kelleher, founder of Southwest Airlines, and Mike Krzyzewski, coach of the Duke University Blue Devils men's basketball team. They combine team member talents and abilities with commitment to achieve the team's full potential. They recognize that a team member can have great skills, but without commitment and teamwork, that team member won't succeed. What matters most is selecting team members who possess the necessary technical skills and abilities to achieve the desired objective — and the personal characteristics required to achieve excellence while working well with others. The best teams are created with a selection strategy that attempts to capture both qualities. When each team member is capable and committed, and brings those qualities together in a way that synergizes with the other members of the team, there's no telling what the team can achieve!

Nurse leaders must surround themselves with team members who have a strong desire to contribute and the capability of collaborating effectively. Effective collaboration requires that the leader and the team members focus on issues instead of positions and be capable of sharing information openly, listening objectively to fellow team members, and bringing out the best in others. Some people simply aren't "wired-up" that way, and there's a delicate balance between respecting individual differences and requiring unity. If the team moves too far toward unity, you can get conformity, groupthink, and the stifling of creativity and divergent thinking. On the other hand, if the group is too conflicted, or has too many identities, it can be immobilized by conflicts of vision and values. The nurse leader must be able to build a team that "fits" together and achieves desired outcomes by simultaneously maximizing the diversity and unity on the team.

Effective leaders in health care today are team builders who understand that all parts of the system are interdependent and that success in one part means success in all. They know the value of genuine teamwork and can bring diverse perspectives together to create work environments in which true collaboration is the norm and in which excellent outcomes are achieved. As the coordinators of health care, nurse leaders are in essence conducting an orchestra, with various instruments and diverse talents and experiences. They must bring them together at the right time and in the right way to create harmony for patients, families, and team members.

To do so requires expert collaboration and demonstrated expertise in systems thinking and managing across complex health care delivery systems. Nurses will go from being primarily providers of total patient care to managers of the delivery of care. Nurse leaders will play more of a facilitative role and will be looked to more as coordinators of care for the patient and his family. This will involve working with new members of the health care team, some of whom may be finance department members, case managers, community service employees, and insurance company employees. In coordinating patient care, the nurse leader must consider the full range of care and establish comfort in working with a variety of team members in various ways. This will require that nurse leaders embrace more global thinking and encourage their team members to think beyond their shift, unit or department, and hospital exclusively, and anticipate patient needs, know which community resources are available and how to access them, and serve as an available resource to the patient and family after discharge.

The most effective leaders and team builders surround themselves with highly competent people and then delegate freely. They align team members with diverse talents and backgrounds and varied perspectives to achieve robust decision making and innovative approaches to problem identification and resolution. Diversity is what brings strength to teams, and it's the effective nurse leader who can coach and align a diverse group around common goals and achieve synergy. Doing so requires that nurse leaders dedicate the time to educate and coach all members of the team, including technicians, secretaries, and other support personnel. Encouraging them to use their skills and to make their optimal contribution to patient care and to the team's effectiveness helps to instill confidence and commitment to the team. With team members aligned and all activities and energy focused on a shared vision, the nurse leader can take on the role of a consultant and facilitator, rather than that of an inspector and enforcer.

A distinguishing feature of effective team builders is their ability to establish and lead by guiding principles. These guiding principles represent what all team members, including the team leader, should expect from one another on a day-to- day basis. Therefore, when building a team, a nurse leader should:[10]

- ➤ avoid compromising the team's objective with political issues
- ➤ exhibit personal commitment to the team's goal
- ➤ not dilute the team's efforts with too many priorities
- ➤ be fair and impartial toward all team members
- ➤ be willing to confront and resolve issues associated with inadequate performance by team members
- ➤ be open to new ideas and information from team members.

The nurse leader who effectively builds and leads teams must live and breathe these guiding principles every day, in every encounter, and with all levels of the organization. In doing so, the team builder leads with consistency, and team members know what to expect from her in any situation. In high-performing teams, team members can substitute for the coach and for each other as needed and develop skills that are transferable and portable. Team members try out different roles and become as flexible and adaptive as possible so they're prepared for any situa-

As geese fly

Perhaps one of the best lessons in teamwork is learned from geese.

➤ As each goose flaps its wings, it creates an uplift for the next one. By flying in a V formation, the whole flock adds 71% greater flying range than if the bird flew alone.

➤ Whenever a goose falls out of formation, it suddenly feels the drag and resistance of trying to fly alone, and quickly gets back into formation to take advantage of the lifting power of the bird immediately in front.

➤ When the lead goose gets tired, it rotates back into the formation and another goose flies at the point position.

➤ The geese in formation honk from behind to encourage those up front to keep up their speed.

➤ When a goose gets sick, wounded, or shot, two geese drop out of formation and follow it down to help protect it. They stay with it until it can fly again or dies. Then they launch out on their own, with another formation, or catch up with the flock.

tion that may arise. On these teams, every member understands every role, therefore if something unforeseen occurs, one team member can step in for another, without losing the team's momentum or missing a deadline. Quality emerges from an environment that's driven by a shared vision, principles, teamwork, and partnerships, and all team members reap the benefits. (See *As geese fly*.)

Building trust

Organizational trust is the extent to which one is willing to ascribe good intentions to and have confidence in the words and actions of others.[11] Employees believe that leaders will be straightforward and that they'll follow through on the commitments that they've made. In an environment of trust, employees believe that organizational actions will ultimately benefit them, and they support the organizational agenda. To achieve such an environment, employees and their leaders must have shared goals, mutual respect, and trust. Leaders who create supportive relationships are more successful because their teams trust and follow them. The simple truth is that leaders can't lead if their followers don't trust them.

It's essential to build trust in an organization and the most effective way to build trust is by sharing information. Trust requires discretion, consistency, fairness, integrity, loyalty, openness, promise fulfillment, and receptivity. These factors have a significant impact on the way employees receive messages and on the support that organizations achieve. Trust influences important organizational factors, such as group cohesion, perceived fairness of decisions, organizational citizenship behavior, job satisfaction, and organizational effectiveness. These factors are critical in today's health care industry, as nurse leaders struggle to retain staff, recruit new employees, and enhance the satisfaction and work life of team members. Without trust, organizational leaders will continue to lose the human resource battle and the people who are the cornerstone of their organization.

Any change initiative or strategic agenda is successful only to the extent to which you've established trust in the workplace. As organizations restructure and reengineer in the name of efficiency and effectiveness, organizational trust is an increasingly important element in determining the organizational climate, employee performance, and commitment to the organization. Most employees will give an idea a chance or get behind a change if they trust the messenger and trust that the organizational leaders have their best interests at heart. It's when trust is lacking that there's the greatest resistance to change and the highest level of employee militancy. These behaviors are nothing short of coping and defense mechanisms that employees feel they must resort to when they don't trust those who are making the decisions.

MANAGER'S TIP

Mistrust results when information is withheld, resources are allocated inconsistently, and employees have no support from management. It doesn't matter if these things have actually happened or not. As long as the perception exists that these situations are real, the climate of mistrust will escalate and employee alienation will grow. ●

All industries suffer from mistrust and disagreement among leaders and employees. In nursing and in health care at large, however, such a climate can have serious consequences. Mistrust of the system can potentially threaten the quality of patient care delivered, as collaboration and communication are hampered, teamwork falters, and response times lag. Lack of trust can also affect productivity, retention, and union vulnerability. Absenteeism, prolonged break times, limited learning, low accountabil-

Positive factors

Nurses in recent focus groups at the American Hospital Association[12] who were most positive about their work environment attributed it to three factors:

➤ They felt that hospital management was committed to communicating with them in-depth about the status of the hospital.

➤ They felt a personal connection with the hospital's leadership.

➤ They were active participants in making tough decisions when finances were tight.

ity, reactionary thinking, low creativity, and the desire for third-party representation are common in low-trust cultures.

The most effective leadership frameworks emphasize high trust as a basis for effectiveness, leadership, principles, people, vision, and a longer-term perspective on profit and development.[13] Effective nurse leaders create a singularity of rhetoric and reality[14] and establish trust among all team members by leading with integrity. Employees can easily see through any facade that leaders create. Honest communication and sharing specific information goes hand in hand with establishing trust. (See *Positive factors*.)

Each of these factors establishes unity between employees and formal leaders and enables them to tackle difficult situations together. Never underestimate the power of trust and its enduring effect on nurse leaders' success. Trust allows team members to stay focused on problems and to be more efficient with time and energy. Team members aren't constantly looking over their shoulders to see who may be stabbing them in the back, so they can commit their attention to the issues of patient care delivery and the team. With trust, there's no suspicion or conflict to divert attention. There may be differences of opinion, but trust allows them to be discussed openly and unemotionally, without personal attack. Trust allows the exchange of ideas and promotes more efficient communication and coordination. There are no ulterior motives. Words and actions can be taken at face value because all members of the team have established trust based on integrity and consistency between what they say and what they do.

The absence of trust diverts the mental concentration and energy of a team away from its performance objectives and onto other issues. In low-trust cultures, there's duplicity, deception, secrecy, hidden agendas, competition, and various personal agendas. The team becomes politicized and alliances and personal agendas take precedence over the team goal. In teams that lack trust, communication is likely to be guarded, ambiguous, distorted, and difficult to understand. There's a lot of maneuvering, denial, defensiveness, and a constant need to refocus. In these environments of care, nurses feel unsafe, unwelcome, unappreciated, and disrespected. They can't identify anyone in the organization who they trust to effectively advocate for them. These low-trust cultures breed the following:

➤ militancy
➤ anger
➤ frustration
➤ hopelessness.

They increase union vulnerability. Every issue seems to be a battle, and decision making takes forever. For leaders, it's time consuming and exhausting to communicate. The emphasis is placed on management, not on leadership. Low-trust cultures wear team members down, and unfortunately, it's often the "right" employees and leaders who leave rather than those who are responsible for breeding the mistrust.

With trust, the nurse leader can create an atmosphere in which people are willing and feel secure to bring problems forward because they're listened to. Trust enables people to take risks (even if they fail) and to state their opinions openly, so decisions are more in tune with what is really happening because team members have been honest. By inspiring trust, nurse leaders improve the quality of collaborative outcomes by having all spokes of the wheel turning in the same direction. One sign that the nurse leader has been effective in building trust is that the team members begin to compensate and pick up the slack for each other. After all, everyone has an off day now and then, and it's an incredible feeling to know that when you do your teammates will support you and help you carry your burden. In high-trust cultures, employees never feel alone and can always rely on the strength of the team for support. With trust, team members are willing to compensate for shortcomings in others and support the development of team members until they're ready to stand fully on their own.

Nurses eat their young

The expression "nurses eating their young" describes the ordeal that the novice nurse experiences at the onset of her profession. For some reason, experienced nurses feel the need to torment the new graduate, almost as an initiation ritual into the profession. This torment is carried out by bombarding the graduate nurse with work and knowledge, or the opposite — by ignoring them.

Either scenario is overwhelming and intimidating. However, with all the incidents of this phenomenon, from nurse-educators to staff nurses, the reason behind it isn't clearly defined. Perhaps it's a wish to show dominance and control. It may also be a *kick back* response, giving back what was received.

Even though many nurses don't realize that they're doing it, with the present nursing shortage, it's a phenomenon that needs to be eliminated in order for the nursing profession to survive.

One rarely sees the "nurses eating their young" phenomenon in high-trust cultures. Such behavior isn't tolerated. The victim-controller paradigm is also rare in high-trust cultures, because team members believe that everyone must share power and succeed if the team is to succeed. (See *Nurses eat their young.*)

With trust as a foundation, communication is easier, camaraderie is greater, and team members are more willing to give each other the benefit of the doubt, even the leadership. The difficult times in health care don't seem to be going away anytime soon, so it behooves nurse leaders now more than ever to do what it takes to establish trust at all levels in their organizations. (See *Creating trust.*)

Celebrating the value set of every team member is one of the most appreciative things you can do. Show your pride and appreciation publicly and often. The level of understanding, teamwork, and camaraderie that will result promotes communication, information sharing, and positive energy. These make up the fabric of a high-trust culture and lay the foundation to establish successful interpersonal relationships that sustain through adversity, chaos, and insecurity — hallmarks of today's health care environment. Establishing a culture of trust and leading in a trustworthy manner is how nurse leaders succeed individually and best support excellence in patient care delivery, collaboration, and human capital fulfillment.

QUESTIONS & ANSWERS

Creating trust

Question: *How do you build trust in your team if it isn't there now?*
Answer: Consider the following helpful hints.[15]

➤ Find out what brings people together. Food usually works well.
➤ Convene when people are ready because timing is everything.
➤ Start meaningful dialogue about things that matter to them and are important to the success of the team.
➤ Cultivate the informal leaders, and invest your time and energy into establishing trust with them. Let them be the messengers and encourage them be the keepers of the new culture as others come on board.
➤ Learn how to host a good gathering, get people together, and acknowledge their contributions.
➤ Involve the whole person and celebrate each person's contributions to team success. Use these times to strengthen the identity of the team, to become one of trust, collegiality, excellence, and vision.
➤ Create meaning in work because that's what is integrated with identity and develops coherence and trust in the organization.
➤ Set expectations and address behaviors that create mistrust.
   Creating trust happens one encounter at a time, and every interaction matters.

Points to remember

The following points summarize the role of team members in the organization:

➤ Leaders need to create an organizational culture that successfully empowers employees to define service standards and create a healthy working environment.
➤ Communication among team members is the vital link in creating a unified, informed team.
➤ A leader's clear articulation of vision and values creates an environment in which team members are expected to do the same.
➤ Nurse leaders must cultivate a workforce that's knowledgeable, articulate, and capable of answering the questions of informed consumers.
➤ Effective nurse leaders surround themselves with team members who have a strong desire to contribute and the ability to collaborate effectively.

➤ Establishing trust among team members allows them to focus on problems, be more efficient with time and energy, commit attention to the issues of patient care delivery and the team, and promote communication of ideas.

References

1. Murray, J. *Think Change.* Aurora, Ill.: Successories, Inc. USA, 1998.
2. Pritchett, P. *The Employee Handbook of New Work Habits for the Next Millennium: 10 New Ground Rules for Job Success.* Dallas: Pritchett & Associates, 1999.
3. Bilchik, G.S. "Organizational Depression," *Hospitals and Health Networks* 74(2):34-36, 38, February 2000.
4. Scott, C., and Jaffe, D. *Managing Organizational Change: A Practical Guide for Managers.* Menlo Park, Calif.: Crisp Publications, Inc., 1989.
5. Larson, C., and LaFasto, F. *TeamWork: What Must Go Right/What Can Go Wrong.* Newbury Park, Calif.: Sage Publications, Inc., 1989.
6. Scott, C., and Jaffe, D. Op. cit.
7. Twain, M. *Life on the Mississippi.* Boston: J.R. Osgood and Company, 1883.
8. Parker, M., and Gadbois, S. "Building Community in the Healthcare Workplace, Part 3: Belonging and Satisfaction at Work," *Journal of Nursing Administration* 30(10):466-73, October 2000.
9. Parker, M., and Gadbois, S. Op. cit.
10. Larson, C., and LaFasto, F. Op. cit.
11. Laschinger, H., et al. "Organizational Trust and Empowerment in Restructured Healthcare Settings. *Journal of Nursing Administration* 30(9):413-25, September 2000.
12. American Hospital Association. *Reality Check III: Searching for Trust Report: America's Message to Hospitals and Health Systems.* Chicago: AHA, August 2, 2001.
13. Johns, J. "Trust: Key to Acculturation in Corporatized Health Care Environments," *Nursing Administration Quarterly* 20(2):13-24, Winter, 1996.
14. Dow, R., and Cook, S. *Turned On: Eight Vital Insights to Energize Your People, Customers, and Profits.* New York: HarperBusiness, 1996.
15. Parker, M., and Gadbois, S. Op. cit.

CHAPTER 6

Motivating your team

Melissa A. Fitzpatrick, RN, MSN, FAAN

> "A leader is not an administrator who loves to run others, but someone who carries water for his people so they can get on with their jobs." — Robert Townsend

Today, nursing is in a state of crisis and in desperate need of leadership. Not just your run of the mill leadership, but the miraculous kind that inspires, motivates, and stimulates others to hang in there and to keep coming back to health care delivery every day. Nurse leaders need to inspire their team members by leading with the heart, staying positive, asking their opinions, and walking and talking pride in the nursing profession.

Leading and coaching

Every day nurse leaders are called on to look beyond the chaos in the environment to find the opportunities that lay dormant, to rediscover the promise that lies within each team member, to draw upon the enthusiasm that led them to nursing, and to re-connect with that strong sense of commitment to caring for people. All of that requires finding a way to regain the joy and satisfaction that comes from making real connections with other human beings — like the last time you asked a patient or team member what you could do for him, and even though it meant jumping through hoops and using precious time, you made it happen. Do you remember that person's gratitude and pleasure

Future empowerment

Question: *How can you begin to move the discipline of nursing toward a future that empowers others and builds upon the strengths that each employee brings to your organization?*

Answer: One place to start is by having all key players embrace a few assumptions for developing leaders:
➤ Leadership skills can be learned.
➤ Leadership potential exists at all levels of the organization.
➤ Progressive responsibility and experience build leadership skills.
➤ Intellectual leadership is the key to future success.
➤ The ability to learn is one of the most important assets that an employee can have.
➤ Self-leadership is the essence of leadership.[1]
    Belief in these leadership principles will guide you in developing new leaders and also provide direction for you in continuing your own leadership journey.

and your own sense of accomplishment? Do you recall the last time you took a new nurse, a respiratory therapist, or a resident under your wing to walk through a procedure? Do you remember that look of awe and gratitude, then of confidence and pride? These are the looks of leadership—and the nursing profession needs more of them. (See *Future empowerment.*)

What does it take to be an effective leader in today's turbulent health care environment? Leadership isn't a title. It isn't about having an office, let alone one with a window. It isn't about how many people report to you or how big a budget you manage. Leadership is about influencing and making decisions. It's about taking appropriate action at the appropriate time. It's about projecting yourself and those around you into a future that's better for patients and families, less costly for society, and more humane for all. Effective leaders influence. They coach. They evoke confidence in others. This kind of leader serves as a role model, enabling her team to see change in a new light. These mavericks know that people change from being led, not from being told. They don't rely solely on authority or information to change behavior, but rather on support, encouragement, caring confrontation, and empathy.

Recognizing leadership potential

The best coaches and leaders have an eye for talent, and accurately predict those with the greatest leadership potential. They look for the following skills:[2]

➤ *Intellectual ability* — is conceptual, analytical, creative
➤ *Results orientation* — works toward outcomes and follows a task through to the end
➤ *Interpersonal skills* — relates to the feelings and needs of others, and conveys interest and respect
➤ *Planning and organizing* — able to schedule time and prioritize for self and others, to handle multiple activities and to meet deadlines
➤ *Team orientation* — able to work collaboratively within a complex organizational structure
➤ *Maturity* — willing to be open and act responsibly when dealing with people and situations
➤ *Presence* — able to create a positive first impression and stand out tactfully (includes verbal and nonverbal communication).

Effective leaders create leaders by mentoring protégés to take their own jobs. As coaches, these leaders encourage growth and risk taking, catch team members when they fall, and celebrate their attempts. They achieve power by releasing the potential of others. The Chinese philosopher Lao Tsu expressed it well when he wrote, "The wicked leader is he who the people despise. The good leader is he who the people revere. The great leader is he who the people say, we did it ourselves."[3]

Nurse leaders who are masters at assessing talent and giving employees progressively more responsibility so that they can grow and achieve their potential in the organization are the ones who develop leaders. (See *Recognizing leadership potential.*)

Effective nurse leaders cultivate these qualities in team members and give them the ability to flex these "leadership muscles" through active use and practice. Succession planning often isn't an issue for these leaders, because they've planted the seeds of leadership excellence in the team. The best leaders foster a sense of family and community so that their people feel they're working for a cause as well as for a company. They identify the best people in the organization and then invest heavily in coaching and developing them. They make it easy for staff to move within the organization and to try new things. If the new things don't work out, the leader welcomes the protégé back with open arms and finds new ways for him to contribute.

Today's nurse leaders employ principles of transformational leadership and achieve results that are sustainable over time. Transformational leaders provide meaningful, clear, consistent communication through multiple forms, act with integrity and are authentic, treat people with respect and dignity, engender trust, and create opportunities for innovation and risk taking that provide the fuel to propel the organization to a new level of effectiveness.[4] They clearly articulate expectations, monitor and reward performance, and live a balanced life engaged in continuous learning. These leaders build relationships with staff and physicians, are visible and sincere, and achieve common ground, involving all stakeholders. They consistently display the right traits that become the predominant elements of the culture.

Transformational leaders recognize the value of teamwork and establish effective partnerships, most importantly with the staff. They excel at delivering key messages and use such tools as newsletters and open forums to communicate milestones achieved, recognize team member accomplishments, reinforce values, and share experiences. They have an open-door policy, enjoy informal chats, round on off shifts, and are committed to listening, action, and caring. These effective leaders focus on their team members and create a learning organization in which education, training, development, and a commitment to learning are core values. This enables them to recognize results and achievements and to honor the important work done every day on their units and in their departments.

These leaders make it personal when they set employee growth and learning as a top priority and truly espouse a participative leadership framework. They consider the impact on staff with every decision made, they find ways for team members to succeed, and they highlight team accomplishments rather than their own. These leaders must manage performance, though, and hold team members to the standards that have been mutually agreed upon. (See *Improving performance.*)

Most leaders and coaches have a bias toward action. They're doers who surround themselves with doers. It isn't much fun to be a doer surrounded by inert colleagues. And it's just as difficult to be a dimly lit bulb surrounded by brightly lit ones. However, nurse leaders see this every day at work—people who can't keep pace with the changes and the demand for continuous improve-

MANAGER'S TIP

Improving performance

One of the biggest complaints that team members have is that many leaders are unwilling to confront and resolve issues associated with inadequate performance or disruptive behaviors by team members.[5]

In providing feedback to improve individual and team performance, the nurse leader should be direct, specific, personal, and honest. The most effective nurse leaders also protect employee self-esteem at all cost. If team members are made to feel that they're failures, feel rejected, or feel that they're being second-guessed, that climate guarantees risk aversion, hesitation, and indecision. True leaders build self-confidence in others and encourage them to be leaders themselves.

ment find themselves "not fitting in." Many simply need to find another workplace to match their energy level and their mindset. The problem today is there aren't many places left for these people to go. Every environment of care is demanding and challenging. The ability of leaders and their team members to adapt and to constantly retool themselves is the only way to stay employed today. Old answers and obsolete methods don't work anymore because the questions and the environment of care keep changing. Nurse leaders must become models of continuous improvement concepts by establishing lifelong learning goals that they diligently work to achieve. This kind of leadership and mentoring will provide the positive example that team members need to become the most flexible and adaptive learners and leaders possible.

Effective leaders assume the coaching role with grace and humility. They have a natural tendency to develop others and are comfortable sharing power and recognition. They treat their team members as well as they treat patients and families. By breaking down the barriers between nurse and respiratory therapist, between nurse leader and lab director, and between nurses on various shifts and in different divisions, nurse leaders create a superior climate of care. By accepting differences among team members and valuing them instead of categorizing coworkers as "step-down nurses, the night shift, or the new manager" they break down more and more barriers. By working to create a shared vision and establishing common goals with all members of the patient care team, they achieve the greatest good for the greatest number. Only when all team members stop focusing exclusively on what's best for them, for their role, and for their department will nurse leaders be able to tap the limitless potential in their environment and truly create a climate of leadership at all levels in the organization.

To achieve this leadership and coaching scenario requires a high level of mentoring and an optimistic outlook. How difficult is it for nurse leaders to be a positive voice in an ocean of negativity? To be a visionary in dark times? Some weeks it may seem impossible, yet many nurse leaders continue to see the hope in nursing and in the world and share that optimism and strength with everyone around them. They continue to recruit friends and neighbors into the nursing profession, sharing heartwarming stories of the lives they've touched over many years of service. They continue to encourage staff leaders to assume formal leadership roles, broaden the scope of their influence, and cultivate the next generation of nurse leaders. They continue to put patients and families first, and they make their team's needs a priority at every decision-making table. These extraordinary leaders magically cut expenses and reduce overhead, doing more with less while never allowing patient care to suffer or employee needs to go unrecognized.

Developing champions

At times, being a nurse leader seems a thankless job. Then a staff nurse you mentored a few years ago sends you an e-mail to tell you that he earned his master's degree. A patient returns for a visit to praise you and your staff for saving her life. A high school student from "shadow" day credits you as her inspiration for entering nursing school. A resident you taught to put in his first central line was just named chief of staff and he stops you in the cafeteria to thank you for coaching him.

There are many examples of world-class coaches. Some work in health care and others in college and professional athletics. The lessons learned from all coaches are the same: to focus on skill development, teamwork, leadership, and preparation. To coach nursing champions, nurse leaders must nurture rookies by partnering them with seasoned staff who can ease their transition. Effective nursing coaches provide adequate time for social-ization, build a shared vision, and truly synthesize a team culture. Championship teams never allow their rookies to wallow in self-doubt after a bad game or an error. Successful nurse leaders sup-port new nurses and new hires through their transition, building safety nets to ensure their success.

Champion nursing teams prepare rigorously for codes, the Joint Commission on Accreditation of Healthcare Organizations surveys, the Occupational Safety and Health Administration in-spections, and disasters. Preparedness is part of the daily routine, not something that occurs every 3 years. Nurse leaders role mod-el it, setting high expectations for our team *and* ourselves.

Those who coach champions measure everything, keeping stats on each player, practice, and game. Nurse leaders must be-come better statisticians, better prepared to measure quality out-comes, team effort, and cost-effectiveness. They must put sys-tems in place for their teams to measure performance so that they can improve.

Great coaches believe that their job isn't to win games: It's to lead, teach, and create future leaders and teachers. The best coaches let their hearts show, take their team members into their families, and teach life lessons. In crisis situations, these leaders show their teams confidence, pride, and their belief in them. The calling of all nurse leaders is to coach champions, but their legacy is to create leaders that exceed patients' expectations.

This level of coaching comes with experience and constant re-finement of one's coaching strategy. There are many resources available to assist you and your teams in such efforts. Stephen Covey's work is over a decade old, but it has stood the test of time and is alive and well in many successful organizations to-day.[6] (See *Covey's principles*, page 142.)

Taking pride in yourself

Whatever strategies you select, they must reflect who you are and the leadership and coaching style that you're comfortable using. As long as you continue to learn, to improve, and to care for yourself and for others, you can enhance your leadership skill and achieve new heights for yourself and your team. Coaching effec-

Covey's principles

Covey's leadership principles,[7] which apply to all team members, encourage you to:
➤ be proactive
➤ begin with the end in mind
➤ put first things first
➤ think win-win
➤ seek first to understand, then to be understood
➤ synergize
➤ sharpen the saw.

tively and bringing out the best in your team members will allow them to achieve their personal and their team goals.

Said another way, "the richer the soil, the greater the harvest." All efforts to enrich the soil of the nursing team foundation will surely reap a much greater harvest than that which is being sowed in many organizations. As a nurse leader, you must commit to provide the tender loving care, the fertilizer and nutrients, and the sunshine and rain to help the harvest to grow. You must commit to tending the fields so that one bad fruit doesn't affect the whole crop. When the plows and tillers are broken or obsolete, you must see to it that they're replaced so that the job gets done and the workers receive the support they need. And when the harvest is in, all who contributed to the bounty should celebrate the fruits of their labor.

Recognizing, rewarding, and appreciating your people

Effective nurse leaders take time to thank their team members and to recognize and reward excellence. They're careful to recognize and to reward attempts, not just achievements. In doing so, employees know that all efforts are valued, whether they're successful or not, and that every attempt to improve the organization and to benefit the team is appreciated. Such appreciation rewards risk taking and creates a culture in which it's safe and valued to try new things. The thank you must be sincere and is best when it's delivered face to face. Certainly, though, written expressions of thanks are better than none at all and can still go a long way in conveying appreciation to the team.

Recognizing excellence

Employee recognition that comes from the top means a lot. A great example of leaders who understand the value of thanking and recognizing team efforts is in the Marriott Hotel organization. Every month, Bill Marriott personally calls the company's top six sales people. Also, Marriott's president, executive vice president, and vice president of sales call six leading performers each month. You can imagine the impact that receiving these personal calls from the company's senior executives has on the employees. Worthy of note is that they do the calling themselves; they don't staff it out to an assistant or someone lower on the ladder. The local and regional leadership teams also perpetuate this practice of appreciation. One manager at a Minneapolis Marriott writes 10 letters a week to people who have been singled out by guests or fellow associates for a job well done. He sends the letter to the employee's home so it can be opened with family present. How gratifying it must be for the employee to open his letter with pride, and with his family sharing in his accomplishment and recognition.

It wouldn't take much for nurse leaders to do the same thing—and what a difference it would make for team members. Have you established an approach to recognizing and appreciating your team members? Is it something that you view as a chore, or as a heartfelt show of gratitude? Team members can see through any demonstration of appreciation that isn't genuine or that appears to be just going through the motions. Appreciative gestures are also less valued by employees when they haven't seen or heard from you all year, and then you show up out of duty sometime during Nurses' Week.

Rewarding excellence

Compensation not only recognizes team members' critical thinking and scope of responsibility but also gives nurses the incentive to remain in the nursing profession, thus ensuring that the next generation of nurses is in place and ready to take over when necessary. Good nurse leaders know their team members so well that they know when a team or an individual makes a tremendous contribution to a patient or to the organization's effectiveness, and they recognize that contribution quickly and in a way that's meaningful to the employee. (See *Making an organization successful,* page 144.)

Making an organization successful

Organizations led by effective nurse leaders compensate for what they care about, reward people only for what they have control over, keep incentive programs clear and simple, and tie customer service results directly to employee compensation.

A key to success is that the nurse leader places a focus on real work and immediate things that people care about. So, keep it simple, and learn by doing. Build from good, expect better, and make it great. Focus on the best, most life-giving forces that are already present, and build on them. Involve people and associate with them. Look for the wellness and wholeness that exists in even the sickest organization and start there.

Provide team members with the essential elements of a satisfying work experience:
➤ work that's interesting and meaningful
➤ a clear statement of the results you expect
➤ appropriate and timely feedback on those results
➤ a reward system for achieving results.

Employees know what's expected and are rewarded when they exceed those expectations. They've participated in establishing goals and targets, and know when they've met or not met them. It's frustrating to staff when they see a one-size-fits-all approach to recognition. In such cases, the mediocre receive the same reward and compensation as the exceptional. Those who abuse the system, are late, call out sick, and have a bad attitude get the same annual increase as those who are leaders and positive role models. Nurse leaders must work closely with Human Resources in crafting compensation plans and incentive plans that reward excellence and that discourage negative behaviors and poor performance.

Appreciating employee potential

Leland Kaiser, a renowned health care futurist, says that only 30% to 40% of the employee genius is tapped in current organizations.[8] Breaking down the walls and empowering others to achieve their full potential is surely a way to begin to realize the genius in our midst. Compensation, recognition, and appreciation can't be left out of this equation. Bringing out the best in your team members requires that you celebrate success with them and support them when things don't go well. It requires that you place attainable targets in sight so employees have realistic goals to which they can aspire. It requires that you invest in nurses in meaningful and substantial ways and not be lulled into complacency by providing artificial and transparent enticements that won't attract or retain the best and the brightest in the profession.

The professional practice model

Nurse leaders must build a professional practice model that supports organizational strategic agendas and that also supports the recruitment and retention of a competent and compassionate team. Attention should be paid to the details of the professional practice model that the team embraces. Will staff be salaried? How will meeting time and governance activities be accounted for and compensated? What are the developmental needs of the team members? How will they be addressed and how will resources be allocated to meet them? How will conflict be handled? What incentives and recognition models are most meaningful to the staff? How will they be administered so that fairness and equity are ensured? Is the incentive plan understood by all team members, and is it attainable?

Start the dialogue with the team about what matters to them and how they can succeed. Show employees all that's being done for them, and make sure you let them know what you're working on and how it will affect their work and their patients. Pay attention to providing the things that make life more convenient for the staff, such as group discounts with local merchants, auto insurance and financial planning, flexible schedules, child care, and on-site banking and dry cleaning. Incentives don't have to be expensive or glitzy. They just have to be meaningful to the recipient, rally team support, and enhance morale.

Give employees who think like leaders and entrepreneurs — those who undertake risk to turn ideas into results — incentives. Entrepreneurs aren't afraid to take chances or to go where others won't. They accept ownership and take responsibility for their ideas and their results. Many nurse leaders have been trained to depend on the hierarchy for stability and direction. However, this mentality is crippling health care organizations. The new era calls for people who are self-directed, self-disciplined leaders, people who know their purpose and pursue it with ownership, passion, and accountability. So, act like you own the place. Stop

CASE IN POINT

Sick day incentive

I saw the entrepreneurial spirit come alive when I worked with a staff group recently that was struggling with absenteeism. Morale was low, staff members were exhausted, and five or six staff members were calling out sick every day.

At a staff meeting, the nurse leader put on her entrepreneurial hat, put the issues on the table, and sought the team's help to address the problem. The staff brainstormed a number of ideas and decided on an incentive plan that went into effect immediately. Every staff member who had perfect attendance in a month had her name entered for a drawing to be held at that month's staff meeting. The team member whose name was drawn would receive a $25 gift certificate to the local mall, a restaurant, or a bookstore. The nurse leader didn't ask anyone's permission to implement this plan: She just did it. She took ownership of her situation with her team and created a solution that everyone thought would work.

The next day, several employees still called out sick. As each day passed, however, a few of the team members got closer to the 1-month mark with perfect attendance. Momentum and excitement began to build on the unit, and at the end of the first month of the incentive program, six nurses had their names entered for the drawing. The first winner received a $25 gift certificate to a local restaurant and was ecstatic. You would have thought she'd won the lottery.

In the months that followed, the incentive plan took on more and more importance, and within a few months, over 90% of the staff had their names entered into the monthly drawings. The unit was abuzz each month on the day of the staff meeting with anticipation of who would win. When a nurse unexpectedly needed a day off, she found someone to cover for her, instead of calling out as she would have done before the incentive program went into effect.

The increased camaraderie and team spirit on the unit was palpable. The impact on the bottom line was substantial, considering the reduction in overtime to cover the sick calls, and the incentive plan cost only $300 per year. This plan led to the development of several others — and to the creation of a high-performing team that exuded entrepreneurial spirit.

asking for permission, and ask for forgiveness only if needed. Ask your team members to list two things they'd do better if they owned the place, and then help them to get them done. Identify niche opportunities, pull together virtual teams, and tap resources that others ignore. Think like an entrepreneur and use your imagination, spirit, courage, conviction, tenacity, responsibility, and resourcefulness to create a positive future for you and your team.[9] (See *Sick day incentive*.)

Motivational factors

In working with diverse groups, it quickly becomes apparent that not all team members are motivated by the same things. When designing a recognition program, the nurse leader must match up personal preference styles and create an awareness of their impact on satisfaction and recognition, all in an effort to make the team as successful as possible so that organizational outcomes will be achieved.

In creating recognition and appreciation models that work, nurse leaders and their team members must focus on those things that are within their control. It causes frustration to continue to long for things that rely on someone else to make them happen. We *can* control how we rely on each other for strength, humor, inspiration, commitment, and recognition. We can create incentive plans and recognition plans that are meaningful, not costly, and that create a culture of pride and teamwork. This recognition and validation builds the nursing profession from within. It celebrates competence and humanity without relying on outside recognition. Sign-on bonuses, free cars, and other incentives don't work to retain staff, and they often alienate the long-term staff in the process. Bringing the best and the brightest into the nursing profession — and retaining them — requires a commitment to rewarding those with staying power, as long as they have the positive attitude and teamwork that create the best work environment and patient outcomes.

At the root of employee recognition is a shared dedication to the patient and family, which draws nurses into the profession and keeps them coming back every day. Patients need nurses. They need their commitment to excellence and to each other. They need their expert communication, optimism, and energy. You know the difference that your work makes. Your patients, their families, and your staff know it, too. Make no mistake — everyone wants to be paid what they're worth. More important, every nurse wants professional recognition. Ensuring appropriate base compensation and benefits is essential, but without sincere and frequent recognition from organizational leadership and peers, the best compensation plan in the world will never be enough.

Empowerment and motivation

Leland Kaiser[10] describes the need for a movement to "quantum nursing," a model of care delivery that blends spirituality and science. In this model, many obsolete notions about health, nursing, and patients go out the window. "Bedside nursing" is no longer a focus. The focus isn't caring for a person in a bed, but rather on caring for a person within a holistic environment in which health can better be attained and supported. Hospitals are no longer viewed as buildings where sick people go, but as places where practitioners can bring their full array of caring practices to assist the care recipient in optimizing his well-being. In quantum nursing, there's no more "it isn't my job." All team members participate in care delivery to the full extent of their capability and are empowered as full participants in leading the organization and in delivering care. All team members add value and do what's needed to support the care recipient.

Achieving such a state of quantum nursing is contingent upon a commitment to staff empowerment and requires exceptional leaders who can motivate staff to participate and to share in the difficult work of managing care delivery. This degree of empowerment requires nurse leaders to let go of many obsolete beliefs about management, being "the boss," decision making, and "who's in charge." It requires them to move away from the paternalistic approaches to leadership and away from "mama" management. In many organizations, to achieve quantum nursing would require a different relationship between employees and formal leaders. This new work contract represents a shift away from dependency and entitlement, from the expectations of security, and toward a more conditional relationship based on mutual maturity. Successfully empowering staff and motivating them to look beyond the rote description of their job opens up a world of possibility for achieving goals that you may never have dreamed possible. In this environment, there's no more "us versus them," but rather "we." The tension that so often exists between staff and managers dissipates and accountability for outcomes is shared by all.

In an environment in which empowerment is nurtured, employees are active participants and change partners. In such a professional climate, employees have:

Positive outcomes of a self-reliant staff

Empowered and autonomous employees enjoy greater job satisfaction, higher morale, and deliver superior clinical care. They view all patients and all aspects of the care environment as their responsibility.

In these workplaces, you never hear "he isn't my patient." You see employees picking up litter from the floor, even though in most places, that's housekeeping's job. You see team members pitching in to help their peers, because they believe that no one gets a break until everyone is caught up. There's no blaming and finger pointing when things don't go as planned. Every team member takes responsibility for team outcomes, good and bad, and works together to continuously learn and to improve care processes.

> greater decision latitude, more need for individual judgment, fewer established policies as guidelines
> broader job descriptions, more strategic responsibility
> individual responsibility to solve customer problems directly
> responsibility for the continuous improvement of processes
> the need to demonstrate team and interpersonal skill
> less certainty and more ambiguity because change is part of the reality.[11]

These factors move employees from a "blue collar" mentality to one of professionalism, accountability, and empowerment. No longer do employees ask permission to solve every problem they encounter. They take necessary action to resolve issues because they're closest to the issues and because they have the authority to do so. Fundamental to establishing such environments is a belief in what Linda Aiken has proven through her research: that "staff accountability and autonomy are linked to job satisfaction, morale, and quality of care."[12] (See *Positive outcomes of a self-reliant staff.*)

Commitment begins with involving the workforce in creating the vision for the future. Visionary leaders recognize that employee involvement increases productivity and don't view involving employees as insignificant and a waste of time.[13] When employees can provide ideas and suggestions directly to senior leaders, employee vulnerability decreases and employee satisfaction increases. Professional practice models that enhance employee autonomy and decision making, such as shared governance or participative leadership, engage employees and create win-win scenarios for them, their patients, and their leaders. Employees feel that their ideas and opinions are valued, and actually see them put into action by the formal leadership. By empowering the staff, the nurse leader unleashes talent and shows a personal interest in each team member. This is accomplished as the nurse leader creates a climate that supports decision making by:

➤ trusting team members with meaningful levels of responsibility
➤ providing team members the necessary autonomy to achieve results
➤ presenting challenging opportunities that stretch the individual abilities of team members
➤ recognizing and rewarding superior performance
➤ standing behind the team and supporting it.[14]

Nurse leaders create leaders through participation and involvement, believing the Native American proverb, "Tell me, and I will forget. Show me, and I may not remember. Involve me, and I will understand." The most effective leaders subjugate their ego needs in favor of the team's goal. They allow team members to take an active part in shaping the destiny of the team's effort. They allow the team to decide, make choices, act, and do something meaningful. This creates the "multiplier effect," as leaders bring out the leadership in others. They give team members the self-confidence to act, take charge of their responsibilities, and make changes occur rather than merely perform assigned tasks. Participation, especially in the planning of strategies for achieving goals, increases motivation, effort and, ultimately, success. Team builders delegate to empower people to act, stretch the abilities of others, and encourage educated risk taking.

The most effective nurse leaders encourage the autonomy of their team members and support their decision making, even if it isn't the way they would have done it themselves. That means that formal leaders don't have to have their hands in every pot. They can stay involved and informed without resorting to micromanagement. By encouraging team members to take risks, to fail as well as to succeed, they learn. To a team member, there are few things worse than being empowered to do something and then having the formal leader hover, be too involved, and try to direct the approach taken. Micromanagers don't empower. They don't have the confidence in themselves or in their team members to truly let go so that the team can be autonomous. Micromanagers haven't successfully learned the art of staying involved and informed without having to know every detail and direct every step of the process. In effect, micromanagers tie the hands of their team members behind their backs and then ask them to be active participants in decision making. Unfortunately, that strategy doesn't work, and it creates tremendous frustration and animosity. Learning to let go is a fundamental concept in empowerment and one that many nurse leaders must work on every day.

Empowerment isn't necessarily every team member's cup of tea either. Some employees have a strong need for structure, identity, defined roles, and low risk taking, as found in traditional organizational structures. Sometimes this is a function of low confidence and self-esteem on the part of the employee. In some cases, the employee has never had the benefit of working with a formal leader who understood empowerment and really knew how to bring out the best in his employees. Sometimes it's laziness or a myopic view of roles and responsibilities and a traditional, blue-collar, and bureaucratic mindset. Many of these employees have become comfortable blaming management as a means of managing anxiety. As one such employee stated, "I'd rather be dead than empowered."[15]

The most effective nurse leaders recognize that involvement and empowerment enhance commitment and know how to work through or around such employees to achieve the greatest good for the greatest number. In many cases, it's actually peer pressure and peer action that most effectively addresses those employees who struggle to embrace the empowerment model. Peer-to-peer feedback and expectations can sometimes be more easily embraced and accepted by the naysayer than that which comes from a formal leader. The effective nurse leader engages the peer group and the informal leaders and involves them in holding all team members accountable to established norms and expectations.

Fortunately, the 80-20 rule usually applies in this situation, as it does to many others. Most team members welcome the chance to be involved, share their ideas, and bring their leadership to bear beyond the clinical realm and into the management realm.

In fact, studies show that most people want to do a good job and wish they could contribute even more.[16] People don't have to be tricked or forced to participate. When leaders give their people the tools, freedom, and trust they need to lead themselves, they'll take care of business with all of the passion and commitment of a CEO.[17] In these environments built on empowerment, the nurse leader acts less as a controller and more as a coordinator, focuser, and facilitator, gaining control by giving it up. The effective nurse leader deploys and disperses power, and it comes back tenfold.

Shared decision making

Once trust and true communication are in place, the ability to foster a participative leadership style is enhanced. The most effective governance in a workplace community is a structure and process that involves dialogue, is shared, and puts decision making closest to the work. Every team should have a built-in balance of power or influence for making decisions about how the work gets done.[18] Managers must believe that staff members have the intelligence to do their jobs and to contribute to the whole. Then, staff and managers must take personal accountability for the outcomes. Too often, managers describe their staff members as incapable of taking on the responsibility that empowerment requires. Such comments can imply that the team members are either not smart enough or not motivated enough to share in decision making. It probably is more the case that the nurse leader hasn't gained staff buy-in and support, and hasn't articulated the benefits of empowerment. Everyone wants to know "what's in it for me"? The nurse leader must be able to state clearly how the staff will reap the rewards of participating and must keep everyone, administrators and staff alike, aware of the progress being made in building community. Leaders must role model and personally take an interest in individuals. They must manage fear and hold everyone accountable to participate.

Fostering employee participation and using empowerment programs to enhance satisfaction will help to avoid unionization.[19] However, that isn't to say that these strategies can't be achieved in a union environment. Community can be established in this type of environment, as long as a balance of power and influence exists. Continuous dialogue based on mutual respect is needed, as is an open door with ground rules followed — and that can be tricky sometimes. Building community and empowerment creates the interconnectedness that can heal fragmentation and begin a shift toward a staff more satisfied with the quality of their work life.[20]

When employees are empowered, everyone benefits, including the patients — and that's the reason empowerment gets so much attention. It's a major component of organizational culture and can make or break the staff's attitude, productivity, and morale. Kanter proposes that an individual's effectiveness on the job is influenced largely by the organizational aspects of the work environment.[21] Leaders who provide access to information, resources, support, and the opportunity to learn and develop empower and enable employees to accomplish their work. Employees sense that management can be trusted, and they're more committed to the organization and more likely to engage in positive organizational activities and to feel autonomy and self-efficacy. Empowered employees become more productive and effective in meeting organizational goals.

The power of perception

Staff nurses' perception of managerial power is important in shaping how they perceive their own positions with respect to power and opportunity. Employees need to see that managers have influence with those above them. Several studies reveal the incredible impact that nurse managers have on the frontline staff. Some go so far as to say that people join companies, but they leave managers and supervisors. Often, deterioration between frontline managers and staff is the impetus for a union campaign and, at the very least, causes a decline in staff morale, productivity, and retention.

Nurse managers must make every effort to stay aligned with their staff members, to know them as people, and to establish trust, rapport, and respect. These lay the foundation for empowerment and for shared leadership and decision making. It's only in truly knowing your people that you can understand what motivates them and how to unleash their potential. One study provides some help in understanding what motivates employees, and also reveals a large perception gap between what employees said

Motivating factors

Do you know what motivates your employees? Using a 10-point scale, with 1 being most important and 10 being least important, managers and staff separately rated staff motivators, as shown below. Managers rated the top three staff motivators as being good wages, job security, and promotional opportunities, yet employees rated the same factors 5, 4, and 7 respectively.

Employees rated their top motivators to be full appreciation for work done, feeling "in" on things, and working for someone who was sympathetic to their personal problems. Managers rated these same motivators 8, 10, and 9 respectively.

Such a disconnect in perception of what motivates employees sets up a scenario in which it's difficult to put recognition plans into place that will be meaningful to the staff. Without knowing what really motivates the staff, the nurse leader is also unable to modify and adapt her leadership and communication style in ways that will meet the staff's expectations and wishes.

	Managers	Employees
Good wages	1	5
Job security	2	4
Promotional opportunities	3	7
Good working conditions	4	9
Interesting work	5	6
Personal loyalty to workers	6	8
Tactful disciplining	7	10
Full appreciation for work done	8	1
Sympathetic to personal problems	9	3
Feeling "in" on things	10	2

motivated them and what managers perceived motivated employees.[22] (See *Motivating factors.*)

If a manager spends all of her time working on a compensation plan when the staff places greater value on face-to-face communication and information sharing, this misalignment of values and priorities will cause dissention on the team. If the manager focuses on communication, but doesn't address issues of job security and flexibility, again, there will be a problem. Such perception gaps must be recognized and understood, and the best way to do so is to collect data and use it to drive decision making. If leaders don't ask their team members what's most important to them, then they'll continue to make judgments that aren't based on fact, but rather on supposition and assumption. This is a recipe for "us versus them" and for continued organizational dysfunction and misalignment. These perception gaps underscore the reason sign-on bonuses and car care are ineffective recruitment and retention strategies. In many cases, these incentives and others like them have been put in place without asking the staff what would be most meaningful to them. In the end, these "incentives" often do more damage than good, because they alienate current staff from those newly recruited.

Perception is very real and must be addressed if nurse leaders and staff are to come together to enhance the quality of work life for nurses and the care environment for patients and families. Thinking influences feelings, which shape behavior and outcomes. Often, managers feel that their employees resist change. However, it isn't change that people resist; it's their perception of the change that motivates the response. Effective nurse leaders take time to tune in to the perceptions that team members have — perceptions of them, their ideas, their vision, and the actions they want the team members to take. What's more, they know that selling positive perceptions sells change.[23] They achieve this understanding through the personal investment of time and energy, and by remembering that leadership is a human process. They also demonstrate a strong work ethic and a tireless commitment to the needs of patients and employees. Nursing's most effective leaders and motivators have the stamina and the endurance to keep going when everyone else has long since faded. They don't tolerate complacency and mediocrity in the culture and set high expectations of themselves and of others. These role models don't ask others to do things that they won't do themselves and certainly aren't afraid to work hard. They maintain expectations of excellence and create new methods for achieving them in the face of challenge and unceasing demands. These characteristics are the essence of effective leaders who through their own work ethic and commitment motivate others to succeed and to contribute.

Charisma: Natural magnetism

Question: *Can you define charisma?*

Answer: Charisma is that personal magic of leadership that arouses special popular loyalty or enthusiasm for a public figure. It's a certain magnetic charm or appeal. Charismatic leaders tap into the hearts of their employees, have a finger on their pulse at all times, and ask what will make a difference for them. They have a "presence" that's engaging, warm, and inviting, and one that encourages participation and involvement. You just know who they are when they walk into the room.

Charisma is often a factor in effectively motivating team members to do things that they really don't want to do. The nurse leader's charismatic pull and heartfelt intentions can often persuade the team to pull together, support change, make do with less, and thrive in chaos. Charismatic leaders know how to deliver bad news, ask the difficult questions, hold people accountable, and take corrective action. The magnetism of charisma draws people to them, inspires trust, and is a motivating force.

Motivating staff and tuning in to their perceptions requires another characteristic that's often used synonymously with leadership — charisma. (See *Charisma: Natural magnetism.*)

People are born with charisma, and some have more than others. However, charisma can be developed and potentiated by connecting with people, sending nonverbal messages of openness and accessibility, possessing excellent "people skills," and above all, learning to be comfortable with our humanity. This means being able to express genuine empathy, humor, and candor — whatever the situation calls for — and even being willing to share our fears, anxieties, and dreams in order to help our team members get to know us as people. It means letting your hair down, being comfortable admitting that you don't have all of the answers, and asking for help when you need it. Charisma is used by effective nurse leaders to motivate others in difficult times and to ask for help and ideas to make a tough situation better.

Effectively motivating team members to succeed and to keep coming back every day is a fundamental responsibility of nurse leaders and a challenge that requires daily attention. For some, meeting this challenge means changing the mental models and assumptions they hold about what motivates people and which priorities are most important. For others, becoming effective

Be a mentor

Throughout my life, most of my role models and mentors have had incredible charisma and used it so effectively that they motivated me to achieve goals I never thought I could. Their magnetic charm and powerful appeal persuaded me to embrace change and challenge even when I didn't want to do so.

These incredible motivators could sell me the shirt off my own back. But they were only able to do so because they had already invested time and energy in establishing trust and getting to know me. They were excellent communicators who were able to motivate not only with charm but also with information and data. They were competent and committed to their work, and it showed. The best motivators I've ever had were those whose motto was "love your work — or do something else." They empowered me to make decisions, gave me the tools and space I needed, and let me fly. I always knew that they would be there to catch me when I fell, and that was all of the motivation that I needed. That's the kind of motivation and charisma we need in nursing, today more than ever before.

Do you have such charismatic leaders and great motivators in your life? Are you such a leader to others?

leaders means taking control of their lives, perfecting the art of stress management, and developing a sense of discovery, innovation, and continuous improvement. Some need to focus on enhancing their charismatic appeal and working with people more on a human level. (See *Be a mentor.*)

Optimism versus pessimism

Before nurse leaders can hope to motivate others to change, they must first be prepared to change their own mindset. After all, the biggest career challenges today are perceptual—psychological—not technical, not even skills based. And, because perspectives heavily influence performance and satisfaction, it's important to tune in to your perspectives on life and work, if you're going to directly and distinctly influence the leader and the person that you're to become.

The best nurse leaders are prepared to challenge their assumptions about their potential and their future. When nurse leaders motivate themselves effectively, they become more effective at motivating others. This requires the nurse leader to use her intuition and her resourcefulness and to confront her own fears as well as the naysayers around her. So do yourself a favor: Identify positive motivators, study them, and learn from them. Formulate a motivational strategy centered on several of the seven Cs: commitment, contribution, communication, cooperation, conflict management, change management, and connections. And don't forget optimism.

Effective leaders and motivators are optimistic. As Colin Powell says, "optimism is a force multiplier."[24] An optimistic leader can motivate the team to multiply its effect exponentially. Optimism is motivating, and it draws people to you. Yes, there's cause for optimism in our future, and the nursing profession needs leaders who believe that. For most of us, we'll need to think differently in order to see the future differently, and our energy level will be a critical factor in our success. Effective nurse leaders learn to generate energy, conserve energy, and channel energy. They stay optimistic and opportunity-minded and use their energy to the most productive advantage.

A negative frame of mind drains your energy and the energy of others. It weakens your confidence and it hurts problem-solving skills. You end up focusing on obstacles and that interferes with your ability to see opportunities. Pessimism drains the joy and happiness out of life, whereas a positive outlook is energizing, empowering, and strengthening. Why would anyone follow a leader who doesn't believe that tomorrow can be better than today? Why would team members rally behind a pessimistic, energy-sucking naysayer who can't even see the glass as half full? Life is too short to listen to negative self-talk and to hang out with negative people. If you are doing so, it's time to make a change.

Start with an assessment. How would your team members evaluate you on this Optimism Barometer?[25]

5. Believes we can leap tall buildings.
4. Believes we can leap townhouses.
3. Believes we can leapfrog.
2. "Leap when I say leap."
1. "No leaping. You'll probably get hurt."

How high did you score? Do you need to focus on honing your optimistic outlook? We all need this once in a while. The question is whether you need it every day. If you do, it may be time to get help or to reevaluate the choices you've made. Is it difficult to remain positive and optimistic today? Yes. But without an optimistic leader, a team won't achieve its maximum potential. It won't feel the positive force of a leader pushing and pulling to achieve a vision. It won't see possibilities, only problems. Optimism can be learned, practiced, and developed. Optimists get paid more, are healthier, win more elections, live longer, and are better at adapting to change. So, choose optimism![26]

The nursing profession desperately needs positive, optimistic role models to point the way toward innovation, creativity, and balance. Effectively empowering and motivating teams results in an energized organization in which the vision, mission, and values are lived and breathed by all, not just left hanging on a plaque in the lobby. Motivation, competence, and influence are palpable. Processes work and the work design supports those with the patients. Leadership is visible, credible, authentic, and focused and motivates and inspires the team to achieve its goals.

Nurse leaders in every corner of this world leave their indelible mark on the health of their community members and on the futures of their team members by motivating them to be the best and by empowering them to own their practice and their environment of care. You are who you believe you are. You become what you believe you'll become. Change your beliefs, change your mind, and you'll change your outcomes for the better.

Points to remember

The following points summarize the power of inspiration in the leadership role:

➤ Effective leaders influence, coach, and evoke confidence in others as well as cultivate this ability in others.
➤ Effective nursing coaches provide adequate time for socialization, build a shared vision, and truly synthesize a team culture.
➤ Recognition and reward are important components in conveying appreciation to the team and its members for efforts put forth to improve the organization.
➤ Visionary leaders recognize that employee involvement increases productivity and strive to enhance employee autonomy and decision making.
➤ Effectively motivating team members to succeed is a fundamental responsibility of nurse leaders and a daily challenge.

References

1. Leider, R.J. "The Ultimate Leadership Task: Self leadership," in *The Leader of the Future: New Visions, Strategies and Practices For The Next Era.* Edited by Hesselbein, F., et al. eds. San Francisco, Calif.: Jossey-Bass, 1996.

2. Larson, C., and LaFasto, F. *TeamWork: What Must Go Right/What Can Go Wrong.* Newbury Park, Calif.: Sage Publications, Inc., 1989.

3. *The Way of Life According to Laotzu: An American Version.* Translated by W. Bynner. New York: John Day Co., 1944.

4. Laschinger, H., et al. "Organizational Trust and Empowerment in Restructured Healthcare Settings," *Journal of Nursing Administration* 30(9):413-25, September, 2000.

5. Larson, C., and LaFasto, F. Op. cit.

6. Covey, S.R. *The 7 Habits of Highly Effective People.* New York: Simon & Schuster, 1980.

7. ibid.

8. Kaiser, L. Address to Duke University Medical Center, Durham, N.C., 1999.

9. Murray, J. *Think Change.* Aurora, Ill.: Successories, Inc. USA, 1998.

10. Kaiser, L. Op. cit.

11. Laschinger, H., et al. Op. cit.

12. Aiken, L.H., et al. "Lower Medicare Mortality Among a Set of Hospitals Known for Good Nursing Care," *Medical Care* 32(8):771-87, August 1994.

13. Terry, D. Effective Employee Relations in Reengineered Organizations," *Journal of Nursing Administration's Healthcare Law, Ethics, and Regulation* 1(3):33-40, September 1999.

14. Larson, C., and LaFasto, F. Op. cit.

15. Jaffe, D., and Scott, C. "The Human Side of Reengineering," *Healthcare Forum Journal* 40(5):14-21, September-October 1997.

16. Scott, C., and Jaffe, D. *Managing Organizational Change: A Practical Guide for Managers.* Menlo Park, Calif.: Crisp Publications, Inc., 1989.

17. Dow, R., and Cook, S. *Turned On: Eight Vital Insights to Energize Your People, Customers, and Profits.* New York: HarperBusiness, 1996

18. Parker, M., and Gadbois, S. "Building Community in the Healthcare Workplace, Part 3: Belonging and Satisfaction at Work," *Journal of Nursing Administrations* 30(10):466-73, October 2000.

19. Payson, M., course leader and partner. "How to Stay Union Free in the 21st Century." Seminar. Jackson, Lewis, Schnitzler & Krupman. Presented by Executive Enterprise Institute, 2000. *www.eeiconferences.com.*

20. Parker, M., and Gadbois, S. "Building Community in the Healthcare Workplace, Part 4: Partnering with Union Members to Create Community," *Journal of Nursing Administrations* 30(11):524-29, November 2000.

21. Laschinger, H., et al. Op. cit.

22. Anderson, M. *Companies Don't Succeed...People Do!* Aurora, Ill.: Successories, Inc. USA, 1998.
23. Murray, J. Op. cit.
24. Powell, C. "Colin Powell's Rules," in *Leadership: An Association Management Supplement for Volunteer Leaders.* Washington, D.C.: American Society of Association Executives, 1995.
25. Dow, R., and Cook, S., Op. cit.
26. Pritchett, P. *The Employee Handbook of New Work Habits for the Next Millennium: 10 New Ground Rules for Job Success.* Dallas, Tex.: Pritchett & Associates, 1999.

CHAPTER 7

Facing challenges

Melissa A. Fitzpatrick, RN, MSN, FAAN

> "The most damaging phrase in the language is: 'It's always been done that way.'" — Rear Admiral Grace Hopper

Each day, nurses are faced with new health care changes, a never-ending list of things to do, a growing number of people who need or want something from them, and expectations of them that grow with each passing moment. Just as the Queen in Alice and Wonderland said, "It takes all of the running you can do to keep in the same place. If you want to get somewhere else, you must run at least twice as fast as that." Some days you may feel as though you're running as fast as you can, and making no progress, but still getting weary from the effort.

Coping with change

Nurse leaders are pulled from many directions, attempting to meet the needs and demands of a growing constituency: patients and families, employees, physicians, fellow executives, the board, the community, and the list goes on. The only constant in the ever changing landscape of nursing, of health care, and of life in general is that of change. We've all heard that before, right? The only thing that you can count on is that change will occur. What feels different in today's health care environment, though, is that more change is of a large magnitude, it involves a broader group of stakeholders who must be involved in the change, and there's

Dealing with organizational change

Question: *What does organizational change mean for nurse leaders?*

Answer: Organizational change requires that nurse leaders do a better job than ever before of building a strong organizational infrastructure to support change efforts. For most, this infrastructure is leaner, although it's also likely to be broader and less one-dimensional than in the past.

It means that nurse leaders must be visible and must communicate like never before so that their partners in change — their team members — trust them and know them and will rally around them during change planning and implementation. It means that they must be more data driven than ever so that they aren't guessing which change is best, but rather using data to support change and to drive effective decision making that maximizes the use of our limited resources.

All of this change means that the team must be able to count on the nurse leader for stability and consistency, even when everything else seems to be up for grabs. If approached with the right mindset, this time of extraordinary change can be one of creativity, innovation, collaboration, and true improvement. If approached with the wrong mindset, it could be one of daily resistance, antagonism, disenfranchisement, and torture.

much less room for error because resources are limited and can't be wasted. Organizations have become more complex, with mergers, acquisitions, and integration, so what once may have seemed like a minor change, now takes on monumental proportions. (See *Dealing with organizational change.*)

Even though most people have read the change literature and understand change theory, some still struggle every day to embrace change or at the very least to adapt to it. Some colleagues still spend energy trying to resist change. What they need to realize is that they can't fight or resist it. More important, though, they need to realize that they have choices to make regarding change and how they respond to it. They can choose to view it as a motivator and as a catalyst for growth and learning. According to Tom Peters, humankind has two basic and equally strong needs: stability and change, and even though change is painful, everyone seeks it. The issue isn't either/or, it's creating a context in which pursuing the novel is cherished, not scorned.[1] The challenge as nurse leaders is to inspire in team members a thirst for change and innovation, and to nurture in them the ability to

Message mapping

One way to evaluate how change is accepted is by message mapping the change from the employee's perspective, and by truly understanding what the change means to the employee.

When presented with a change, the employee considers the facts in ways different from the manager, as illustrated in the chart below.

Consideration of the change

Initially, the employee uses his head to understand cognitively what's happening.
Next, he tries to understand the implications of the change, using his heart affectively to understand the change. Finally, the employee focuses on the impact behaviorally, "with his hands."

The facts	The implications	The impact
➤ "What is changing?"	➤ "How does this affect me personally?"	➤ "What should I do as a result?"
➤ "Why is it changing?"	➤ "Am I better or worse off?"	➤ "What will the organization do to help me through this change?"
➤ "How were decisions made?"	➤ "Who can I talk to about this?"	➤ "How do I take advantage of this?"
➤ "What does the organization have to gain from this?"	➤ "Why change?"	
➤ "What do I have now?"	➤ "How does this fit with other messages that I'm hearing?"	
➤ "Why are these the right changes?"	➤ "How do I feel about this?"	
➤ "When will all of this happen?"		

Once the employee has walked through the facts, implications, and impact of the change, he'll start to draw conclusions as to whether he can support the change. It's in this decision-making process that leadership is essential.

The nurse leader must listen to the employee describe the personal implications of the change. When she can walk through the change in the employee's shoes, she can help him consider all sides of the issues and present the possible implications objectively. Then she can discuss how she can best support the employee regarding those implications.[2]

maximize the opportunities that change presents. (See *Message mapping.*)

If such leadership support were to be made available when changes are introduced in organizations, resistance, drama, and emotion that tends to result during change would be decreased exponentially. Again, leadership takes time and energy, and requires that nurse leaders tend to the people side of the equation in order to be successful. In truth, people change from being led, not from being told.

People don't normally change their behavior simply from information. Just look at smokers for example. It's far more common for people to change because of the support, encouragement, caring confrontation, and empathy of a relationship. Nurse leaders who create supportive relationships are more successful change agents because their team members trust them and will follow them.

It starts at the top. Top leaders commonly believe that sponsoring change means making the decision, hiring a consultant, signing the checks, and giving a pep talk. No deep change is successful if the leaders aren't deeply involved in the effort. If you're leading the change, the first changes that have to take place are those in your own behavior. If you don't change, how can you expect others to change? If you don't change, can the organization really change? True leaders are role models of adaptability and flexibility and are comfortable in an environment of constant change. They don't ask their team members to respond well to change if they don't do so themselves. The health care industry is in dire need of new thoughts, ideas, and approaches to change management. Such new leadership creates change; it doesn't just react to it. It commits people to action, prompting movement away from the status quo and toward a better way of delivering care and supporting employees. It creates an environment in which people *want* to — not *have* to — do their jobs and adapt to change.

Effective nurse leaders understand employee response to change and create scenarios in which employees can successfully move through the change cycle. (See *Responding to change*, page 166.)

Every team has a few copers, adapters, and exploiters. The key for nurse leaders is to surround themselves with those who have the energy and fortitude to build the team and the environment needed to achieve their positive vision. They must create a mix on the team that facilitates change and that moves employees successfully through the stages of change. To propel nursing from its current crisis mode to one of creativity and adaptability, nurse leaders must envision their future with optimism and create those changes — *on purpose.*

A key concept here is that nurse leaders have to view themselves and their roles differently if they're to succeed in the fu-

Responding to change

There are four options for handling change.[3] They include:

➤ *coping with change* — Those who merely cope with change exude a victim mentality, helplessness, pessimism, dependency, resistance, anger, blame, and fear. They think that "change will pass," and they wait and hope for a return to normal. While they're waiting, their productivity drops, they focus on "me issues," and they do all they can to protect the status quo. The intent is to survive the change and the chaos, not to lead it. This approach to change damages both personal and organizational effectiveness.

➤ *adapting to change* — Those who adapt to change go with the flow, taking on an adjustment mentality. They don't, however, put forth any effort to help drive the change. Often, they show grudging compliance or a cut-your-losses attitude, which, although unfortunate, is less of a drain on the organization than their coping counterparts.

➤ *exploiting change* — Exploiters of change possess an opportunity-focused mentality. They try to turn change to their advantage and search for positive personal benefits. Change is actively embraced as a potential opportunity that should be seized. Those who exploit change readily contribute their energy and attention to the cause, even though they don't create the change up front.

➤ *creating change* — Those who create change — the best leaders — have a "possibilities mentality" and remain proactive, not reactive. These are the true leaders who make change happen. They are architects of their own future and are energizing and fun to be around. They demonstrate optimism, faith, purpose, adventure, curiosity, and innovation. They move with a true sense of urgency. This is where the best nurse leaders live, and when truly successful, their teams live there, too.

ture. As Albert Einstein said, "The significant problems we face cannot be solved at the same level of thinking we were at when we created them." Every workplace has employees who are still waiting for things to go back to the "good old days." They think that if they hold their breath long enough, that these demanding times will go away, that the pace of change will slow, that what they know today will be enough to last them until retirement, and that they can hide out with their patients and exempt themselves from the rest of the health care delivery system. These employees can keep wishing for those things, but the reality is that it's yesterday's approaches that created today's problems — the exorbitant cost of care, the lack of true collaboration in the workplace, the need for patients and families to demand care that they define, and the lack of leadership preparation. So, it becomes crucial that nurse leaders help these employees to change their mindsets, to help them think and act differently, to acquire the skills that they need, or to help them into alternative opportunities in which there's a better fit for them.

An optimal climate

With an effective team in place, the nurse leader creates a climate in which decision making is fostered. Think about the relationship between vision, change, decisions, and leadership:[4]
➤ To achieve a goal or vision, change must occur.
➤ For change to occur, a decision must be made.
➤ For a decision to occur, a choice must be made.
➤ To make a choice, a risk must be taken.
➤ To encourage risk taking, a supportive climate must exist.
➤ A supportive climate is demonstrated by day-to-day leadership behavior.

Effective leaders promote and initiate change and galvanize team members around the change at hand. They're aware that change invites chaos, complexity, employee dissatisfaction, and the threat of unionization, and they do everything in their power to communicate well and to be visible to the team as it navigates through the change process. Reengineering has been a popular strategy for dealing with change, and it has also been a catalyst for unionization.[5] When done well, change is orchestrated by the nurse leader in a way that's inclusive, instructive, and productive. (See *An optimal climate.*)

The nurse leader creates change on purpose and doesn't wait for change to be imposed. In doing so, she becomes a positive role model and change agent, enabling her team to see change in a new light. (See *Bringing your team along,* page 168.)

When you take on a new project or decide to revamp a current system or process, be sure to reengineer the right way. Reengineering efforts that use an employee-centered approach produce better results and sustain them for a longer period of time. An employee-guided approach minimizes divisions between management and staff and decreases union vulnerability. Tune into the response of your team members to the proposed change and get them involved from square one. Too many times change processes miss the mark because they change a symptom of a problem rather than the real problem. Use those closest to the issue or problem to truly dissect it into its component parts so that real resolution and improvement occur.

Seek input from all constituents and remain open-minded and flexible. No one knows for sure what the best systems for health care delivery will be. Some predict specialization, whereas others

QUESTIONS & ANSWERS

Bringing your team along

Question: *How do you start bringing alive the potential that each team member has to be a leader and change agent? How do you know which approach will work best for you?*

Answer: First, you need to recognize and acknowledge everything that you know and everything that you're already doing. Then you need to build on that. You need to choose one quality or area that you'd like to improve and make small consistent changes. Behaviorists say it takes 21 days to establish a new habit. You need to give yourself that time.

predict generalization. Some foresee the use of assistant personnel diminishing, whereas others predict a growing need for their services to support the professional nurse in new ways. Because no one can predict every aspect of the future, prescribe precisely what jobs will require, what social circumstances may involve, or what supports may exist, nurse leaders will need to be flexible in their mindset and to give new meaning to the terms *adaptive* and *go with the flow*. The best shot at success that nurse leaders have is to keep learning and changing, to continue to hone their interpersonal skills, and to approach their work and their lives with a flexible mindset and a can-do attitude, always seeing the glass as half full, rather than half empty.

Hope for the future lies in the ability to embrace change and to galvanize others to do the same. Florence Nightingale said, "Nursing is a progressive art in which to stand still is to have gone back."[6] Nurse leaders don't have the luxury of standing still. To do so would lose immeasurable ground for patients and for the nursing profession.

Conflict management and toxic leadership

Much has been written on the topic of conflict management. It's a prevalent issue today, as pressures within the health care industry rise and resources shrink. Often, advice in the literature is aimed at helping nurse leaders cope with difficult peers or physicians, but not as much has been written about the conflict that involves a "boss." The following text is based on personal experiences with toxic bosses as well as on current literature regarding toxic leadership. It may hit close to home for you, as you remember experiences you've had with a psycho boss. Read it with your antennae tuned in to see if you, as a nurse leader and boss, exhibit any signs of toxic leadership. If you do, just remember that acknowledging that fact is the first step toward resolving the issues.

Reasons for toxic leadership

The term *psycho* congers up visions of the shower scene in the movie *Psycho* and of Jack Nicholson in *The Shining* with a crazed look in his eyes. For some, it may also conger up certain employee-boss relationships, like poor Bob Cratchit and his boss Scrooge, or the Dilbert cartoons about management incompetence, or Dagwood Bumstead and Mr. Dithers.

Most people at sometime in their career have worked for someone who could easily be described as a "psycho" — simply stated, someone who is stressed out, too demanding, difficult to communicate with, unlikable, not trustworthy, or downright mean. Most of these bosses aren't clinically psychotic, but they sure can act that way, which is why the term "psycho" has gained such familiarity in the popular press.

According to a recent Internet poll, more than half of Web-surfing employees surveyed rated their bosses as "toxic." The terms *psycho* and *toxic* have been used interchangeably here to describe a syndrome that's growing more prevalent in leaders today and that requires both humanity and humor to address it effectively.

So why are there so many psycho, toxic, lousy, impossible bosses out there today? Well, it may go without saying, but many workplaces aren't environments of care in which the boss or other employees feel secure and nurtured. They're places of stress, burnout, fatigue, frustration, cutbacks, turnover, and insecurity. The demands placed on bosses continue to grow, yet the resources to address these demands continue to shrink. Not only are there more demands, but there are also competing demands that force bosses to make difficult choices and render them unable to create the win-win scenario. Paul Babiak, an organizational psychologist from New York, says that "industrial psychopaths are the result of the chaotic environments of the modern workplace."[7]

The financial imperatives in health care today have placed immeasurable stress and conflict on the boss's shoulders. Doing more with less, working employees harder, and still trying to meet the vision of quality patient care often place the boss in the middle of ethical dilemmas. Bosses must also answer to many people and thus may feel themselves pulled between the demands of the board, their own boss, their peers, and their subordinates, not to mention the customers, both inside and outside the organization.

For many bosses, an absolute fear of failure and risk aversion contribute to the psycho syndrome. Job insecurity is a reality, as is turnover in the leadership ranks. One Director of Nursing in Philadelphia has had three different CEOs in the past 2 years. With each CEO change came an entirely new senior leadership team. The result for those who remain has been chaos and job insecurity, and a lack of loyalty to the organization.

Too many bosses walk around just biding their time, trying to stay off the radar screen, in hopes that they can hang on until retirement, until the kids are out of college, until the car is paid off, until, until, until. In the meantime, their personal fear of losing their job, or failing at it, creates chaos and craziness for everyone with whom they work. In today's economy, most people "need to work," and that financial imperative makes some bosses say or do anything to keep their job, whether at the expense of their ethical principles or at the expense of others.

Then, there's the Peter Principle: those in positions of power and influence who either aren't qualified for the job in the first place or who aren't capable of performing the job effectively. Many got there on the coattails of someone else and were promoted up the ranks because of that friendship or personal relationship. Others, who live the Imposter Syndrome, talk a good game and are great performers when they have a script in hand. However, they must always consult with someone else to answer a question, they can't make decisions without running it by a colleague, and they don't have the work experience to draw from to be effective in their roles.

Those bosses who are the product of the Peter Principle and who are Imposters are classic examples of psycho bosses. But it really isn't their fault. They've gotten in over their heads because of lack of leadership in other levels of the organization, and the situation is miserable for everyone. Their own insecurities and "secrets" cause them to constantly second guess themselves and others, and their team members see them for what they are, causing conflict and questioning of their positional power, all of which leads to signs of the psycho boss.

Signs of toxic leadership

How do you know when you're working for a psycho boss? Unfortunately, you may not have any warning signs at all. Your interview process may have gone extremely well. It may have been open, with two-way dialogue, and you may have felt very comfortable asking in-depth questions about how you'd work with the boss. In some scenarios, the boss may have given all of the "right" answers. She may have stated that she isn't a micromanager, when in fact she is. She may have stated that she has great delegation skills, when in fact she doesn't. And, she may have stated that empowerment is great, yet in reality she's controlling.

The best course of action in the interview phase is to be open and forthright and to put all questions and issues on the table. Ask questions such as, "Tell me about your management style." "How would we communicate with each other?" "If you have concerns about my performance, how will you bring them to my attention?" "What's your leadership philosophy?" "What's your vision for our team, and how do you define our roles on it?"

If your gut says that the boss isn't being truthful, keep probing and be specific. Unfortunately, many psycho bosses lack self-awareness and may not even know that they're controlling, micromanaging, or deceptive. The only thing you can do in the interview phase is to put your needs on the table and to use your intuition and best judgment to ensure that you'll be a good fit with this boss. Remember, it's a two-way decision, and to be an effective team, both of you must support the relationship and bring your best selves to it.

Once you're hired — whether as a staff nurse, nurse manager, or chief nurse executive — your job becomes making your boss look good. The goal of all bosses should be to surround themselves with excellence and to let the team shine, whereas your goal should be to communicate effectively, keep your boss informed, and never let your boss be caught off guard or taken by surprise. After all, there's nothing worse than looking uninformed, uninvolved, and out of the loop. This is a bad thing, and one that could start your boss down the psycho path.

Although things usually go well for at least the first few months with a new boss, they could go awry more quickly, depending on what's going on in the organization. Most bosses try their best to nurture and mentor new team members and to offer them information, support, and coaching to help them to integrate into the new role or organization and to be successful. In the meantime, you're also building relationships with peers, subordinates, physicians, and other department members and establishing your competence and value to the organization. All feedback should find its way back to your boss and continue to strengthen your relationship with her and to build confidence in your abilities. Your success is testimony to your boss's ability to hire good people, to promote good people, and to build a strong team. For most bosses, these are all good things.

How will you know when things have started to go awry? Assuming that you're doing all the right things — such as meeting deadlines, achieving your goals, communicating effectively, and being a strong team player — when things go wrong in your relationship with your boss, it may be your boss. Some symptoms may surface insidiously, so you may not recognize them right away. Some may be demonstrated just to a greater degree or with heightened intensity than you've seen before in your boss. Others may be brand new symptoms or behaviors in your boss. The key for you is to be aware at all times.

Micromanagement

A classic sign of a psycho boss is micromanagement. Whether it stems from the Peter Principle, the Imposter syndrome, or other causes of insecurity, ineffective bosses feel the need to have their hands in everything. They're unable to empower their team members to do their jobs, they lack trust that the team members will keep them adequately informed, and they're terrified of being caught off-guard or without every answer on the tip of their tongue. It isn't uncommon to find psycho bosses doing the work of everyone on the team along with their own work. One of

Nursing Management journal's 1,200 respondents to the 2000 annual salary survey stated, "My VP of Nursing is such a micromanager that we can't be autonomous." You may find a chief nurse executive mired in the minutiae of staffing plans for the patient care units or a leader spending hours at executive team meetings deliberating over the color of brochures to be distributed and whether to give out turkeys at Thanksgiving.

Most of these bosses are just trying to do a good job. What they fail to see is that micromanagement depletes team members of ambition and motivation. It causes them to feel incompetent and unvalued, and breeds frustration and contempt for the boss. If you start to feel micromanaged, talk with your boss about it. Ask, "Are you not getting the amount of information from me that you need?" State your expectations about having sufficient space to do your job, and clarify boundaries with your boss. She may not change, but at least you've started to put your concerns on the table.

Another approach comes from the author of "Messing with the boss' head,"[8] who suggests drowning micromanaging bosses in details, documents, and information until they back off. This approach may or may not work, but it might be worth a try!

Dysfunctional communication

Another sign of a psycho boss is dysfunctional communication, which may take any number of forms. A psycho boss typically acts pleasant and supportive to your face, but otherwise behind your back. For example, you may leave a meeting with your boss thinking that all is well, only to return to your office to find a scathing e-mail, voice mail, or memo about a topic that never came up during the meeting. At the root of such psycho behavior is the boss's inability to confront issues directly and to provide direct feedback. Psycho bosses often jump to conclusions, without ever seeking clarification or inquiring about the situation. They're notorious for not using inquiry skills, but rather being reactive and taking an "off with their heads" approach to management.

What should you do if you receive a psycho communication from your boss? Keep a copy for your files, and take the other copy to your boss and sit down calmly to discuss it. Do so immediately, but at a time when you can discuss the situation without emotion, or the psycho behavior may well escalate.

A common finding in psycho communications is lack of specificity. A psycho boss may use phrases such as "the team thinks" or "I've heard rumblings" or "everyone says that you do such and such." Your goal in the discussion is to clarify ambiguity and get details. Most often, the psycho boss won't have any—otherwise, she would have brought them to your attention directly. Without any details or specifics, you'll be unable to work on the issues being raised, and you must state that. You must also state your expectation that these issues be brought to you directly so that you can respond to them appropriately. Keep copies of all correspondence and document the discussion that you had about them.

Sending of others to do "dirty work"

Another common sign of a psycho boss is the sending of others to do their dirty work. Generally, psycho bosses create a small inner circle, the members of which have been brought up on their coattails to be the boss's confidantes, snoops, or "hatchet men or women." Sometimes the psycho boss sends others out so that later she can say that you're also having problems with the team. These folks may approach you with the same nebulous feedback that your boss does. They may make innuendoes at meetings about your performance or raise questions about your integrity or loyalty to the organization. Your approach must be the same as with the boss: direct, calm, unemotional, and seeking information and clarification. Ask for specifics, and don't become defensive or make it personal, even if the other person does so. Document these encounters as well. Disprove any false allegations through your professional conduct and competence without ever having to say a word in your own defense.

Sabotage

In the extreme, some psycho symptoms constitute sabotage, the third most common behavioral issue in women-dominated workplaces.[9] Sabotage is often the only method that the psycho boss can use to derail the employee who has done nothing wrong. The psycho boss may use lying, slander, and ethical breeches to sabotage the employee, or she may have one of the inner circle do so.

Many employees who work for a psycho boss use the term "passive-aggressive" to describe the boss's behaviors. They never know what to expect, sometimes being treated like the boss's best friend, other times getting the absolute cold shoulder and isolation treatment. The psycho boss often uses this method to keep an employee off-guard and to exert control in the relationship. She may change your job responsibilities for no good reason, or may remove you from a work group, all to keep you off-guard and to exert control.

Another method of exerting control is to withhold information necessary for the employee to make good decisions or to avert problems. Information is power, and the psycho boss will hold on to power at all cost. Psycho bosses may be late in their responses or not make decisions at all in an effort to ostracize the employee. Things may get lost on the boss's desk, messages may never get received, and deadlines may be unfortunately missed because the psycho boss needs to be in control and to let you know who is in charge. The psycho boss may "forget" to give the employee key information or to let the employee know of a deadline before the very last minute. The psycho boss may give a plum assignment to one of your peers, even though it was initially promised to you, because she must have "forgotten" the earlier promise. Such a memory of convenience and indecisiveness are most common with employees and support staff only. Psycho bosses usually put a much better foot forward for their own bosses.

Petty jealousy

Petty jealousy is another sign of a psycho boss, whether male or female. One male executive noticed that his extremely overweight boss developed psycho signs after the executive lost weight and started an exercise program. A female employee noticed psycho signs in her infertile boss after the birth of her child. A female, unmarried boss turned psycho with an employee after the employee returned from her honeymoon.

Whether the underlying cause of the boss's jealousy is appearance, wealth, national recognition, popularity, competence, or just that the employee is happy in general, the results are the same. A jealous boss can't look past the issue at hand, and everything becomes personal. Oftentimes a jealous boss will outright deny that the issue exists — for example, the overweight boss stated to the newly trim employee that she was glad the employee lost weight, but that she could do that too if she wanted to. That's a sign that the boss does have an issue and that she's making it personal, and that the employee needs to be on the lookout for jealous behaviors and comments.

Narcissism

Another classic sign of a psycho boss is narcissism. The traits of a narcissistic leader include being emotionally isolated, highly distrustful, preoccupied with himself, grandiose, self-involved, paranoid, driven to gain power and glory, need to be admired, not loved, and desire to leave behind a legacy.[10] (Think of Napoleon Bonaparte.) Although everyone possesses some degree of narcissism, when taken to the extreme, narcissistic leaders are impossible to work for and can bring the organization to its knees. Oftentimes, narcissistic leaders are charismatic, skillful orators, and visionary. The problem is that narcissistic leaders need adulation, don't listen, have major insecurity issues, are unimaginably thin skinned, and are relentless in their pursuit of victory. This is demonstrated in meetings with subordinates, in which the narcissist must dominate. They can be very abrasive with employees who doubt them or who are tough enough to fight back and to hold them accountable. Narcissistic leaders really want a group of yes-men. They are overly sensitive to criticism, and easily feel threatened or attacked, even by innocent questions. Narcissists create enemies where there are none. Oftentimes, the more independent-minded team members leave or are pushed out, so succession planning is a particular problem for narcissistic bosses. Narcissistic bosses lack empathy, find intimacy uncomfortable, typically have few regrets, and aren't restrained by conscience.

These traits make it difficult for narcissists to mentor or to be mentored. They want their protégés to be pale reflections of themselves, and are more interested in instructing than coaching. Evaluations don't help, because narcissistic bosses don't want to change and take little heed from feedback that they receive. (See *Dealing with narcissism.*)

QUESTIONS & ANSWERS

Dealing with narcissism

Question: *What is the best way to deal with a narcissistic boss?*

Answer: When dealing with a narcissistic boss, always empathize with the boss's feelings, but don't expect empathy back. Learn to get your strokes from other places. Don't expect her to boost your self-esteem, but praise her achievements and protect her image. You can't praise and flatter her shamelessly, or the narcissistic boss will see through that and will likely retaliate against you for blatantly seeking favor. Be careful in giving honest feedback to your boss or threatening her inflated self-image. This too may result in retaliation.

Give the boss ideas, but always let her take credit for them. Disagree only when you can demonstrate how she'll benefit from a different point of view. Hone your time management skills, because narcissistic leaders often give subordinates many more orders than they can possibly execute. They feel free to call you at any hour of the day or night. Make yourself available, or be prepared to change bosses. Be prepared to look for another job if your boss becomes too narcissistic to let you disagree with her. [11]

Dealing with toxic leadership

Many signs of toxic leadership are flagrant, whereas others sneak up on you. It's essential that you maintain close enough contact with your boss to assess how your relationship is faring. You must have face-to-face meetings with enough frequency to determine if your relationship is healthy or if adjustments are needed. There's a great risk in communicating mostly by e-mail, which is all too common today, because it's often difficult to read the inflection and get the true meaning behind it. In person, you can read body language, seek clarification, and get timely feedback. If your boss demonstrates psycho symptoms to any degree, your goal should be to get closer to her, not withdraw. If you become isolated from your boss, her symptoms will only become more severe as her insecurity and paranoia worsen.

Personal reactions to the psycho boss

How does it feel to work for a psycho boss? The symptoms tend to be the same, whether the employee is at the frontline or in an executive position. The first inkling of trouble is the employee's gut telling her that something is wrong. Red flags will go off when she interacts with the boss, and she'll have a jittery feeling in her stomach. Many symptoms are visceral, in response to being treated badly or unjustly. Many employees describe the inability to sleep as well as nightmares about the boss and her inner circle. Other physical responses include nausea, vomiting, diarrhea, headaches, and "knots in the stomach."

The employee may not be herself and family and friends may sense impatience, crankiness, and lashing out. Some employees, as they feel more hopeless and powerless, become isolated and withdrawn and retreat into themselves. The employee's confidence may be shaken, and she may start to second-guess her decisions and intuition. Fear and job insecurity may immobilize her, and the employee may feel unable to move past where she is. Some employees speak of feeling betrayed and emotionally depleted because of continual violations of trust. Employees are usually frustrated and most times can't put their finger on what went wrong or what they could have done differently.

Some employees develop extreme anger and hostility toward the boss, and describe the desire to bring the boss down, to go public with the issues, and to seek revenge. These feelings may lead to a lack of organizational loyalty and commitment on the part of the employee, and may well extend to other team members who witness the mistreatment and who begin to fear for their own job as long as the psycho boss stays in place. If left unchecked, these problems can lead to depression, both at the individual employee level and at the organizational level.

Organizational depression

Organizational depression can result from many factors, but when those in positions of power and influence misuse them, treat others poorly, and fail to role model true leadership and integrity, the organization is ripe for depression. Organizational depression is a pervasive attitude,[12] and just one psycho boss can start the negative cascade of hopelessness, impotence, confusion, frustration, denial, and malaise within an organization. Many labor actions and unionization efforts result from organizational depression, so it's important to identify and address the root cause of the problems—and that includes seeking out psycho bosses and dealing with them effectively.

Looking out for yourself

Once you identify signs of toxic leadership—whether you identify them in your boss or in yourself—you should take active steps to free your workplace of such leadership practices for the future.

COMMUNICATE, COMMUNICATE, COMMUNICATE! Start with communication. Clarify expectations and deadlines, and restate agreements and expectations—for example, "What I hear you saying is...."

Make sure face-to-face meetings are held regularly with your boss, and don't cancel them, even if you don't have a specific agenda item to discuss. Use the one-on-one time to check in and get ongoing feedback. If you aren't routinely getting feedback from your boss, ask for it.

DOCUMENT, DOCUMENT, DOCUMENT! Keep notes from all meetings with your boss. Put all deadlines in writing. Send an e-mail restating your understanding of agreements that were made at your meeting. Keep copies of all correspondence in a file, preferably at home. Seek feedback from others, and document it. Evaluate your boss, but recognize that a narcissistic boss won't value your feedback. Get feedback in writing, and make sure that examples of your performance—whether good or bad—are specific and detailed.

ENGAGE A THIRD PARTY IF NEEDED. Human resource personnel can be helpful, as can those who have been trained in mediation. Know up front that your request for a third party to participate in your meetings with your boss will probably push her over the edge. In general, psycho bosses aren't open to mediation and aren't honest enough during the meetings with the third party to really get to the issues and the truth.

FIND A SAFE HAVEN TO VENT YOUR FEELINGS AND FRUSTRATIONS. Know who your trusted colleagues are. It may not be safe for you to discuss these issues in your workplace at all. Seek advice and counsel from family, friends, clergy, counselors, or anyone else who will be able not only to listen and support you but also to give you career guidance.

SEEK LEGAL COUNSEL IF NEEDED. In some cases, psycho bosses cross the line by discriminating against employees, slandering or harassing employees, or breaching the ethical code of conduct. If your boss is guilty of any such action—and if you can prove it—you may be able to have her removed from her role, and you may win monetary damages as a result.

Before entering into any legal action, however, know that the organization will in most cases mount a significant defense on behalf of the boss. You don't want to be labeled as someone who sued her boss, unless there's no other recourse.

FIND EFFECTIVE AND HEALTHY OUTLETS FOR YOUR ENERGY AND FEELINGS. Exercising, eating well, and not overindulging in harmful substances (like drugs, alcohol, nicotine, and caffeine) are important ways to stay healthy and to prepare for fight or flight. You don't want to dim your senses while you're trying to determine your best course of action. You need to be in tune to your feelings so you can work through them and come out stronger in the long run.

ATTEND PROFESSIONAL DEVELOPMENT SEMINARS. Start thinking about the future, and your role in it. Reaffirm your leadership skills and competence if the psycho boss has placed any seeds of doubt in your mind about them. Attend classes or seminars that will cultivate skills that you can use in the future, in case you need to look for a new job. Use professional development seminars as a positive outlet and as a means to engage your mind in something other than the toxic leadership practices of your boss. Broaden your professional network, and make new contacts that may be able to help you down the road if needed.

KNOW WHAT YOU WANT. You won't be able to negotiate for it if you can't articulate it. If it's clear that your psycho boss isn't going anywhere, you may need to negotiate a change in job, department, or organization. If your relationship with the psycho boss has deteriorated to the point at which you can't have productive conversation, then you need to negotiate with her boss and use

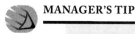

MANAGER'S TIP

The bottom line

Life is 10% what happens to you and 90% how you respond to it. Stay on the high road at all cost. Don't burn bridges with anyone at your workplace, including your psycho boss. Be professional and courteous in every encounter, and never "lower" yourself to your boss's level. Always rise above it. As much as you may want to slander and defame her, and put the organization through the wringer, don't. It will always come back to haunt you, and you don't want to be that kind of person or be known as that kind of employee. If you choose to leave the organization, you'll be able to walk out with your head held high and with your integrity intact.

human resources leadership to assist you. Depending on your role and the circumstances, you may be eligible for a severance package, or for some financial assistance or economic bridge to your next job. Most importantly, never sign anything or agree to anything on the spot. Take time for your family, counselor, or lawyer to review the information with you so that you're assured the best result possible.

KNOW YOUR BOTTOM LINE. One colleague worked for a boss who consistently breeched confidentiality, slandered other team members, and demonstrated most of the psycho boss signs described above. She realized that these breeches went against her core values and felt that if she continued to work for this boss, that she would be compromising her own personal and professional integrity. She chose to leave the department and work for someone else, and felt as if the weight of the world had been taken off of her shoulders. Therefore, you must know what your bottom line is and when it's being jeopardized and challenged. Then it's all about choices: No one is handcuffed to a job, and although most employees say that they "need a job," you don't need *that* job. You can find another job and hopefully find some sanity with it. (See *The bottom line.*)

Avoid talking about the details of your situation and the specifics of your departure, if you choose to leave. Negotiate the ability to craft an appropriate message about your departure, and try to make it positive and healthy. Those who know you will know the situation, and you'll find support and reassurance that you never knew existed as long as you stay on that high road. Leaving such a situation is difficult, so make sure you have people around you who can help you stay on the high road, and with whom you can let your true feelings show and let your hair down.

Finally, ask yourself what you would do if you weren't afraid. Then, turn your response into strategies to help you achieve that. After all, you may be clear about what you want but need to get past the fear of failure in order to make it happen.

Turning the negative into a positive

Many positive things can result from going through negative experiences with psycho bosses. You may now be able to explore opportunities that you would have never even looked twice at before these experiences. Your dealings with your boss may be just the push you needed to try new things and to branch out in new directions. Go back to school, go into consulting, change hospitals or health systems, change roles, work part-time, write more, spend more time with family. The possibilities are unlimited if you're open to them.

Most people go through life afraid of losing their job. Even if you aren't terminated and you leave by your own choice, you may still feel like you failed. Once you've experienced this challenge, you'll understand what it entails and you won't be afraid of it any more. Eleanor Roosevelt said it well: "Every time you meet a situation, though you think at the time it is an impossibility and you go through the tortures of the damned, once you have met it and lived through it, you find that forever after you are freer than you were before."

Facing reality

Although it's human to believe that your department or organization will disintegrate without you, the fact is most organizations can carry on "business as usual" in the face of even the most dramatic changes—and you must do the same. Get on with your life and start new relationships. Remember that you can't control what others say or what changes are made after you leave. You know the truth, and the truth will always prevail. Rest assured, your psycho boss most likely exhibited those questionable behaviors in other circles and at other levels in the organization, but her boss may not have been able to address the situation in time to save your job. Just remember that psycho bosses are usually found out and dealt with in time.

Also, be very careful with whom you share information. Keep in mind that it's best not to share the details of your circumstances with people at work, unless they work in Human Resources or the Legal Department. If your situation takes you to court, you have no idea who may be called upon to testify or to provide testimony on behalf of your boss. The less you've shared the details with coworkers, the better.

Undoubtedly, this situation will enable you to test out your life priorities and gain clarity about who you are and who you do or don't want to be. Going through personal or professional struggles can teach you a lot about what you're made of and how much you can endure. It also validates the values that you espouse and what you are or aren't willing to sacrifice in order to be true to those values. When faced with these choices, you'll quickly see just what caliber human being you are. The choice is always yours to make. Make the right one.

Being magnanimous

Don't seek revenge or be vindictive: It corrodes the spirit and is beneath you. If your boss gets fired soon after you leave, it's human to feel vindication, satisfaction, and happiness, but don't lower yourself in the eyes of others by gloating or finding pleasure in the toxic boss's loss. When you resist the opportunity to gloat and to be vindictive, it shows others just how wrong the toxic boss really was and keeps your professional and personal integrity intact in their eyes.

You realize how courageous you are, and you grow from the experience. You find strength and resolve that you might not have known that you have. Then comes the time for discernment; the time to see what comes next and what choice will be the most healthy and satisfying for you. Most people don't go through a day at work feeling courageous. Surviving the toxic boss syndrome can be an experience that tests you in many ways and reinforces the courage of your convictions. In going through such an experience and coming out on the other side, you realize the inner strength that you have and the support and resources that are available in your profession and in your life to deal with adversity in a positive and healthy way.

Lesson from a child

The most powerful lesson that I learned in researching change didn't come from a valued and trusted nurse colleague. Rather, it came from a child. One Sunday, on the way home from church, my husband and I were discussing the sermon that had been about forgiveness. I was in the middle of a professionally challenging time with a toxic boss and stated that I hoped that I would be able to forgive this boss one day for all that I was being put through.

From the backseat, my son Brian asked, "Mommy, are they being mean to you at work?"

My husband and I looked at each other, and I said, "No, honey. Sometimes grown-ups just don't treat each other as well as they should, and Mommy is trying to work all of this out right now."

Brian thought for a moment and then said, "Mommy, did you use your words and then walk away?" He was remembering what we had told him countless times before. If someone is bullying you or being mean, use words to describe how you feel and what you want. If the bully persists, then just walk away.

With emotion welling up, I turned to the backseat and said, "Yes, Brian, Mommy used her words, and now I'm going to walk away."

It suddenly had become crystal clear to me that it was time to make a change. I had talked until I was blue in the face. I had used all of the words that I could, to no avail. I had tried every strategy to deal with the situation at work, and nothing seemed to make it better. I had sought advice from wonderful colleagues and resources, and still had not been able to draw my own conclusion. I was afraid to make a change and to have others think that I had failed. It took a preschooler to make it all abundantly clear to me. The time had come to walk away, and that was what I was going to do.

I realized that if I couldn't look my young son in the eye and explain why I would tolerate such behavior and how I could let it interfere with my life and family, then I needed to do something different. I did, and it turned out to be the greatest gift of my career. It opened up worlds of possibility and professional opportunities that I had never considered before. It reinforced every value that I had and validated that I was marketable and would always land on my feet. Above all, it reminded me that work is work, and that it isn't the only thing in life. Yes, most of us need to work, but we don't need to subject ourselves to torture on a daily basis and compromise who we are and who we want to become. Going through this situation gave me great stories to tell to help others through it and also allowed me to walk my own talk with my son. If I wouldn't want him to be in a situation with a toxic boss, then I knew I shouldn't be either.

Let it go

Even the best nurse leaders can learn a lesson from Mother Teresa's writing. This is called "Anyway."

People are often unreasonable, illogical and self-centered; Forgive them anyway.

If you are kind, people may accuse you of selfish, ulterior motives; Be kind anyway.

If you are successful, you will win some false friends and some true enemies; Succeed anyway.

If you are honest and frank, people may cheat you; Be honest and frank anyway.

What you spend years building, someone could destroy overnight; Build anyway.

If you find serenity and happiness, they may be jealous. Be happy anyway.

Give the world the best you have, and it may never be enough. Give the world the best you've got anyway.

You see, in the final analysis, it is between you and God. It was never between you and them anyway.

Trust in a greater plan. You may never understand why bad things happen to good people, or why you must face some of the challenges in life that are placed in your path. Coming out on the positive side of this challenge restores faith and helps the survivor to find lessons in the journey. (See *Lesson from a child.*)

There isn't always an easy answer to explain why people act the way they do. The author of the book *Nasty People*[13] explained that usually people are mean for one of three reasons:

➤ to get their way
➤ because someone was nasty to them
➤ because they don't feel good about themselves.

For some toxic bosses, all of these factors may be in play; for others, just one. Understanding what's driving someone's behavior is the first step to dealing with it effectively. (See *Let it go.*)

Recognize that your commitment to your vision and your leadership values may be challenged every day by naysayers and cynics, by the unenlightened and the uninformed, who find it easier to criticize and belittle your efforts than to participate, support, and learn. True leaders stand above their critics. They have the courage to take the criticism, learn from it, and keep moving forward. Commitment to leadership values means taking small steps every day and learning how to respond to difficult and challenging situations, instead of reacting to them. Commitment means learning how to healthfully detach yourself from the emotion and chaos, so team members know they can count on you as a stabilizing force, even when they're dealing with a toxic boss themselves.

The challenges you face today force you to make important choices. Choices to be good people and good leaders. Choices that aren't based in fear. Choices that allow you to be true to yourself, maintain your integrity, and be effective in your roles. Continue to cultivate leadership excellence at all levels and make choices that eliminate the psycho boss syndrome. Create environments of care in which it's safe to challenge each other, disagree, shine brighter on a given day than the boss or a team member, and truly value the diversity that each employee brings and the unique contributions that each employee has to make. By giving this syndrome a name, you've already begun to resist the toxic boss and give voice to the backbone and life's blood of our organizations: the employees.

Employee relations and union vulnerability

Health care administrators typically whisper the word *union* in dark hallways or behind closed doors. They find themselves in the thick of trying to stave off unions, while the Norma Rae types of their hospitals bargain for better pay, better work environments and, above all, more respect. Although administrators prefer to work directly with employees to solve problems and to improve conditions, nationally, union activity in health care organizations is on the rise. Issues such as staffing, workplace safety, the environment of care, and inadequate leadership plague us and are driving many in our workforce to seek solutions from a third party. Other key issues of nursing's union movement include protesting layoffs and raising quality of work-life issues. Nurses want a voice in decisions that affect the patient care environment and their ability to deliver quality care. As they ponder the prospects of unionization, they fear for their jobs, worry about picket lines, and sicken at the thought of a strike.

Certainly, unionization has different meanings for employees than for managers. Most executives feel that union-free status gives them a competitive advantage. Regardless of the role you play in health care delivery, it's essential to cultivate a high degree of awareness regarding union vulnerability within your organization.

Nurse leaders play a pivotal role in assessing union vulnerability because they're closest to the staff, patients, and issues. However, just as important is an organization-wide assessment that crosses roles, service delivery units, and disciplines, because all health care professionals face the possibility of unionization these days, including physicians. Human resource professionals usually take the lead in assessing vulnerability. Most assessments cover two primary areas: organizational values and communication and the environment of care. It's been said that health care administrators and nurse leaders need to pay more attention to the "soft side" of the organization. The drivers of human capital — that is, those things that affect employees as human beings — are often linked to union vulnerability. Many of these drivers have been discussed throughout this chapter, such as trust, team building, conflict management, and coping with change. Each of these "people" issues plays a fundamental role in determining the likelihood that a nursing organization will unionize.

Is your organization vulnerable to unionization? As a nurse leader, which signs of union vulnerability should you look for? What role must you play in creating an environment of care and of professional excellence in which unions aren't perceived as necessary? (See *And the survey says...*, page 188.)

Union vulnerability is low when staff satisfaction and morale are high, so the better job that managers and executives do in knowing their staff, communicating with them, and solving problems together, the higher morale will be, the greater retention will be, and the less likely that staff will feel the need for a third party to represent their issues to the leadership team. Administrators must learn which things satisfy their staff and ensure that those things dominate the workplace. In many health care organizations, employee satisfaction surveys aren't done at all or with sufficient regularity to deduce meaningful, timely data to support change. Those who falsely assume that interviewing supervisors can determine the sentiment for unions among hourly employees may pay the price for that when the campaign begins. Asking the staff directly and regularly yields the best results. Creating a successful employee relation culture is essential not only to staving off a union but also to establishing the foundation and culture of employee excellence and organizational loyalty.

And the survey says...

Look at the findings from the following surveys, and see how your organization and staff compares.

Health Affairs Study of Nurses' Perception of Their Workplace and Care[14]

This 1998-1999 survey of 43,000 nurses in 700 hospitals in the United States, Canada, England, Scotland, and Germany revealed the following:

➤ More than 40% of nurses working in hospitals reported being dissatisfied, compared to 10% to 15 % of workers in general.

➤ Less than one-third of U.S. nurses felt that their management is responsive to their concerns. Linda Aiken stated that "this should be of great concern to the public" as an indicator of attention to patient needs. Nurses are really the voices of patients.

➤ Nearly 60% of U.S. nurses felt their salary was adequate. Nurses were more likely to be dissatisfied with working conditions than salary.

➤ Half of U.S. nurses cited verbal abuse from patients and families in the past year.

➤ One of every three U.S. nurses younger than age 30 planned to leave hospital work within a year.

ANA staffing survey[15]

This survey by the American Nurses Association garnered responses from 7,300 nurses. Of these, 70% worked in hospitals, 48% were staff nurses, 39% had over 21 years in nursing, 61% worked full time in nursing, and 66% were older than age 41. The survey revealed the following:

➤ 56% said their time available for patient care has decreased.

➤ 75% reported increased patient care load for registered nurses leading to a decrease in quality of patient care over the past 2 years.

➤ The majority described inadequate staffing, decreased registered nurse satisfaction, delays in providing basic care, and an increase in floating.

➤ The use of assistant personnel was a concern (and is often an organizing issue).

➤ Workplace violence and stress-related illnesses were perceived to be on the increase.

➤ Staff had no time for meals and breaks and felt increased pressure to accomplish their work.

➤ Respondents felt forced to work voluntary overtime.

➤ They left work exhausted, discouraged, and saddened that they couldn't provide for their patients.

➤ They felt powerless to affect change necessary for safe, quality, patient care.

➤ They were frightened for their patients.

➤ They described decreased support and reimbursement for continuing education activities.

➤ 42% of respondents wouldn't feel confident having a loved one cared for where they work.

➤ 55% wouldn't recommend nursing as a career for their children or friends.

➤ 23% would actively discourage those close to them from entering nursing.

The environment of care

A critical area in assessing union vulnerability is the environment of care. All health care leaders should strive to create patient care environments in which nurses can practice safely and professionally as they deliver high quality care to patients and families. Essential to staff satisfaction and retention is establishing a workplace in which collegiality is fostered and flexible work arrangements and schedules are the norm.

In a survey of nurses that asked "Should nurses unionize?" 66% of respondents either strongly agreed or agreed, and 34% disagreed or strongly disagreed.[16] Respondents who favored unions most likely faced one or several of the issues that detract from staff satisfaction and increase union vulnerability:

➤ inadequate staffing
➤ mandatory overtime
➤ floating
➤ abuse (verbal or physical)
➤ feelings of incompetence
➤ public humiliation
➤ sexual harassment
➤ being undervalued as a person
➤ feeling overloaded, overwhelmed, or unsupported
➤ unfair pay
➤ lack of attention or recognition
➤ deception
➤ leadership by fear and intimidation.

Many of these factors come from the all-too-common victim-controller paradigm and create environments of care in which nurses feel unsafe, unwelcome, unappreciated, and disrespected. These employees look up the organizational chart and can't identify anyone who they feel can effectively advocate for them. These environments breed militancy, anger, frustration, and hopelessness and increase union vulnerability.[17]

Only when nurse leaders exert their exceptional people skills and commit to team building, coaching, and all of the other strategies discussed in this chapter will the threat of unionization in nursing be diminished and will a culture of "we" be established.

The issues facing health care providers today—and, in particular, those affecting nurses—aren't going away in the near future. In fact, you can expect greater regulation, higher expectations from your health care consumers, and very real challenges presented by the workforce supply issues. The underlying cause of turnover is dissatisfaction with the job, the supervisor, or career prospects. It's these very same turnover indicators that go hand-in-hand with increased union vulnerability for your organization. These significant threats to employee satisfaction and to quality of care place every health care organization at risk for unionization.

Unionization in nursing often causes polarization when discussed. Nurses must be able to articulate who they are, what they want, and what difference they make for their organizations. They must do so in ways that bring all nurses together, not in ways that further divide us. What's more, nurse leaders must exert their considerable influence over the cultures, environments of care, and communication strategies in their health care organizations. When done well, the chasms between "us and them" and between "victim and controller" will close for good, and nursing will be able to solve our problems internally.[18]

Points to remember

The following points summarize the role of challenge for a manager:

➤ The nurse leader is challenged to inspire a thirst for change and innovation in team members as well as to nurture an ability to maximize the opportunities that change presents.
➤ The nurse leader should seek change rather than wait for it to be imposed.
➤ Micromanagement depletes team members of ambition and motivation and causes them to feel incompetent, unvalued, and frustrated. Successful leaders avoid this management style.
➤ Toxic leadership causes employees to develop anger and hostility toward the boss and lead to a decline in organizational

loyalty and commitment. Take active steps to free your workplace from such leadership practices.

➤ True leaders have the courage to take criticism, learn from it, and keep moving forward.

References

1. Peters, T. *Thriving on Chaos.* New York: Harper Collins Publishers, 1987.
2. Mercer, W.M. "Attracting and Retaining Registered Nurses: Survey Results." Chicago: William M. Mercer, 1999. *www.mercerHR.com.*
3. Pritchett, P. *The Employee Handbook of New Work Habits for the Next Millennium: 10 New Ground Rules for Job Success.* Dallas, Tex.: Pritchett & Associates, 1999.
4. Larson, C., and LaFasto, F. *TeamWork: What Must Go Right/What Can Go Wrong.* Newbury Park, Calif.: Sage Publications, Inc., 1989
5. Terry, D. "Effective Employee Relations in Reengineered Organizations," *Journal of Nursing Administration's Healthcare Law, Ethics, and Regulation* 1(3):33-40, September 1999.
6. Nightingale, F. *Notes on Nursing.* Philadelphia: J.B. Lippincott, 1859.
7. Babiak, P. "When Psychopaths Go to Work," *International Jou rnal of Applied Psychology* 44(2):171-88, 1995.
8. Vinzant, C. "Messing with the Boss' Head," *Fortune* 141(9):329-31, May 2000.
9. Briles, J. "Solving Sabotage and Betrayal in the New Millenium." Seminar. The Briles Group, Inc. Aurora, Col. *www.briles.com/programs.html.*
10. Maccoby, M. "Narcissistic Leaders: The Incredible Pros, the Inevitable Cons. *Harvard Business Review* 78(1):68-77, January-February 2000.
11. ibid.
12. Bilchik, G.S. "Organizational Depression," *H&HN: Hospitals and Health Networks* 74(2):34-36, 38, February 2000.
13. Carter, J. *Nasty People: How to Stop Being Hurt By Them Without Becoming One of Them.* Chicago: Contemporary Books, 1989.
14. "Study of Nurses' Perception of Their Workplace and Care," *Health Affairs,* May 7, 2001. *www.healthaffairs.org/archiveslibrary.htm.*
15. American Nurses Association. Analysis of American Nurses Association Staffing Survey. February 6, 2001. *www.nursingworld.org/survey/staffreport.pdf.*
16. "Should Nurses Unionize?" *Nursing2000* 30(6):52, June 2000. *www.springnet.com.*
17. Fitzpatrick, M. "Collective Bargaining: A Vulnerability Assessment," *Nursing Management* 32(2):40-42, February 2001.
18. Fitzpatrick, M. Op. cit.

CHAPTER 8

Creating balance

Melissa A. Fitzpatrick, RN, MSN, FAAN

> "A healthy attitude is contagious, but don't wait to catch it from others. Be a carrier." —Unknown

The new millennium has brought several challenges for the nursing profession as well as tremendous opportunities to solve some longstanding problems. Various factors play heavily in assessing strategies to maximize recruitment and retention of nursing professionals. The data are clear and will help to direct action. However, the incredible impact that "people" issues have on the ability to attract and retain nursing professionals can't be underestimated. Each of these issues — including trust, team building, conflict management, recognition, and others — has a significant impact on those already working in nursing and on those who may consider nursing as a career. Therefore, the better job that nurse leaders do resolving the "people" side of the industry, the better they'll do ensuring that they have enough nurses to meet the growing needs of the patients and families that they serve.

Recruitment and retention

When thinking about the issues at the heart of the nursing profession, consider the following statistics:

➤ Nursing remains the single largest professional group of health care providers in the United States.

Potential solutions to your nursing shortfall

A long-term, multifaceted approach is needed to retain and recruit nurses, including:
➤ encouraging associate degree nurses to continue their education
➤ offering loan forgiveness programs
➤ providing nursing scholarships and improved financial aid to nursing students
➤ advertising and promoting nursing through radio and newspapers
➤ educating youth about nursing careers through activities such as nursing camps and "shadow" days for high school students, scout troop activities, and career days at elementary schools
➤ targeting underrepresented and nontraditional groups for nursing, specifically males, minority students, and faculty.

➤ Employment for registered nurses will grow faster than the average for all U.S. occupations through 2008.
➤ In the past 5 years, the average age of registered nurses increased from age 42.4 to 44.
➤ The average registered nurse age will peak at age 45.4 in 2010, then slowly decline.
➤ Registered nurses in their forties outnumber registered nurses in their twenties four to one.
➤ Nurses younger than age 24 have the highest turnover and many leave the profession altogether.[1]

The aging nursing workforce and increased competition for qualified registered nurses have compounded the problems of recruitment and retention. Chief causes of the nursing shortfall include expanded career opportunities for women and a lingering belief that nursing isn't a secure job, a hangover from previous reports of hospital cost cutting and registered nurse layoffs. As a result, this nursing shortage is deeper than past shortages and more resistant to short-term fixes, such as sign-on bonuses, international recruitment, cross-training programs, lawn service, maid service, dry cleaning, auto care, and shoe repair, among others. (See *Potential solutions to your nursing shortfall*.)

The nursing shortage places increased pressure on the profession to address society's needs. The tremendous societal implications of this shortage tug at the heart of nursing. If society loses confidence in the nursing profession, it will lose all confidence in the health care system. However, several initiatives are underway to boost public awareness of nursing contributions to the well-being of society. Nursing is more vocal and unrelenting in its efforts to positively influence inpatient work environments, create effective workforce planning models, and enhance the public's grasp of the importance of professional nursing to society's health outcomes.[2] A significant legislative effort has been mounted, and substantive legislation has been passed to address some of the major dissatisfactions in the profession. More focus in the legislative arena is necessary to gain momentum and to address nursing's issues for the long haul.

A major thrust of the profession in ensuring the next generation of nurses and nurse leaders is to provide leadership development, mentoring, ongoing education, and support for nurse-managers in order to enhance retention.[3] Supporting frontline nurse leaders in their efforts to ensure patient and staff satisfaction, manage the bottom line, and foster an environment in which healing can occur is paramount to our long-term success. Without effective leadership at the frontlines of patient care, nurses will never feel the support and encouragement needed to continue to do this demanding work every day. Nurturing the kind of nurse leaders who tend to the people who provide the care is as important as tending to those receiving the care. If nurse leaders don't support the care providers, there will be no care delivery systems.

Compensation issues

Compensation undoubtedly plays a role in nursing recruitment and retention. Over the past several years, nursing salaries have increased, and certainly base compensation must be constantly assessed to ensure that the profession is keeping pace with the market. However, most nurses are more likely to leave the profession over satisfaction issues — such as flexible schedules, respect, collaboration, autonomy, and leadership support — than they are over base compensation.

Market issues and the shortage make it relatively easy for nurses who are unhappy in one organization to find work in another. Although market demand makes it easier for employees to find a new job, it generally doesn't make them unhappy enough to start looking. In today's market, nurses are less likely to jump from hospital to hospital for a dollar an hour raise as they might have been in the past. That being said, an emphasis of nurse leaders on some of the intangible aspects of recruitment and retention is paramount. As one nurse-manager who fully understands this said, "I no longer take care of patients. I take care of nurses." This philosophy and approach is one that goes a long way to providing the support and stability that nurses need to keep them satisfied and in the profession.

Retention issues

Retention of experienced nurses will continue to be a dominant concern, and nurse leaders will reverse the flight of nursing talent by focusing their attention on frontline retention. Nurse leaders are using various methods to slow the exodus of nurses from health care organizations and from the nursing profession. Some methods have proven more effective than others in addressing nurse recruitment and retention over the long haul. Providing nurses with dry cleaning, lawn care, and car care might make nurse leaders feel as though they're making progress on the retention curve, but are these incentives addressing the root cause of the problems, or are they merely temporary fixes?

The slippery slope of sign-on bonuses and spa incentives is one that may entice nurses to an organization and keep some for the short-term. These approaches don't, however, satisfy over time. Nurse leaders know this in their hearts, yet many are out of innovative solutions to address the recruitment and retention problem. One facility is giving up to $6,000 bonuses to nurses who stay employed for 3 years. Do these organizational leaders really believe that nurses will stay that long when faced by the daily realities of short staffing, workplace violence, and mandatory overtime? Three years may seem like a small price to pay for such a bonus, but for those living at the frontlines of direct patient care every day, 3 years may be an impossible eternity to endure. Applying those bonus dollars to solve issues in the care environment and to provide true support to nurses in ways that they deem meaningful would be far more effective.

Successful leaders pay daily attention to strategies that help them to keep their top talent,[4] making sure to focus on the factors that significantly impact retention. They use some of the highest rated tactics to decrease turnover and enhance satisfaction, such as new clinical advancement programs, enhanced continuing education, flexible scheduling and shifts, and enhance-

MANAGER'S TIP

A success story

At Delnor-Community Hospital in Geneva, Illinois, they're rerecruiting their best employees, knowing that satisfied employees provide better patient care.[5] They overtly reward, recognize, and praise team members. Patient praise brings a mini-celebration at the nursing station, with public recognition. Management sends out thank you notes. Employees recognize each other with "Best of the Best" awards ($5 gift certificates; 300 per month awarded).

The goal is to nurture, cherish, and promote customer service and enthusiasm for work. Each employee received a bonus last year when the margin was made. The excitement at the hospital is palpable, and employees want to work there. The result: Nursing turnover dropped from 17% to 10%, and patient satisfaction scores are up.

So remember, many of the best recruitment and retention plans aren't expensive and don't require laborious strategic plans to bring them to fruition. It all comes back to establishing a culture in which effort is appreciated and rewarded and in which commitment to values is supported.

ments to supplemental pay plans such as shift differentials.[6] They tend to the critical issues that are common front-runners of unionization, such as reassignment, work hours, and longevity recognition. To many, a pleasant work environment means as much as the pay. Employees want lifestyle benefits and flexible work schedules. Employees want to feel connected to the place at which they work and to have an employer who knows them, respects them, and understands their concerns.[7]

Leading the market

Have you developed a reputation as a market leader so that your employees will see moving to a competitor as a step down? Have you figured out how to find and keep good help in a tight labor market? How well do you communicate the benefits of working at your facility, including the monetary and nonmonetary rewards? Have you asked your team members what the most important recruitment and retention variables are to them, and do you have concrete plans articulated to address them? Are you data driven in your recruitment and retention efforts? Do you have an accurate baseline of data regarding turnover rates; exit interview data; retention data by unit, department, and manager;

and data providing a competitive analysis with other organizations? Without data, it's difficult to assess when progress is being made and what the cause and effect relationship between changes that you've implemented and their impact on improvement in the recruitment and retention arenas is. Using data to drive decisions helps nurse leaders to resist knee-jerk reactions and the slippery slope of some incentive and bonus plans.

Energized environments of care do exist, and there are many recruitment and retention success stories from which you can learn. (See *A success story*.)

Karlene Kerfoot, a renowned nurse leader, describes management as a sacred trust and a privilege. She encourages nurse leaders to have a vision of what's possible and to be guides, healers, and trust builders. Nurse leaders must celebrate their achievements and demonstrate their compassion by creating sanctuaries of healing and caring for patients and for each other. They must put their best efforts to preserving humanity and sanity at work by growing their souls at work and outside of work. Nurse leaders must mentor others to develop those who can move the human heart, not just count money.

Some believe that management is taught but that leadership is learned through experience. Nurse leaders must continue to cultivate positive experiences for their protégés and to create approaches to recruitment and retention that tend to the full array of issues, those on the money side of the equation and those on the people side, too. When effective, the results will be positive for nurses and for patients, because improving staff satisfaction improves patient satisfaction. What's more, nurse leaders will make the greatest strides in the recruitment and retention of nurses when they achieve the caring bottom line and focus on the heart of nursing: people.

Achieving and fostering balance

Each day, the demands on nurse leaders grow. Personnel shortages, leadership turnover, higher patient acuity, and increasing regulation require more time, energy, and focus. More than ever, the nursing profession needs nurse leaders who lead balanced lives, generate energy, conserve energy, and channel energy.

The most effective nurse leaders lead balanced lives and encourage their employees to do the same. They make the commitment to start less and to finish more. They flex their "no muscle" and say no, especially to themselves. In being open to new ideas, the best nurse leaders are able to break bad habits and to handle themselves with care. They focus not on keeping busy, but on getting results.

Nurse leaders who understand balance seek simplicity and have figured out how to stop cluttering their lives with things that don't matter and to set limits. They create a pleasant work environment and one that's comfortable in which to work. It's difficult to think clearly when surrounded by clutter. What's more, a cluttered environment is neither inviting nor welcoming to others on the team. So, take time to clear out your workspace and you'll feel an immediate clearing of your mind. Then, the trick is to keep the area uncluttered and comfortable to enhance your productivity every day and to create a warm, welcoming, and safe zone for your team.

In today's turbulent health care workplace, nurse leaders must take care of the caregivers. Supporting one another is more important today than ever before because work and life are more complex. Most nurse leaders wear many hats every day:

➤ parent
➤ significant other
➤ nurse leader
➤ sibling
➤ child
➤ neighbor
➤ parent-teacher association member
➤ church member
➤ caregiver
➤ student
➤ professional association member.

Even pets and plants demand time and attention. Recognizing the conflict between work and personal life for team members and working with them to resolve this conflict is one of the greatest gifts you can give them.

Most people only think about balancing their lives when they hit rock bottom or face a crisis. Don't wait until your heart attack to eat right and exercise. Don't wait until your spouse walks out

QUESTIONS & ANSWERS

The key to balance

Question: *What is the key to maintaining balance in my life?*
Answer: To maintain balance, you must do something energizing with enough frequency to keep your mind, body, and relationships healthy. Everyone has a passion that brought happiness and respite long ago, but nobody can find the time anymore.

Find the time. What's your passion? Reconnect with it. Take time out for self-discovery and find out what works best to help you rest, relax, play, and stay healthy. And when you define what that thing is that brings you joy, make it part of your daily routine. Schedule it and regard it as important as the time you spend with your team and your patients. It's the only way you can continue giving to your team members and family and maintain a high level of commitment and energy for your work.

the door to have a relationship with your family. Continuous renewal, constant retreat, and recurrent time-out are critical. John O'Neil, author of *The Paradox of Success* and president of the California School of Professional Psychology says, "We live our lives so tightly wound, our souls can't breathe. To retreat is to let our souls breathe."[8] Nurse leaders who lead balanced lives take time for themselves and their team members to refresh their minds, recharge their spirits and, as a result, become more effective. They recognize that all work is relational and that nurturing and sustaining relationships between themselves and their work, themselves and their boss, and themselves and themselves is the key to health and success.[9] (See *The key to balance.*)

The nursing profession needs you for the long haul. You can't have empathy and energy for others unless your own reservoir is filled and unless you take time out to replenish and rejuvenate yourself. On empty? Recharge, fill up your tank, and keep your eye on that gauge! Your body, mind, family, and team need you.

Once you've achieved balance, you'll never want to go back to the way things used to be. Then you can help others to achieve health and balance in their lives and spread a renewed energy and commitment to the work at hand. People caring for people is what nursing is all about. Tending to your own need for balance is the first step in tending to the "people" needs of those you serve.

Points to remember

The following points summarize the importance of support in nursing practice:

➤ Supporting frontline nurse leaders is paramount to the long-term success of the nursing profession.
➤ Nurse leaders provide support and stability to nurses in their care to keep them satisfied and active in their profession.
➤ The most effective nurse leaders lead balanced lives and encourage their employees to do the same.

References

1. U.S. Bureau of Labor and Statistics. 2000. And "AON...Insure Your Vision." *Healthcare at Work 2000: Creating a Reason to Stay.* Chicago: AON consulting, 2000.
2. The Kiplinger Washington Editors, Inc. "What's Ahead for 2001 and What You Can Do About It." Washington, D.C.: (Suppl) The Kiplinger Letter, 2000. *www.kiplinger.com.*
3. U.S. Bureau of Labor and Statistics. 2000. And "AON...Insure Your Vision." *Healthcare at Work 2000: Creating a Reason to Stay.* Chicago: AON consulting, 2000.
4. The Nursing Executive Center Nursing Watch Issue #5. "Investing in a Pivotal Role: Strategies for Nurse Manager Skill Enhancement. Washington, D.C.: The Advisory Board Company, 1999, 1-15.
5. Dow, R., and Cook, S. *Turned On: Eight Vital Insights to Energize Your People, Customers, and Profits.* New York: HarperBusiness, 1996.
6. The Nursing Executive Center Annual Membership Meeting. "Reversing the Flight of Talent: Nursing Retention in an Era of Gathering Shortage." Washington, D.C.: The Advisory Board Company, 1999, 1-165.
7. Mercer, W.M. "Attracting and Retaining Registered Nurses: Survey Results." Chicago: William M. Mercer, 1999. *www.mercerHR.com.*
8. O'Neil, J.R. *Paradox of Success: When Winning at Work Means Losing at Life: A Book of Renewal for Leaders.* New York: G.P. Putnam, 1993.
9. Pritchett, P. *The Employee Handbook of New Work Habits for the Next Millennium: 10 New Ground Rules for Job Success.* Dallas, Tex.: Pritchett & Associates, 1999.

PART THREE

*B*udgeting and finance skills

CHAPTER 9

Staffing for inpatient care

Pamela S. Hunt, RN, MSN

> "It is as impossible in a book to teach a person in charge of sick how to manage as it is to teach her how to nurse. But it is possible to press upon her to think for herself." — Florence Nightingale

You'll soon be fluent in what may seem like a foreign language — *finance*. And finance begins with budgeting. Have you ever wondered why you should bother budgeting? Even though your departmental budget is likely an educated guess, the primary purpose of budgeting in your facility isn't unlike the purpose of budgeting in your own life. Both budgets serve as a method to plan for services that you want to provide or purchase, to manage ongoing expenses, and to control spending.

The planning phase is to ensure that your resources are being used to meet the strategic plans of the facility — or, in the case of your personal budget, the goals for your household. Planning forces you to look at future services and the direction health care is moving to make educated and sound business decisions. For example, in your personal budget, you must compare your income to your expenses to determine and prioritize how much you can afford to spend on other things. In your facility's budget, you must include information that enables you to predict incoming revenue and evaluate your health care environment to help you plan where to best allocate those dollars.

The second function of the budget involves management of ongoing activities. This includes comparing the actual spending to the budgeted amounts and making adjustments accordingly.

Reports are generated that compare what was budgeted for staffing and operational supplies in comparison to what was actually spent. Nurse leaders must receive this information in a timely manner so they can justify any variance between the two and make necessary adjustments.

The final function of the budget is to control spending. When you've predicted what revenue you'll be generating and how you'll spend it — and you've compared what was spent with how much was predicted — then you must use that information to control excessive spending or to justify additional services and spending during the year.

In terms of your department budget, say volume and revenue are up due to a strong marketing program and strong contract negotiations by materials management. The department's actual revenue is way ahead of the budgeted amount. Now is the time to use this information to justify the upgrade on your monitoring equipment that you've been wanting to do but didn't feel you had the additional dollars to justify.

Remember, the department budget should always be consistent with your facility's mission and should always consider the services your department provides now and what it may provide in the future. With thorough strategic planning, management of ongoing expenses, and control of spending, you can position your department and the entire facility to be the competitive leader in the market, providing the right services and the revenue to maintain those services.

Another very important factor to keep in mind is the facility's accountability to the governing board. An accurate budget reflects management's ability to plan and budget appropriately. It also provides the governing board with a tool to measure management's performance compared to the plan and reflects management's plan to adhere to the board's policies.

The staffing budget

Staffing has been and always will be one of the greatest challenges for nursing management. Not only is it a challenge to find qualified people to fill positions; it's difficult to communicate and prove to the finance department how many people it actually

The staffing challenge

Staffing has many facets, including:
➤ determining the number of staff members needed
➤ obtaining the appropriate skill mix
➤ providing coverage for the number of hours and days per week that the department is open
➤ determining the impact of nonproductive benefit time.
   Using a step-by-step approach, you can build a staffing plan that includes all the variables necessary to ensure adequate staffing coverage and, therefore, effective patient care.

takes to staff a nursing department to provide safe, patient-oriented care. (See *The staffing challenge.*)

About 15 years ago, requests for additional staff were usually granted with little discussion. A new job posting would go up, but no numbers or statistics were used to justify the request.

Today, however, the nursing environment operates differently. No longer can nurse leaders justify how much staff or additional staffing they need with broad statements. Instead, they must come to the table with specific data, based on statistics that are understood and have validity with the finance department, to justify the numbers they're requesting.

The discussion and examples in this chapter are for traditional inpatient nursing units. Following chapters cover outpatient and surgical departments.

Calculating full-time equivalents

Most staffing plans are built using the full-time equivalents (FTEs) needed for each unit. An FTE is one or more persons who work a total of 40 hours per week or 80 hours per 2-week pay period. One FTE equals 2,080 hours/year of work, provided that they take no vacation or holiday. To calculate what percentage of an FTE each staff member in your department is consuming, you'd divide the hours/day that the person works, multiply the number of days worked per week, and divide that number by 40 hours/week.

Although an employee may be receiving full-time benefits, she may not be consuming a full FTE of your staffing budget. For example, an employee who works 8 hours/day, 3 days/week,

Calculating FTEs

Use the following method to calculate the appropriate percentage of time that your employees work, to obtain accurate full-time equivalents (FTEs) for your nursing unit.

To calculate the percentage of an FTE that each staff member in your department fills, divide the hours per day that the person works, multiply the number of days worked per week, and divide that number by 40 hours/week.

Examples

$$\frac{8 \text{ hours/day} \times 3 \text{ days/week}}{40 \text{ hours (FTE)}} = \frac{24 \text{ hours/week}}{40 \text{ hours (FTE)}} = 0.6 \text{ FTE}$$

$$\frac{12 \text{ hours/day} \times 3 \text{ days/week}}{40 \text{ hours (FTE)}} = \frac{36 \text{ hours/week}}{40 \text{ hours (FTE)}} = 0.9 \text{ FTE}$$

works 24 hours/week. Divide 24 hours/week by 40 hours, which is an FTE's weekly workload, and you arrive at the fact that this person is consuming 0.6 FTE of your staffing plan. However, an employee who works that same 3 days/week but instead of 8 hours/day works 12 hours/day is most likely receiving full-time benefits but is actually only working 36 hours/week. Using the same formula, 36 hours divided by 40 hours/FTE means that this individual is consuming 0.9 FTE of your staffing plan. (See *Calculating FTEs.*)

You can easily see that if you had just 10 employees in one department who worked 12 hours/day, 3 days/week and you counted them as 1 FTE instead of 0.9 FTE, you would actually be shorting yourself 1 FTE, or 80 hours every 2 weeks. It's important to separate the percentage of FTE each person in your department is consuming from the amount of human resource benefit that they're receiving. When predicting staffing plans for unit coverage, focus only on the amount of time you can count on these individuals to be on the unit, providing patient care and services.

How many staff do you need to adequately cover your department for the number of days you're open and the number of hours per day you need coverage, giving consideration for nonproductive time such as vacations, sick leave, and holidays?

After understanding how finance calculates an FTE, the director of the department must go through several steps to logically predict how many FTEs are needed to adequately staff the department, based on average daily need, allowing for vacation and sick time coverage. The next section takes you through specific steps to come up with the number of FTEs needed, in a logical format that finance can understand.

Step 1: Determine average daily need

For inpatient units, average daily need is usually determined by the average daily census and nursing hours per patient day (NHPPD). The average daily census is driven off of the midnight census. NHPPD should include everyone who's charged to your staffing budget or whose hours show up on your department financial report, which may include professional and nonprofessional staff. For example, some facilities have employees in ancillary services (such as housekeeping, respiratory therapy, and food service) reporting to a nursing unit and included in that unit's budget. If this is the case, then the NHPPD for that unit should include those employees. However if those same employees work on your unit but don't come out of your budget, then you shouldn't include them in your NHPPD. (See *Determining NHPPD.*)

Benchmark data that give best practice or most productive number for NHPPD are available. When using benchmark data, just make sure you're comparing the same skill levels, the same job classifications, and the same region of the country. Patient care is typically driven by the expectations of the patients and their physicians. Therefore, comparing NHPPD in the midwest to NHPPD on the east or west coast may not be a realistic comparison. Likewise, comparing a nursing unit that includes ancillary services in its budget with a unit that doesn't would definitely skew the comparison. Both departments may be equally as productive, but the reported NHPPD would be different.

So how do you use benchmark data? Obtain data from a region and environment similar to yours. Next, make sure comparable job classifications are used in reporting NHPPD. Then, if the benchmark data are considered "best practice," use the data as a target to bring your unit's NHPPD closer to this number.

Although acuity of patients may vary significantly between specialty units, the acuity of patients on any one unit varies little. The type of patients cared for on a specific nursing unit can be justification for a higher or lower NHPPD. For example, a step-down neurologic unit would be expected to have a higher NHPPD than

Determining NHPPD

Question: *How do you determine your unit's nursing hours per patient day (NHPPD)?*

Answer: If your finance department doesn't have this information readily available, try doing a retrospective record of your unit's current activity. For a 31-day period, keep track of how many licensed and nonlicensed employees are needed in a 24-hour period.

NHPPD			**Unit:** 2 East **Month:** August
Number of FTEs			
Day	**Licensed**	**Nonlicensed**	**Total hours**
1	8.0	8.0	128
2	7.0	5.0	96
3	6.0	5.0	88
31	9.0	6.0	120
Averages	8.6	6.5	121/average daily census

Multiply the total number of employees by the number of hours per day that they work, then divide that number by the midnight census for that day. This gives you the NHPPD. This number may or may not please you and your finance department, but it's a place to start when determining where you are and where you want to be.

a short-stay, surgical unit. What does all this mean for nursing leaders? Establish the NHPPD based on the work demands and patient needs of the patients on each unit. When this is established, then the demand for staffing is based on patient census. If you're consistently feeling that the staffing plan isn't meeting the needs of the patient population, then you should evaluate the NHPPD and the patient population acuity that was considered when the staffing plan was developed. Most nursing leaders today find that they need to consider patient acuity when developing a staffing plan; however, daily assessment of acuity is no longer necessary because of the overall stability from day to day within the department. After department acuity is assessed and NHPPD developed, unit census becomes the driving force for staffing need.

In the examples in this chapter, the inpatient medical-surgical unit has an NHPPD of 8.5 and an average daily census of 20. Therefore, 20 × 8.5 produces a 24-hour staffing need of 170 hours. (See *Calculating daily staffing needs*, page 208.)

Calculating daily staffing needs

This example illustrates how to compute full-time equivalents for an inpatient medical-surgical unit with an average daily census (ADC) of 20 and nursing hours per patient day (NHPPD) of 8.5.

$$ADC \times NHPPD = 24\text{-hour needs}$$
$$20 \times 8.5 = 170 \text{ nursing hours per 24-hour period needed.}$$

Step 2: Calculate productive hours

When you've determined your 24-hour need for clinical staffing, you need to divide that number by the number of productive hours per shift. (See *Differentiating productive and nonproductive hours.*) The best assumption is that the staff are productive for the number of hours they're scheduled minus the time allowed for paid breaks. If your staff works 8 hour-shifts, they would be totally productive if they worked 7.5 hours; if they work 10-hour shifts, 9.5 hours. The half an hour taken out of each shift accounts for paid breaks in the workday. The lunch break isn't taken out because it's nonpaid time. Using the example of the medical-surgical unit given, the 170 hours needed to staff this inpatient unit for 24 hours/day divided by 7.5 productive hours for an 8-hour shift results in 22.6 FTEs needed. If staffing this unit with a 12-hour staffing pattern, you'd need 14.8 FTEs (170/11.5) (See *Computing productive hours,* page 210.)

Step 3: Allocate FTEs to shifts by skill mix

Skill mix has been debated and discussed for years. California has current legislation that now dictates minimum staffing requirements, including skill mix.[1] Although health care cuts have forced nurses to use all skills to the best of their abilities, every director should pay close attention to skill mix and quality in their facility. Nursing research has documented proof that as the percentage of registered nurses increases, the number of undesirable outcomes decreases. Undesirable outcomes include falls, medication errors, infection rates, patient and family complaints, and death.[2] With that said, you must now take the number of FTEs that your unit needs on a daily basis and divide them into

Differentiating productive and nonproductive hours

Productive hours are hours worked at the bedside or in the department. These hours include regular hours, overtime hours, hours worked when called in, and emergency called-in hours. They don't include hours paid for being on call but not working.

Nonproductive hours are hours that are included in the 2,080 hours that a full-time equivalent is counted upon but hours that aren't worked in the department. They include vacation, sick, holiday, funeral, jury duty, and education time and other benefits that your organization gives to employees that allow them to be away from the department.

the number it needs on each shift and the job classification needed for the patient population that the unit services.

Determining shift percentages should be based on the work distribution on the unit. A high-acuity unit, such as a critical care unit, is more likely to have a flatter, or more equal, need for staff numbers on each shift. In such a unit, the nursing care required for these patients is consistently high and doesn't vary greatly among days, evenings, and nights. For this medical-surgical unit example, 45% of the total need is allocated to days, 35% to evenings, and 20% to nights, assuming that most physician activity and the two patient meals occur on days and that both days and evenings share the brunt of admissions, discharges, and transfers. Although some facilities have similar practices, many don't. Therefore, making informed, intelligent decisions based on the specific practices, processes, and procedures of your unit—and not using a standard benchmark norm—is imperative to the success of your staffing plan. (See *Dividing skill mix,* page 211.)

The next step is to take the calculated numbers and create a staffing plan using whole numbers of people and not partial numbers. At this point, decisions have to be made based on what you know about your unit. What types of patients do you care for and what is the workload for these patients? Depending on those considerations, you'll either round the numbers in the example up or down. When making these decisions, you need to stay close to the total number of FTEs (22.6) so that you don't create an overbudget staffing plan. Using the numbers in this example, develop a staffing plan that includes 24-hour coverage and outlines the skill mix needed to adequately care for the patient population on your unit.

Computing productive hours

Use this formula to calculate productive hours per 24-hour needs:

Step 1: If your employees work 8-hour shifts, they would be totally productive if they worked 7.5 hours; if they work 10-hour shifts, 9.5 hours; and so on.

Step 2: 24-hour needs/productive hours per shift

8-hour shifts: 170/7.5 = 22.6

OR

12-hour shifts: 170/11.5 = 14.8

Step 4: Consider the number of days to staff

Did you think you were done? 22.6 FTEs would be enough staff if this department were open 5 days/week and closed on weekends and all holidays. Unfortunately, that isn't the case in most inpatient facilities. Therefore, step 4 considers the number of days that you need to provide this staffing level on the unit. The formula is as follows:

$$\frac{\text{for each 1 FTE needed, multiply by the number of days you need to staff}}{\text{number of days the FTE works/week}} = \frac{\text{factor to account for}}{\text{additional days to staff}}$$

Because this medical-surgical unit is open 7 days/week and functions on 8-hour shifts, the first example below is the equation you would use to calculate what impact covering the schedule 7 days/week would have on each job class needed. For every FTE needed in your proposed staffing plan, you need that FTE 7 days/week to staff this inpatient department. An FTE who works 8 hours/day works 5 days/week; therefore, for every one FTE needed, multiply by 1.4 to arrive at a number in the staffing plan that allows you enough FTEs to accommodate the 7-days/week staffing need. Look at the example below for 8-hour shifts, 7 days/week:

$$\frac{1 \text{ FTE} \times 7 \text{ days to staff}}{5 \text{ days/week worked}} = \text{factor of } 1.4$$

In this example unit, for every one FTE needed on the staffing plan, multiply that FTE by 1.4 to cover the schedule

Dividing skill mix

Allocate full-time equivalents (FTEs) to shifts by skill mix in the following way. In the example given, you'll note the skill levels across the top. The one FTE unit-director position in the example is spread out over all three shifts. Why include the director position in your staffing plan, but spread the FTE equally over all shifts in the department? Sharing the director FTE among the shifts is necessary so that the clinical day shift allotted FTEs aren't adversely affected, which they would be if the director's FTE were included in the clinical day shift staffing. Also, the director's work should support the work necessary to all three shifts. The example shows the number of FTEs needed (23.2) divided into skill mix and shifts.

	Percentage	Dir	RN	LPN	NA	UC
D	45%	0.33	3.9	2.9	1.9	1.0
E	35%	0.33	3.0	2.9	1.5	0.8
N	20%	0.33	2.2	1.3	0.8	
Totals	100%	1.0	9.1	7.1	4.2	1.8

Key: D-day, E-evening, N-night, Dir-director, RN-registered nurse, LPN-licensed practical nurse, NA-nurse's aide, UC-unit clerk

7 days/week. This is a critical step to adequate staffing coverage, so let's take another example to again illustrate the point of 7 days/week coverage.

Using the popular 12-hour staffing pattern would make a big difference in the factor needed to determine 7 days/week coverage. Here again, for every one FTE needed on the staffing plan, you need that FTE 7 days/week. However, the 12-hour FTE works only 3 days/week. Therefore, you would divide the formula by 3 days/week instead of 5 days/week, which results in a much higher factor of 2.3. Look at the example below for 12-hour shifts, 7 days/week:

$$\frac{1 \text{ FTE} \times 7 \text{ days to staff}}{3 \text{ days/week worked}} = \text{factor of } 2.3$$

When you're developing a staffing plan, you must multiply each skill mix by the appropriate factor (1.4 for 8-hour shifts, in these examples) to provide adequate coverage for 7 days/week on all three shifts. This brings the total FTE needed to staff this until to 31.8. (See *Developing a staffing plan*, page 212.)

Developing a staffing plan

This staffing plan includes 24-hour coverage and outlines the skill mix needed to adequately care for the patient population on this unit.

	Percentage	Dir	RN	LPN	NA	UC
D	45%	0.33	4	23	2	1
E	35%	0.33	3	2	1	1
N	20%	0.33	2	2	1	2
Totals	100%	1.0	9	7	4	4

Key: D-day, E-evening, N-night, Dir-director, RN- registered nurse, LPN- licensed practical nurse, NA-nurse's aide, UC-unit clerk

You'll notice in *Developing the staffing plan* that the director position is only included in the day shift because it doesn't affect the percentage of clinical staff per shift. Also, the director position isn't multiplied by the 7 days/week coverage factor. Why? Although you probably feel like you work 7 days/week, someone else probably doesn't do your work when you aren't in the office on the weekends. Similarly, when you're in the office on the weekends, you probably aren't getting paid extra dollars for that extra time. Therefore, the director position isn't multiplied by the 1.4 factor and for simplification is included in the day-shift position only. (See *Staffing for the 7-day week.*)

Step 5: Account for productive and nonproductive hours

Accounting for productive and nonproductive hours in your staffing plan can allow staff who have accrued vacation hours to actually take a vacation. Accounting for nonproductive hours also means that the staff who aren't on vacation and are left behind aren't overworking themselves to compensate for vacationing employees. Both measures foster staff satisfaction.

Most medical-surgical units experience a high percentage of staff turnover. From a budgeting standpoint, that can be beneficial because the staff aren't around long enough to accrue many hours of vacation time. On the other hand, such units as obstetrics, critical care, and the operating rooms are typically blessed with long-term seniority—and along with that comes competence, low turnover rates, and 3 to 4 weeks of vacation per year.

Staffing for the 7-day week

Using the information from *Developing a staff plan* on page 212, multiply by the appropriate factor (1.4 for 8-hour shifts — see text for information about calculating) to provide adequate coverage for 7 days/week, on all three shifts.

	Dir	RN	LPN	NA	UC
D	1.0	5.6	4.2	2.8	1.4
E		4.2	2.8	1.4	1.4
N		2.8	2.8	1.4	
Totals	1.0	12.6	9.8	5.6	2.8

Total 7-day full-time equivalent (FTE) needed = 31.8

Key: D-day, E-evening, N-night, Dir-director, RN-registered nurse, LPN-licensed practical nurse, NA-nurse's aide, UC-unit clerk

Satisfied employees who can take vacation time and who aren't left behind to labor with many overtime hours when others are on vacation is a big key to retention. (See *The impact of nonproductive time,* page 214.)

If you have a paid time off (PTO) pay structure, instead of individual vacation, holiday, and sick time, you still need to determine the average PTO per FTE in your department. The formula would be the same; however, you wouldn't have each individual time-off component to calculate. Total PTO paid in the department divided by the total number of FTE = average lost time per FTE.

Now that you know the number of staff you need to adequately cover the department, it's time to focus on daily staffing so you can accommodate and adjust to variations in patient census and patient needs.

Daily staffing

The first issue needing to be addressed in daily staffing is acuity and a method to measure it and therefore the level of care needed by patients. The patient acuity of a general medical-surgical unit may be different than the patient acuity of a step-down critical care unit. For the most part, however, patients of like groups on like units vary little from day to day in total acuity needs.

The impact of nonproductive time

To determine how many nonproductive hours you have per staff member, take a look back at your department totals. Take the hours of nonproductive time paid out in the most recent 12-month period, and divide that by the number of full-time equivalents (FTEs) in the department. For example, if in a 12-month period the department paid 3,749 vacation hours to 31.24 FTEs, that would average about 120 hours/FTE. Proceeding down the list of nonproductive hours, calculate the average time lost per employee for each nonproductive benefit your organization allows time off to the employee.

Nonproductive hours

Vacation = 15 paid days × 8 hours = 120 hours
Sick = 10 paid days × 8 hours = 80 hours
Holidays = 8 paid days × 8 hours = 64 hours
Funeral = 2 hours
Jury duty = 8 hours
Education = 2 paid days × 8 hours = 16 hours
Total = 290 hours

Next, determine what impact this nonproductive time has on your staffing. Divide the average number of nonproductive hours per FTE by 2,080 (number of hours 1 FTE would work in 1 year without taking any benefit time). The resulting number (for the example, it's 14%) is the percent of lost time.

Calculating FTE loss from nonproductive hours

2,080 annual hours for 1 FTE
− 290 hours of nonproductive time
1,790 hours available for productive time

290/2,080 = 14% lost time
31.8 FTE + 14% = 36.2 FTEs needed

You must increase each job category needing a replacement during out-of-department hours by 14%. Again, just like the weekend coverage, employees who are on vacation need to be replaced, or the work of the department can't continue. The department in the example, which started out needing 23.2 FTEs, ends up needing 36.2 FTEs to cover the staffing for 7 days/week and 24 hours/day and to have enough coverage for nonproductive time.

	FTE need	Benefit factor	Total FTE need
Director	1.0	14%	1.0
RN	12.6	14%	14.4
LPN	9.8	14%	11.2
NA	5.6	14%	6.4
UC	2.8	14%	3.2
Totals	31.8		36.2

Key: RN- registered nurse, LPN- licensed practical nurse, NA-nurse's aide, UC-unit clerk

What does this mean for practice? It means that each nursing unit should be assessed for a 20- to 30-day period with an acuity tool that you've chosen. Then, based on that data, the NHPPD is established for each unit. The patient acuity should be spot checked about once every 6 months, to ensure that patient severity hasn't changed significantly, and as needed if the staff on the unit express feelings of being overworked and understaffed.

After the acuity for the patient population is established — and therefore the NHPPD — the main variable that drives the need for staffing becomes patient census. The need for staffing on the unit is the NHPPD multiplied by the census. However, to stay within your budgeted NHPPD, you must consider a couple of things before using the above formula to calculate how many clinical staff you can put on each shift. Remember the NHPPD includes everyone on the unit's budget and all hours that they're paid productive time. Therefore, to stay within the budgeted NHPPD, you must deduct administrative hours before calculating clinical staff hours. Administrative hours include hours for the director and the nonclinical time given to other staff members, such as the performance improvement leader, the charge nurse for evaluation and time card activities, staff meetings, and mandatory education events, such as cardiopulmonary resuscitation and standard precautions, as well as pathway meetings. Although 1-hour meetings may not seem like enough time to worry about in the big picture, if 30 employees on a 40-employee unit attend a 1-hour staff meeting, that adds up to 30 hours that will be clocked as productive hours worked — but 30 hours that those staff members weren't on the unit providing care and support services for the functioning of the unit. Taking that a step further, if the average wage of these 30 employees is $17/hour, the unit budget has just spent $510 for a staff meeting. (See *Making meetings productive,* page 216.)

When you have those meetings under control, how do you go about predicting how many administrative hours will be needed? You have to guess what nonclinical activities your unit is required to attend and make an educated guess as to how much time each activity will take away from your clinical staffing plan.

For example, a staff member is given 1 day/month for performance improvement activities on the unit. This results in 8 hours multiplied by 12 days/year, or 96 hours. To account for this lost time evenly over the year, you need to divide those 96 hours by

Making meetings productive

Keeping meetings productive can be challenging for any nurse leader. The next time those hours start adding up into dollar signs for you, consider the following tips to help keep you and your staff on track.

➤ *Always have an agenda.* Agendas help you keep on track and give definite starting and ending times for the meeting.

➤ *Distribute written information before the meeting.* Avoid spending group time with reading activity. Make sure written information is distributed before the meeting and expect that staff will read it.

➤ *Schedule meetings strategically.* What's the best time to schedule a meeting? It's 1 hour before lunch or 1 hour before quitting time. Why? Most participants will have a greater motivation to keep the meeting on track and not stall or offer unrealistic suggestions if they have lunch or free time waiting on them.

➤ *Master the sophisticated send off.* The sophisticated send off is necessary when someone won't leave the meeting or your office. You begin by summarizing the results of the meeting, thanking the person for their participation, stand up, shake hands, and open the door for them.

365 days, which results in a loss of 0.26 hour/day. A charge nurse is given one office day per pay, for evaluations. There's a charge nurse on each of the three shifts. To account for the lost clinical time, you need to multiply 8 hours/day by three charge nurses by 26 pay periods and divide by 365 to calculate the clinical productive time lost per day. (See *Predicting nonclinical hours.*)

Not shown in the table are the nonclinical director's hours, which, because they're in this budget, must also be taken out of the hours allowed for clinical staffing. Therefore, if the department has 8 to 12 administrative hours (a director, assistant director, supervisor) not devoted to clinical patient care, these hours must be added into the administrative hours and subtracted before creating a clinical staffing plan. These few hours may seem inconsequential, but could end up totaling 15 administrative hours per day. If you don't consider this number when developing a staffing plan, you could end up being overbudget in your NHPPD.

The clinical staffing equation now becomes:

$$\frac{(\text{NHPPD} \times \text{patient census}) - \text{administrative hours} \times \text{percentage desired on the shift for which you're calculating}}{\text{hours per shift worked}}$$

Predicting nonclinical hours

To predict nonclinical hours, make a list of nonclinical activities on your unit and assign a time element to it. Do this for each staff member.

Performance improvement time	$8 \times 12/365 = 0.26$
Office time	$8 \times 3 \times 26/365 = 1.71$
Mandatory education	$60 \times 4/365 = 0.66$
Basic life support training	$60 \times 2/365 = 0.33$
Staff meetings	$45 \times 1 \times 12/365 = 1.48$
Pathway meetings	$2 \times 1 \times 2 \times 12/365 = 0.13$

Look at this example for the day shift:

$$\frac{(8.5 \times 30) - 15 \text{ administrative hours} \times 40\%}{8 \text{ hours/shift}}$$

$$255 - 15 = 240 \text{ hours}$$
$$240 \times 40\% = 96 \text{ hours}$$
$$96/8 \text{ hours per shift} = 12 \text{ staff on day shift for 30 patients.}$$

The staffing matrix

To avoid going through lengthy calculations for every shift, learn to use the staffing matrix. (See *Using a staffing matrix,* page 218.) The staffing matrix is developed using the formula above for every combination of patient census that the unit may have. Hours approved per shift are then divided into job classifications based on percentages calculated from the type of unit, the level of care needed by the patients on this unit, and any regulations that may govern your staffing plans such as state legislation.

The first number in the total column represents the number of hours approved according to the formula. The second number represents the number of hours that the matrix plan adds up to. The matrix number may be a little higher or a little lower, depending on the decision of the nurse-manager making out the plan and her knowledge of the patient population.

With a matrix plan already laid out, the nurse-manager can easily look at the number of staff and the skill mix required based on the number of patients to determine how many staff are

Using a staffing matrix

Census	RN 40%	LPN 30%	NA 20%	UC 10%	Total
26	4	3	2	1	82.4/78.5
28	4	3	2	1	89.2/78.5
30	5	3	2	1	96.0/86.5
32	5	4	2	1	102.8/94.5

Key: RN- registered nurse, LPN- licensed practical nurse, NA-nurse's aide, UC-unit clerk

needed. She should have the critical thinking skills and the authority to adjust the number of staff needed from the matrix number if she feels it would be in the patients' best interests.

Calculating productivity

Being able to prove to the finance department that you're going to keep all the people on the staffing plan in a productive mode is essential. Unlike an industrial production line, it isn't easy for nursing to justify productivity. After all, the work isn't measured in widgets made or wires soldered. In both areas, however, productivity is a factor of volume versus hours worked.

To define productivity you must first establish what the target or goal of what 100% productivity would be and then compare actual hours worked to that number. The midnight census is a variable number. The NHPPD is a number that your administration has determined based on your unit's current NHPPD, or based on benchmark data, or perhaps a combination of the two. If your current NHPPD is unfavorable, but the benchmark NHPPD is too much of a difference, use a number that's acceptable to you and administration as an interim goal to work toward.

The equation for the goal or target is:

$$\text{measurement of work (midnight census)} \times \text{NHPPD} = \text{required hours}$$

Calculating productivity and comparing the required hours to the actual hours worked is essential in helping the finance department understand that you're being a responsible manager with all the FTEs you have calculated that you need.

Productivity based on workload

When determining productivity, use only productive hours or hours worked, which includes regular hours, overtime hours, emergency called-in hours, and regular call hours worked. Don't include hours that are paid but not spent at the bedside, such as hours paid for on call but not worked, vacation hours, sick time, and workshop hours, which are paid hours but not hours that should be measured against your volume of work.

Only including worked hours is critical to being able to prove, improve, and respond to productivity at the bedside. If nonproductive hours are included in the productivity calculation, then there isn't any way you as a manager can determine if something should be changed based on the incorrect information.

To determine the productivity of your department for each pay period, use the following sample facts: in a 2-week period, you have 325 patient days, thus 2,850 actual worked hours.

Step one: Determine required hours based on pay-period volume

$$325 \times 8.5 = 2{,}763 \text{ required hours}$$

$$2{,}763 \text{ hours} = 100\% \text{ productivity}$$

Step two: Compare required hours to actual worked hours

$$\frac{2{,}763 \text{ required hours}}{2{,}850 \text{ actual worked hours}} = 97\% \text{ productivity}$$

For this 2-week pay period, the staff who worked were 97% productive. By comparing the required hours based on census and NHPPD to actual hours worked, you can arrive at a number that speaks to the finance department that you're being responsible with the number of FTEs assigned to your unit.

Certain factors can create a variance in your productivity without meaning that you were necessarily nonproductive. For this reason, make it a practice to write down possible reasons for a productivity variance at the end of every pay period. Examples include attending staff meetings, following through with mandatory education, being sent to employee health for a needlestick, being away from the clinical setting for 2 hours but still being on the time clock, and orienting new staff members who are clocking worked hours but can't be expected to be as productive as a senior staff person. In justifying these variances, write down how many hours the variance took up. For example, if 30 people attended a staff meeting for 1 hour each, that would mean there were 30 hours of clocked time that weren't spent at the bedside.

Earlier in the chapter when you were calculating your staffing need and NHPPD, staff meetings were included in the total. However, you can use staff meetings, performance improvement time, and so on to justify variances in your productivity on a per-pay-period basis. Over time, either a 4-week pay period average or a 12-month average, factors such as staff meetings and mandatory education can't be used to justify variances because the pay periods that you didn't have staff meetings even out with the pay periods that you did have them. Frequent orientations, outside workshops, and increased volume are all examples of variances that aren't always planned for and therefore could be used to justify a 4-week or a 12-month average variance.

Keep in mind that 4-week productivity figures can and should be used when requesting additional or replacement staffing. Included in the justification should be your latest 4-week pay period average of productivity, along with a statement that tells if the position that you're requesting is included in those hours and some discussion about whether this is a positive or negative variance. Use productivity calculations as a positive — not a negative — tool to justify staffing and to prove the department's use and ability to respond to fluctuations in patient census.

Percentage of overtime

Overtime is another important measurement that nurse-managers are asked to control on a constant basis. Percentage of overtime is the calculation used to compare, pay period to pay period, whether overtime is excessive and how it's being controlled. The formula for this calculation is:

$$\frac{\text{overtime hours paid}}{\text{productive hours worked}}$$

Refer to the sample medical-surgical unit. The worked hours for this unit were 2,850. Say the overtime paid for this pay period was 125 hours. Here's how the formula would look:

$$\frac{125 \text{ overtime hours worked}}{2,850 \text{ productive hours worked}} = 4\% \text{ overtime paid}$$

There's always going to be some overtime paid in health care. Situations arise, patients' needs change, families have questions, and coworkers call in sick. The goal is to control your overtime so that it averages somewhere around 2% to 3% per pay period.[3] If you're consistently experiencing a percentage higher than 3%, you should look at your practice as well as your staffing patterns.

Percentage of nonproductive hours

The final calculation that may help justify use productivity is the percent of nonproductive hours paid compared to the total paid hours per pay period. This can help you evaluate how much of your budgeted wages are consumed in nonproductive time paid.

A department with a high retention rate can be a curse and a blessing. It's a blessing because you're more likely to have clinically competent staff at the bedside and you'll spend fewer orientation dollars than units that are constantly orienting new staff. However, along with longevity comes benefit hours, such as more sick time and more vacation time. If you have a department with a high retention rate, you can easily be within your budgeted FTEs worked, but over on budgeted paid dollars. This comes from having a high percentage of nonproductive paid time, such as vacation time and sick time. It's calculated as follows:

$$\frac{\text{productive hours}}{\text{total paid hours}} = \begin{array}{c} \text{percentage of} \\ \text{productive hours paid} \\ \text{subtracted from 100\%} \end{array} = \begin{array}{c} \text{percentage of} \\ \text{nonproductive} \\ \text{hours paid} \end{array}$$

Using the same example unit, say that for the same pay period there were 2,850 productive hours worked and 3,100 hours paid. The equation would look like this:

$$\frac{2{,}850 \text{ hours worked}}{3{,}100 \text{ hours paid}} = \frac{91\% \text{ subtracted}}{\text{from } 100\%} = \frac{9\% \text{ of the hours}}{\text{paid were}}_{\text{nonproductive}}$$

Although you can do little to control nonproductive paid time, you can use this figure to justify variance in the budgeted wages.

Admissions, discharges, and transfers

Nurse-managers commonly struggle to explain to the finance department what admissions, discharges, and transfers (ADTs) do to their need for staffing. ADTs account for the activity level on patient care units that isn't reflected in the midnight census. It accounts for a significant number of nursing hours, unit confusion, and movement of patients, beds, papers, and other items associated with patient care.

As length of stay has dropped across the country, ADTs have become a bigger drain on nursing hours. Patients no longer stay in the bed assigned for days before being dismissed. ADTs are also elusive because, for most departments, nurse-managers have to capture the number of ADTs manually.

A possible solution is to keep track of the number of ADTs on your unit for at least 30 days. Compare the number of ADTs in that same 30-day period to the total midnight census.

ADTs compared to midnight census

The number of ADTs in a pay period divided by the midnight census for that same pay period gives you the ADT index. Next, you should determine for your unit what is expected activity, or what the expected ADT index for your unit will be. This number may vary from unit to unit. For example, in a telemetry, step-down unit, the ADT should be higher than in an orthopedic surgical unit. If the average ADT for your unit is high, use that number to justify additional staffing in the original staffing plan or to justify a higher NHPPD. When the expected ADT is established and taken into consideration on the staffing plan, you can use the expected level to justify variances above that level. For every additional ADT that the unit has above what the expected number is, the unit should be given one earned hour to be added onto the required hours for the pay period. For example:

Medical-surgical unit
2-week pay period
Total patient days: 500
Total ADTs: 303
Expected ADT index: 50% (The number is
predetermined based on the history of the unit.)

Fifty percent of the patient census is 250 ADTs. This figure represents what this unit would expect to have based on their ADT expected threshold, which is determined based on historic data for the unit. For this sample pay period, the unit had 303 ADTs, or 53 ADTs above their expected threshold. This unit is entitled to 53 earned hours for the 2-week pay period above what their normal target or required hours calculated to be.

If this were the same unit that was used in the example for productivity, these 53 hours would be added to the required hours of 2,763, to make a new total required hours of 2,816. If you remember, 2,850 productive hours were worked in this sample pay period. Therefore, the adjusted productivity use, taking into consideration the added ADT above the expected index, is:

$$\frac{\text{required hours plus added ADT (2,816)}}{\text{productive hours worked (2,850)}} = 99\% \text{ productivity}$$

Remember, the productivity without considering the ADTs was 97%. Keeping a record of ADTs and their impact on the staffing need (and therefore the productivity of the department) is a great way to justify variance in the staffing plan.

Points to remember

The following points summarize the role of budgeting for a nurse manager:

➤ Budgeting serves as a method to plan for services needed to effectively run your unit and should be consistent with your facility's mission.

➤ Budgeting not only involves ongoing activities but also requires planning for future services that may develop with health care changes.

➤ A staffing plan includes those variables necessary to ensure adequate staffing coverage and effective patient care.

➤ You should consider patient acuity and census when developing a staffing plan, as this may supply justification for established nursing hours per patient day.

➤ To foster staff satisfaction, make sure the staffing plan accounts for productive and nonproductive hours.

References

1. "Nurses Embrace Lay in Staffing Requirements," *San Diego Union-Tribune* A:3, October 14, 1999.
2. Blegen, M.A., et al. "Nurse Staffing and Patient Outcomes," *Nursing Research* 47(1):43-50, January-February 1998.
3. Dennis, C. Delta Health Systems, Inc. Personal communication with the author, West Palm Beach, Fla., April 1999.

Selected readings

Cappelli, P. "A Market-driven Approach to Retaining Talent," *Harvard Business Review* 78(1):103-11, January-February, 2000.

Coile, R.C. "Magnet Hospitals: Ten Strategies to Becoming a Model Nursing Employer," *Russ Coile's Health Trends* 11(7):8-12, 1999.

Hunt, P. "Speaking the Language of Finance." *AORN Journal.* 73(4):774-76, 779-82, 785-87, April 2001.

Keeling, B. "How to Allocate the Right Staff Mix Across Shifts: Part 1," *Nursing Management* 30(9):16-17, September 1999.

Kobs, A. "The Adequacy of Nurse Staffing," *Nursing Management* 28(11):16, 20, November 1997.

Nelson, B. *1001 Ways to Reward Employees.* New York: Workman Publishing, 1994.

Strickland, B., and Neely, S. "Using a Standard Staffing Index to Allocate Nursing Staff," *Journal of Nursing Administration* 25(3):13-21, March 1995.

Walker, D.A. "'Bottom-Line' Approach to Nurse Staffing," *Nursing Management* 27(10):31-32, October 1996.

McClung, T.M. "Assessing the Reported Financial Benefits of Unlicensed Assistive Personnel in Nursing," *JONA* 30(11):530-34, November 2000.

CHAPTER 10

Staffing outpatient departments

Pamela S. Hunt, RN, MSN

> "There are moments when everything goes well, but don't be frightened—it won't last." — Jules Renard

Staffing outpatient and surgery departments remains an ongoing challenge. If you're responsible for one of these departments, you'll use a step-by-step approach to determine overall department staffing needs, daily staffing needs, and productivity similar to that used by those responsible for inpatient departments.

Step 1: Determine staffing needs

Although inpatient units determine their daily need according to average daily census and nursing hours per patient day (NHPPD), outpatient and surgery departments don't have such statistics. Determining staffing needs for outpatient departments requires multiplying the average number of patient visits by the average clinical staff time per visit. (See *Calculating outpatient FTEs,* page 226.)

You can easily determine the average number of patient visits by looking back at the clinic records. Determining the average clinical staff time per visit may require a 1- to 2-month "real time" monitor to effectively arrive at the number of minutes spent with each patient, which should include direct patient contact as well as any activities associated with that patient's total visit. For example, checking the patient in, taking his vital signs, and assessing his condition are considered activities included in his visit as well as

Calculating outpatient FTEs

Use the following formula to calculate full-time equivalents (FTEs) in the outpatient setting: average number of patient visits × average clinical staff time per visit.

Example

40 patient visits × 25 minutes = 1,000 minutes/60 = 16 hours/day

mixing medications, documenting the visit, and communicating with the laboratory, pharmacy, and physician.

Staffing the presurgical admission and ambulatory surgery department

Another department that doesn't have an NHPPD is the presurgical admission and ambulatory surgery department. Here again, it's necessary to determine the average number of minutes required to prepare that patient before surgery and the average number of minutes necessary to recover and dismiss the average ambulatory surgery patient. It isn't uncommon to have both of these patient populations in the same unit.

For example, all surgery patients are admitted and prepared for surgery. If the patient is an inpatient, then he's taken to an inpatient room postoperatively. If the patient is an outpatient, then he's returned to and dismissed from the same unit. In this type of setting, one patient may account for two patient encounters. The unit is given credit for the initial admission encounter and also for the second admission postoperatively until dismissal.

For a unit such as this, plan for 2.1 nursing hours for every patient encounter, which includes all activities necessary to care for the average patient preoperatively and the average dismissal for ambulatory patients. Again, this number is based on a retrospective review of the unit, the type of patients served, the average length of stay, and the amount of nursing time required for all activities associated with the patient's care.

Now what do you do with this information? For example, tomorrow's surgery schedule has 15 patients, all of whom are morning admissions. Of these 15 patients, 8 of them are outpatients. Therefore, this unit has a staffing need of 15 + 8 = 23 patient encounters × 2.1 nursing hours per patient encounter = 48.3 nursing hours to take care of this patient population.

Staffing the PACU

In a department, such as the postanesthesia care unit (PACU), staffing need is predicted in much the same way but using a different nursing hours per patient encounter number. The following factors are used to come up with the number in this area:

> ➤ minimum number of nurses required
> ➤ average length of stay in the PACU
> ➤ average time it takes to prepare for the patient's arrival, transfer the patient, and prepare for the next patient.

Therefore, if the standard is a minimum of two nurses in the department, the average length of stay is 60 minutes, and the average time for preparation, transfer, and clean-up is 20 minutes, then the answer is 2.8 nursing hours per patient encounter.

To predict the staffing need for the PACU, multiply the number of patients on the operating room schedule by 2.8 to find the total number of nursing hours needed for the day's schedule. Predicting nonscheduled, add-on cases can certainly be a challenge. Your best bet is to keep track of averages. Trend add-on cases by the day of the week and the surgeon on call, and look at each day's schedule for breaks to fit in add-on cases should they occur. These tools for predicting staffing need should be used with a combination of good sense and professional judgment.

Staffing the surgery department

Other facility areas, such as the surgery department, require yet another method to calculate daily staffing needs. In the operating room, the calculation is based on the number of operating rooms, the number of hours the room is available for scheduling, and the average number of paid staff per room.

At this point, you may have to break down your total department into "like rooms" to calculate staff. For example, your facility has a four-room operating room. Two rooms for 8 hours per

Calculating operating room FTEs

Use the following formula to calculate full-time equivalents (FTEs) for the operating room: number of operating rooms × number of hours per room × average number of paid staff per room.

Examples

2 rooms × 8 hours × 3.5 staff = 56 hours

2 rooms × 10 hours × 3.5 staff = 70 hours

Total = 126 hours

day and two rooms for 10 hours per day. Because you have a high inpatient and anesthesia classification of patients, upon record review you determine that the average number of paid staff per room (registered nurses, certified surgical technicians [CSTs], licensed practical nurses [LPNs], and nursing assistants [NAs]) for all four operating rooms is 3.5. When your calculations are completed, you see that you need an average of 126 staff hours per day to staff two rooms for 8 hours and two rooms for 10 hours. (See *Calculating operating room FTEs.*)

The number of rooms you wish to staff should be a straightforward number. The number of hours the rooms are available is a calculation you may want to evaluate according to your facility's climate. You may use (as in the example) the number of hours the rooms are available, or the number of hours the rooms are used on an average day. Several factors specific to your facility may determine which factor you use: the amount of administrative support you have to make rooms available based on use data, the surgeon climate, the percentage of add-on versus scheduled cases (the higher your add-on percentage, the more likely you'll need to staff using available and not utilization averages), or anesthesia availability.

As with inpatient NHPPD, nursing journals and consulting firms cite benchmark data on the average paid staff per room. Just make sure if you're using benchmark data that you're comparing like practices, procedures, and responsibilities. The number (3.5) used in the example was derived from a retrospective

6-month record review. Each procedure was evaluated by clinical staff to determine the minimum number of staff needed to complete the procedure safely and efficiently for the patient and the surgeon. The number of clinical staff needed in a room is subjective and depends on many variables. In the example, judgments were based on procedure type, hospital climate, administrative support to the surgeons regarding additional staffing, and number of staff that would be required if this case were done on call.

It's no secret that many times procedures are completed on call with less staffing than would be required during administrative hours with no adverse patient outcomes. Just remember that your staffing need per room should be based on your specific environment. Whereas a nonteaching facility with over 75% of its patient population inpatient (longer and more labor-intensive cases) and over 35% of its surgical population Medicare (older, higher-anesthesia classification patients) may have a clinical staffing need of 3.5 per case, your staffing need per room may be different because the needs of your environment are different.

When calculating staff needs for inpatient units, all clinical job classifications are included in the NHPPD. A major difference in outpatient and surgical departments is that clinical staffing is only calculated using the average number of visits or procedures. Support staff, such as the scheduling secretary and inventory clerk, are added onto the clinical staffing need after it's determined because these jobs usually don't depend on patient census. The scheduling secretary needs to be accepting calls, regardless of the number of patients on the current day's schedule.

Step 2: Calculate productive hours

After you've determined your 24-hour need for clinical staffing, you need to divide that number by the number of productive hours per shift. (See *Differentiating productive and nonproductive hours*, in chapter 9, page 209.) Staff who work 8-hour shifts would be totally productive if they worked 7.5 hours; staff who work 10-hour shifts, 9.5 hours. The half-hour taken out of each shift accounts for paid breaks in the clinical staff workday. The lunch break isn't taken out because it's nonpaid time. Using the above example for the surgery department, the 56 hours needed to staff two rooms for 8 hours would be divided by 7.5 (7.5 FTEs), and the 70 hours needed to staff two rooms for 10 hours per day would be divided by 9.5 (7.4 FTEs). The total clinical FTE need for this department is 14.9 FTEs per day.

Step 3: Allocate FTEs to skill mix

Although health care cuts have forced nurse leaders to use all skills to the best of their abilities, every director should pay close attention to skill mix and quality in the facility. Nursing research has documented proof that as the percentage of registered nurses increases, the number of undesirable outcomes decreases. Undesirable outcomes include falls, medication errors, infection rates, patient and family complaints, and death.

The Association of Operating Room Nurses standards currently support one registered nurse immediately supervising each operating room. Use this standard to justify skill mix if challenged. With that said, you must now take the number of clinical FTEs that you need on a daily basis and divide them into skills needed. For this example, the skill mix will be 50% registered nurse, 30% CST, and 20% NA. (See *Allocating skill mix.*)

Step 4: Allocate FTEs to shifts

Now that you have the total clinical FTE need divided into skill mix, the next step is to divide them into shifts. For this example, 50% are allocated to the 8-hour shift and 50% are allocated to the 10-hour shift. (See *Allocating skill mix to shifts.*)

Step 5: Consider the number of days to staff

Staffing this example department for 5 days/week would require 14.9 clinical FTEs divided into 2 shifts and skill mix. However, if the department were open more than 5 days/week for scheduled cases, the FTE need would increase to accommodate the added days worked. To explain this additional need to the finance department, use this logical, critical thinking formula:

Allocating skill mix

Starting with 14.9 clinical full-time equivalents needed, allocate skill mix as shown below:

RN	50%	7.5 hours
CST	30%	4.5 hours
NA	20%	3.0 hours

Key: RN-registered nurse; CST-certified surgical technician; NA-nursing assistant.

$$\frac{\text{for each 1 FTE needed, multiply by the number of days you need to staff}}{\text{number of days each FTE works per week}} = \text{factor to account for additional days to staff}$$

For example, say this department staffs two rooms 6 days/week for 8 hours and two rooms 5 days/week for 10 hours. Example: 8-hour shifts

$$\frac{1 \text{ FTE} \times 6 \text{ days to staff}}{5 \text{ days per week}} = 1.2$$

Example: 10-hour shifts

$$\frac{1 \text{ FTE} \times 5 \text{ days to staff}}{4 \text{ days per week}} = 1.25$$

Allocating skill mix to shifts

The table below shows skill mix and shift allocation.

	RN hours	CST hours	NA hours
8-hour shift: 50%	3.7	2.3	1.5
10-hour shift: 50%	3.7	2.3	1.5
Totals	7.4	4.6	3.0

Clinical need

	RN hours	CST hours	NA hours
8-hour shifts	4.4	2.7	1.8
10-hours shifts	4.6	2.8	1.9
Totals	9.0	5.5	3.7

Total clinical need = 18.2 full-time equivalents

Key: RN-registered nurse; CST-certified surgical technician; NA-nursing assistant.

In the 8-hour example, for every FTE needed, you multiply by 6 days and divide by 5 days/week because an FTE who works 8 hours/day works 5 days/week. In the 10-hour example above, for every FTE needed, you multiply by 5 days and divide by 4 days/week because an FTE who works 10 hours/day works 4 days/week. Thus, each skill mix must be multiplied by the appropriate factor (1.2 for 8-hour shifts, 1.25 for 10-hour shifts) to provide coverage for two rooms running 8 hours/day for 6 days/week and two rooms running 10 hours/day for 5 days/week. This brings the total clinical need to 18.20 FTEs. (See *Clinical need.*)

Step 6: Add fixed and nonclinical job classes

Usually you think of fixed staffing as only those who are paid a salary. When creating a staffing plan, fixed positions are those positions whose work isn't dependent on census. Examples in the operating room include the director, charge nurse, scheduler, inventory clerk, and housekeeper. For the most part, even when the schedule is light, these positions have work that's done so the department can continue running smoothly. These positions perform job functions that support the work in each room but aren't included in the clinical staffing calculated in steps 1 through 5. It's now time to add these positions into the total department need. In the example shown, the director splits her FTE consumption between multiple departments and has determined that half of her hours are spent supporting functions in the surgery department. (See *Fixed and nonclinical job class needs.*)

Fixed and nonclinical job class needs

Job class	Full-time-equivalents needed
Director	0.5
Charge nurse	1.0
Scheduler	1.0
Inventory	1.0
Housekeeper	1.0
Registered nurse	9.0
Certified surgical technician	5.5
Nursing Assistant	3.7
Total	22.7

Productive versus nonproductive hours

One of the blessings of most operating rooms is long-term seniority—and along with that comes competence and low turnover rates. However, long-term employees are also the ones rewarded with 3 to 4 weeks of vacation per year. If you aren't taking nonproductive hours into consideration when developing a total department staffing plan, you may have difficulty when trying to cover vacations for the department. Just keep in mind that satisfied employees able to take their vacation time earned and who aren't left behind to labor with many overtime hours when others are on vacation is a big key to retention. The question becomes, "How do I determine how much nonproductive time I have per employee in my department, and how does that impact the overall staffing need?"

To determine how many nonproductive hours you have per staff member, take a retrospective look at your department totals. Figure out how many hours of nonproductive time you paid out in the most recent 12-month period, and then divide that by the number of FTEs in the department. For example, if in a 12-month period the department paid a total of 2,724 vacation hours to 22.7 FTEs that would average 120 hours per FTE. Proceeding down the list of nonproductive hours, calculate average time lost per employee for each of the nonproductive benefits

Adjusting total full-time-equivalent (FTE) need

Job class	FTEs needed	Nonproductive time	Total FTE need
Director	0.5	11%	0.5
Charge nurse	1.0	11%	1.11
Scheduler	1.0	11%	1.11
Inventory	1.0	11%	1.11
Housekeeper	1.0	11%	1.11
Registered nurse	9.0	11%	9.9
Certified surgical technician	5.5	11%	6.1
Nursing assistant	3.7	11%	4.1
Total	22.7		25.1

your facility allows time off to the employee. (See *The impact of nonproductive time,* in chapter 9, page 214.)

The next step is to determine the impact that this nonproductive time has on your staffing, dividing the average number of nonproductive hours per FTE by 2,080 (total number hours one FTE would work if no benefit time was taken). Notice the big difference in the nonproductive hours for outpatient areas versus the inpatient area is that you can't account for nonproductive time, such as holidays, if the department is closed on holidays and you aren't required to provide regular staffing coverage for that period. With this in mind, the resulting number is the percentage of lost time (for the example below, it would be 11%):

$$\frac{226 \text{ example benefit hours}}{2080} = 11\% \text{ lost time per FTE}$$

Therefore, you need to increase each job category that needs replaced when that FTE is out of the department by 11%. When the director of the department is on vacation, someone else usually doesn't do her work; however, all other job categories would need to be temporarily replaced or the work of the department couldn't continue. The department in the example, which started out needing 14.9 FTEs, ends up needing 25.1 to cover the staffing for two operating rooms 5 days/week for 10 hours and two operating rooms 6 days/week for 8 hours as well as coverage for nonproductive time. (See *Adjusting total full-time-equivalent (FTE) need.*)

Points to remember

The following points summarize the challenge of staffing various types of clinical departments:

- ➤ For staffing any department, a step-by-step approach can help determine the overall staffing needs.
- ➤ If you're using benchmark data to develop a staffing plan, be sure to compare similar practices, procedures, and responsibilities.
- ➤ Skill mix represents an important factor in any department when determining staffing needs because it affects quality of care and patient outcomes.

Selected readings

Finkler, S., and Kovner, C. *Financial Management for Nurse Managers and Executives,* 2nd ed. Philadelphia: W.B. Saunders Co., 2000.

Fralic, M., ed., and American Organization of Nurse Executives. *Staffing Management and Methods: Tools and Techniques for Nursing Leaders.* San Francisco: Jossey-Bass, 2000.

Keeling, B. "How to Allocate the Right Staff Mix Across Shifts: Part II," *Nursing Management* 30(10):16-18, October 1999.

Malloch, K., et al. "Patient Classification Systems, Part 2: The Third Generation," *Journal of Nursing Administration* 29(9):33-42, September 1999.

Strasen, L. *Key Business Skills for Nurse Managers.* Philadelphia: Lippincott Williams & Wilkins, 1987.

CHAPTER 11

Enhancing productivity

Pamela S. Hunt, RN, MSN

> "Start by doing what's necessary, then do what's possible, and suddenly you are doing the impossible." — St. Francis of Assisi

Productivity isn't as easily defined in health care as it is in industry, where assembly-line workers are counting parts. In both places, however, productivity is a factor of volume versus hours worked. In the operating room, the number of procedures — or because cases vary so greatly, the number of operating room minutes — can define volume.

For example, a freestanding outpatient surgery center opens across the street from its affiliated hospital. Within 18 months, 25% of total case volume moves to the surgery center. However, nursing staff doesn't feel as though they have 25% less work, so the proportionate 25% downsizing of the full-time equivalent (FTE) budget leaves them feeling constantly overworked.

Why? The cases that went across the street were quick, low-acuity cases that produced high volumes with short turnover times. The cases that were left at the hospital were longer and required complicated setups and turnovers. Therefore, using operating room minutes (patient in to patient out) as volume during this same 18-month period shows that the hospital actually only decreased its volume by 13%, not 25%.

Calculating productivity

To define productivity you must first establish a target or a goal of what 100% productivity would be and then compare actual hours worked to that number. The equation is:

measurement of work (# of operating room minutes) × nursing hours per operating room minute = required hours

Determining nursing hours per operating room minute can be based on your current practice, benchmark data, or a combination of both, to arrive at a number that you and your administration feels is a reasonable number to strive toward.

Carrying through the example in the staffing plan above, the hospital needs 3.5 clinical staff per room as well as 4.5 fixed staff for supportive functions of the department. The nursing hours per operating room minute for this staffing pattern is then:

$$\frac{8 \text{ staff/hour}}{60 \text{ minutes/hour}} = \frac{0.13 \text{ paid hour worked}}{\text{per operating room minute}}$$

For every operating room minute, you should have 0.13 worked hour.

For an outpatient clinic, this calculation is the same concept with a slightly different twist. To calculate required hours, the formula is:

$$\frac{\text{measurement of work time in minutes per visit}}{60 \text{ minutes/hour}} = \text{required hours}$$

Example:

$$\frac{25 \text{ nursing minutes per patient visit}}{60 \text{ minutes/hour}} = 0.42 \text{ hour worked per patient visit}$$

For every patient visit you should have 0.42 worked hour.

Calculating productivity based on workload

You can now determine how productive your department is for each pay period by the following steps:

In a 2-week period, you have, for example:

12,000 operating room minutes
1,680 actual worked hours

Step 1: Determine target hours based on pay-period volume.

$12,000 \times 0.13 = 1,560$ target hours

Step 2: Compare target hours to actual worked hours.

$$\frac{1,560 \text{ target hours}}{1,680 \text{ worked hours}} = 93\% \text{ productivity}$$

In this example, operating room minutes were used as the measurement of work, which can then be compared to the productive hours worked by the staff in the same pay period.

Make sure you're using only productive worked hours — that is, regular hours, overtime hours, and worked call hours — in this calculation. You don't want to count nonproductive hours against work volume to calculate productivity.

The outpatient clinic's example would be as follows:

In a 2-week period you have, for example:

400 patient visits
175 actual hours worked

Step 1: Determine target hours based on pay-period volume.

$400 \times 0.42 = 168$ target hours

Step 2: Compare target hours to actual worked hours.

$$\frac{168 \text{ target hours}}{175 \text{ worked hours}} = 96\% \text{ productivity}$$

Calculating percentage of overtime

Another important measurement of productivity is the percentage of overtime in the department on a per-pay-period basis. Health care is always going to require some overtime hours. Increased volume of operating room minutes or an increased number of patient visits should justify overtime, calculated as follows:

$$\frac{\text{overtime hours paid}}{\text{productive hours worked}} = \% \text{ overtime}$$

Example:

$$\frac{50 \text{ overtime hours}}{1,860 \text{ hours worked}} = 2.7\% \text{ overtime}$$

When calculating overtime hours, don't include hours that are "worked on call," which may be paid at an overtime rate but aren't the same as the potentially unnecessary overtime hours that can occur at the end of the shift. Removing the worked-on-call hours from the total overtime will give a clearer indication of end-of-the-day overtime. You can expect 2% to 3% overtime per pay period. If it's consistently higher than 3%, you should look at your practice as well as your staffing patterns.

Calculating percentage of nonproductive hours paid

The final calculation that's helpful in justifying productivity is the percentage of nonproductive hours paid compared to the total paid hours per pay period. This calculation can help you evaluate how much of your budgeted wages are consumed in nonproductive time paid. In a department such as surgery, which has a high retention rate, you can easily be within your budgeted FTEs worked; however, finance may show that you're overbudgeted paid dollars. Why? You may have a high percentage of nonproductive paid time, such as vacation time and sick time. These hours are calculated as follows:

$$\frac{\text{productive hours}}{\text{total paid hours}} = \begin{array}{c} \text{percentage of} \\ \text{productive hours paid} \\ \text{subtracted from 100\%} \end{array} = \begin{array}{c} \text{percentage of} \\ \text{nonproductive} \\ \text{hours paid} \end{array}$$

Example:

$$\frac{1,860 \text{ hours worked}}{2,020 \text{ hours paid}} = \begin{array}{c} 92\% \text{ subtracted} \\ \text{from } 100\% \end{array} = \begin{array}{c} 8\% \text{ of the hours} \\ \text{paid were} \\ \text{nonproductive} \end{array}$$

Although you can do little to control nonproductive paid time, you can use this figure to justify variance in the budgeted wages.

Explaining variance

Productivity is merely a comparison of number of hours expected (target) and number of hours worked. Make yourself a spreadsheet to keep track of these data on a pay-period basis. Trend it and constantly ask yourself, "What is going on in this department to cause this variance?" (See *Tracking variance.*)

Additional FTEs versus overtime

Because of the benefits and risks associated with hiring new employees, it's usually more cost-effective to pay the additional hourly amount for overtime work than to hire another employee.

In health care, many hospitals experience seasonal highs and lows, resulting in a volume fluctuation that's difficult to staff. That same question of when you should hire more staff as opposed to having the current staff work overtime becomes important, from both financial and human resource perspectives. Financially, you can determine the break-even point for how many overtime hours you can pay before hiring a new employee becomes more cost-effective.

Additional nurse

1 FTE nurse at $17.00/hour × 2,080 hours
+ 20% (benefit factor)

Additional nurse cost = $42,432.00

Tracking variance

Here's an example of a spreadsheet that can be set up to more easily account for variations on a per-pay-period basis. This example uses a census of 325 and nursing hours per patient day (NHPPD) of 8.5. It's important for the nurse-manager to understand the formulas that make up the spreadsheet and that prove the variances. However, knowing how to create the spreadsheet isn't necessary; use secretarial or other support staff to help with this task if they're available.

Productivity tracking

Pay period ending		5/04/02	5/19/02	6/02/02	6/16/02	7/02/02	7/16/02
Target hours	(A)	2,763					
Productive hours	(B)	2,850					
Use (%)	(C)	97%					
Reasons for variance							
Orientation hours	(D)	80					
Workshop hours	(E)	0					
CPR/ACLS/Mandatory	(F)	0					
Other	(G)	0					
Other	(H)	0					
Other	(I)	0					
Total variance justification	(J)	80					
ADT –Actual for pay period	(K)	215					
ADT –Threshold	(L)	162					
ADT-Adjustment	(M)	53					
Adjusted target	(N)	2,816					
Adjusted productive hours	(O)	2,770					
Adjusted use	(P)	101%					
Running average use		101%					
Overtime							
Overtime	(Q)	110					
Call hours worked	(R)	60					
Core overtime	(S)	50					
Overtime percentage	(T)	2%					

Worksheet explanations

(A) Target hours = measurement of volume multiplied by measurement of work (midnight census multiplied by NHPPD)

(B) Productive hours = all worked hours

(C) Use = A/B (target hours divided by productive hours)

(D-I) Reasons for variances expressed in hours

(J) Total variance justification hours (D + E + F + G + H + I)

(K) Admissions/discharges/transfers (ADT) = number for pay period

(L) Formula = threshold percentage expected multiplied by actual unit census minus actual ADTs

(M) ADT adjustment = earned credit hours (K – L)

(N) Adjusted target = M + A (add only ADT credit to target hours required)

(O) Adjusted productive hours = B - J (actual productive hours minus variance justifications)

(P) Adjusted use = N/O (adjusted target hours divided by adjusted productive hours)

(Q) Overtime = overtime hours

(R) Call hours worked = if paid as overtime, will be in overtime hours but need to be taken out of pure overtime

(S) Core overtime = overtime without call hours worked

(T) Overtime percentage adjusted = S/B (overtime hours divided by productive hours)

Overtime:

$$\$17.00/\text{hour} \times 1^{1}/_{2} = \$25.50/\text{hour}$$
$$\$42,432.00/25.50 = 1,664 \text{ hours/year,}$$
or an average of 64 overtime hours/pay period

In the above example, you pay not only an hourly wage for an additional full-time nurse but also a benefit factor. The amount of benefit factor depends on the facility; your human resources department should be able to give you this percentage. Benefit factor includes time paid away from the bedside, such as vacation and sick time, and such things as life insurance, health benefits, and retirement costs. You also need to consider the amount of risk that the facility takes on by hiring an additional employee — for example, the cost of workers' compensation and the potential risk of a large claim against the heath or life insurance benefit.

On the other hand, the overtime nurse doesn't incur additional benefit costs, which is why in this example you could actually average 64 paid overtime hours per pay period and be more cost-effective than hiring an additional employee. This formula should be used only as a guideline.

Keep in mind that every leader should evaluate individual employees and the department workload. Errors in health care due to fatigued employees is unacceptable. Each department should be evaluated with employee input as to how much overtime they can tolerate and not become exhausted and start looking for another job. For today's evolving workforce, overtime may not be considered a motivating factor, which is why employee satisfaction and patient safety should always be taken into consideration when developing a staffing plan.

Scheduled shifts versus call staffing

If you have a department that requires 24-hour emergency coverage but doesn't require 24-hour staffing, you may ask yourself, "At what point is having a scheduled staff more cost-effective than paying call staff wages?" The following formula allows you to answer the question of where the break-even point is, based on your current pay scale and call pay wages.

Calculating cost per hour for scheduled staff

Average wage + shift differential + 20% (The 20% is the assumption that you would have to hire new employees who would require benefit factor to cover this additional shift.)

Example:
Registered nurse $17.00 + 10% + 20% = $22.44
CST $12.00 + 10% + 20% = $15.84
NA $ 9.00 +10% +20% = $11.88
Total cost is $50.16/hour.

Calculating cost per hour of worked call time

Average wage x call premium + shift differential (No 20% benefit factor because these are already employees.)
Example:
Registered nurse $17.00 $\times$ $1^1/_2$ + 10% = $27.20
CST $12.00 $\times$ $1^1/_2$ + 10% = $19.20
NA $ 9.00 $\times$ $1^1/_2$ +10% = $14.40
Total cost for call crew per hour is $60.80

Comparison:
8-hour scheduled crew: $50.16 $\times$ 8 hours = $401.28
Call crew costs per hour = $60.80

Scheduled staff would need to work 6.6 hours consistently to be more cost-effective than covering the hours with a call crew.

Full-time versus part-time employees

Full-time employees are easier to orient: They attend staff meetings regularly because they're in the department when the meetings occur and they're informed of changes more easily. Having staff who are consistently on the unit when new equipment is brought in and when changes are made makes for improved consistency in workflow and patient care. Thus, using a balance of part-time and full-time employees is essential to improving your weekend and call coverage. Although employees work part-time, they're still required to fulfill weekend and call commitments.

Example: Inpatient unit

$$\frac{18 \text{ FTEs}}{\text{all full-time}} = \frac{18 \text{ people}}{2 \text{ weekends}} = \frac{9 \text{ people/weekend}}{(3/\text{shift})}$$

$$\frac{18 \text{ FTEs}}{\text{some part-time}} = \frac{24 \text{ people}}{2 \text{ weekends}} = \frac{12 \text{ people/weekend}}{(4/\text{shift})}$$

Example: Surgery department "on call" employees

$$\frac{14 \text{ FTEs}}{\text{all full-time}} = \frac{14 \text{ people}}{7 \text{ call nights/week}} = \frac{\text{on call every}}{2 \text{ weeks}}$$

$$\frac{14 \text{ FTEs}}{\text{some working part-time}} = \frac{21 \text{ people}}{7 \text{ call nights}} = \frac{\text{on call every}}{3 \text{ weeks}}$$

This example clearly demonstrates the advantages of using a balance of full-time and part-time employees to achieve greater coverage. The other factor is the improvement gained with employee satisfaction. Few people want to work weekends and holidays, especially if patient care is going to be inadequate because of staffing. By finding the right mix of part-time and full-time staff, you can more adequately cover the unit during weekends and holidays and spread out the call commitment as well.

Tips for improving productivity

Finding the right nursing hours per patient day and matching that to the patient census is always going to improve your productivity. Fluctuating staffing volume is the best method for maintaining productivity.

Evaluate your busy times. When do you receive the most admissions, discharges, and transfers? When are physicians making rounds and generating orders to be completed? It's for these times that you need to schedule additional staff.

There's no hard-and-fast rule that says every nurse on the unit has to report at 0700 hours. If most of your admissions, discharges, and transfers are occurring between the hours of 1100 and 1900 hours, then why not bring some staff in for a 1100 to 1930 shift, instead of the traditional 0700 to 1530 shift? Match the staffing plan to the workflow — even for the operating room.

Once a year in staff meetings, require everyone on your staff to complete the following statement, "If I had an extra hour at work, I would...." Actually require them to write their answers on a piece of paper to turn into you. This creates an instant work list of things to do. When you come to those times in your staffing plan that one less nurse could result in a burden, but keeping everyone you have makes you look a little overstaffed, require the team to get out that work list and find something on it to do in addition to their patient assignment for the day.

Floating staff within clusters

Another frequently used but seldom popular method to ensure productivity is to float nurses from one assigned area to another. Floating has been used for many years in nursing as a means to move nurses to where the patient need is.

Few nurses really like the idea of floating. Being assigned to a unit that's unfamiliar, with a patient population that may be unfamiliar as well, is frustrating for the nurse who is reassigned as well as the patients, physicians, and other nurses on the unit. Furthermore, the acuity and specialty of many patient areas today implies that, "a nurse is not a nurse is not a nurse." In other words, just as physicians have specialized skills, so do nurses. Floating an adult critical care nurse to a pediatric unit can be frustrating and dangerous.

That said, there are days when patient census fluctuates and nursing reassignment is necessary to provide patients with care and nurses with wages. The solution? Try the cluster method of floating. Nurses are floated from one unit to another, based on census and patient and nurse needs within a similar department cluster. For example, the intensive care, coronary care, and telemetry units are like units. The obstetrics, gynecology, nursery, and pediatric units are like units. The surgery department, postanesthesia care unit, endoscopy suite, and presurgical admissions unit are like units. Nurses are cross-trained for a minimum level of competency and unit orientation within their cluster.

A cluster must be a large enough group to have options for re-assignment. The departments within the cluster communicate with one another when there's a need for additional staffing and when there's a need to shed staffing because of low census on one of the units. Floating staff within a cluster allows for response to patient census, it provides a more controlled level of competency to be maintained, and it eases the burden of the unknown for the nursing staff who are reassigned.

Additional staffing options

One final thought on staffing patterns. You should evaluate your volume trends by day of the week and use part-time staff on high-volume days. If you can demonstrate a consistently higher census in the middle of the week, with a lower census on the weekends (a common scenario for most acute-care facilities), then it makes sense to use your part-time staff to boost the number of staff on those predicted high-census days. Achieving the right staffing patterns keeps nurses, physicians, administrative staff, and patients happy.

Another area to evaluate for optimal productivity involves asking yourself, "Who's doing what?" Are nurses transporting patients, passing meal trays, and traveling to the pharmacy and other supply areas frequently? Is there enough of this work to hire a lower-cost patient care tech to save nursing time? The hourly wage is different for these two job classes, and a nurse's time may be better spent performing another function.

Determine whether things on your unit are where they need to be. Evaluate whether certain products, supplies, and errands consistently take staff away from the unit — and whether budget dollars would be better spent bringing those items (for example, a copy machine) to the unit.

Justifying your requests

After you've determined that you do need additional staffing, what next? Top-level administration wants bottom-line information with supporting documentation for most requests. (See *Making a proper request.*)

Making a proper request

The front page of the request should clearly and concisely state what is being requested, and it should include the following points:

➤ *Job class description:* List the description that human resources uses to identify the job classification. Human resources establishes a position control for all positions in the facility. Each position is assigned a job class description.

➤ *Job class code:* List the job class code that human resources uses for this position. Like the job class description, each job class is associated with a job class code.

➤ *Department:* List the actual department where these hours are to be budgeted.

➤ *Start date:* Estimate the start date for this position.

➤ *Hourly rate:* Estimate the hourly wages to be paid.

➤ *Scheduled hours per pay:* Estimate the normal scheduled hours to be worked each pay period.

➤ *Department director's signature:* Make sure the director of the department requesting the new position signs the request.

The supporting documentation—for example, all work you've done to go through the step-by-step calculations, show volume trends, or show overtime climb—should be attached as supporting documentation.

The same documentation should be included for positions that need to be eliminated. This documentation enables finance to plan in the staffing budget to eliminate this salary for the remainder of the fiscal year and not include it in future years.

Just good ideas

Recurring schedules are always easier to work but sometimes not as staff friendly. One of the biggest keys to staff retention is making sure they can have a life outside of work. If you have a staff member who works into the evening shift but wants to participate on a bowling league, work the schedule and do what it takes to allow that person to have off work on bowling night. Allowing staff to have requested days away from work and negotiating with them for those days not only allows them to have a life outside of work but also establishes loyalty, trust, and a sense of collaboration.

Building teamwork and continuity of care is important not only for staff retention but also for patient care competency. In the clinical inpatient areas, staff who are assigned to work on the same weekend seem to develop a natural bond over time. Due to little or no administrative involvement on the weekends, the weekend team learns each other's strengths and weakness and seems to do well capitalizing on each person's strengths. This learned dependence — and therefore team independence — is a great asset during nonadministrative hours. One of the characteristics of an effective team is that every member identifies and capitalizes on each member's strengths and weaknesses. Building a sense of relationship and community among team members can be the bond that keeps them in the department.

Many departments are now using a self-scheduling method. If you're in one of these areas, or if you still have one person doing the traditional scheduling, make sure you educate your staff on overtime regulations and other staffing requirements so that they can independently trade days and shifts if necessary. Educate staff on the 8/80 rule verses the 12/40 rule. With this knowledge, staff can trade among themselves, increasing the need for them to communicate and help each other out as well as protecting the time of the nurse-manager.

Per diem staffing has become a popular way to respond to an increased demand of patient census. Agency staffing can be expensive, and the competency of staff who arrive on the unit to work is uncertain. Many facilities have had success with creating their own per diem resource pool. The facility benefits by having staff who go through their own orientation, agree to a written level of commitment, receive no benefit time, and know that they're the first to be canceled if the census drops. Plans are typically broken into two or more options: Option one might include working at least 16 hours per pay, 16 hours of weekend time per month, and 2 minor holidays per year. Option two would have a higher hourly wage but would require a higher level of commitment, including more hours per pay, more weekend hours, and working some major holidays as well as some minor holidays. The employee benefits by not having to work benefit hours and receiving a significantly higher dollar-per-hour wage.

It's always good management to allow employees who have worked overtime or come in extra to have the first chance at going home should the census drop later in the week or in the pay period — however, they shouldn't be forced to go home if they don't want to lose the hours. Be sensitive to those staff members who go the extra mile for the department, the patients, and you. Be financially smart, but remember that losing a nurse because of 5 or 6 hours of overtime isn't nearly worth the cost of recruitment and orientation of another nurse.

In the past 10 years, the health care industry has tried to turn its focus from a illness model to a wellness model. Companies are putting more dollars aside to provide their employees with preventive care benefits and hopefully save dollars and save lives later on by creating a plan that leads to early detection of serious problems. What is your facility doing for healthy incentives? Providing fitness club memberships, promoting healthy food selections in the cafeteria, and other incentives for living a healthy lifestyle are important to employees and the facility. Some facilities give a monetary bonus to employees who control their weight and have normal blood pressure and cholesterol levels. Others have wellness programs that award employees with quarterly, semiannual, and annual monetary incentives to achieve a point total. Healthy lifestyle points can be earned by not smoking, exercising regularly, wearing a seat belt, and attending educational programs. The thought is that employees who meet these criteria are less likely to require sick time and are less likely to access the health care plan. A wellness plan should provide incentives to employees who choose to live a healthy lifestyle, not punish those who don't. Remember, it's a choice!

The final "good idea" is to celebrate with your teams on a *regular* basis. Celebrating special designated days such as Nurse's Day should be included every year in your celebration, but don't forget to celebrate other successes with the team. Are you encouraging them in your leadership to always do their best and telling them when they do? When your team hits a new high for productivity, treat them to a special box of candy, hang a banner, or buy lunch with the department budget. Tell your team when they do a good job. Encourage them when times are tough, and lead by example. You'll greatly decrease your staffing turnover.

Points to remember

The following points summarize how calculating and optimizing productivity can benefit your facility:

> ➤ Building a staffing plan requires a well-thought-out step-by-step plan to ensure that adequate numbers of staff and the right skill mix are at the bedside taking care of patients.
> ➤ Measuring productivity is valuable for proving that employees are functioning in a productive mode.
> ➤ Finding the right number of staff for your department and then proving that they remain productive becomes imperative in providing safe, effective patient care.

Selected readings

Blegen, M.A., et al. "Nurse Staffing and Patient Outcomes," *Nursing Research* 47(1):43-50, January-February 1998.

Buerhaus, P.I. "What is the Harm in Imposing Mandatory Hospital Nurse Staffing Regulations?" *Nursing Economics* 15(2):66-72, March-April 1997.

Cleland, V. *The Economics of Nursing.* Norwalk, Conn.: Appleton and Lang, 1990.

Katzenbach, J. *Peak Performance: Alighting the Hearts and Minds of Your Employees.* Boston: Harvard Business School Press, 2000.

Malloch, K., and Conovaloff, A.J. "Patient Classification Systems, Part 1: The Third Generation," *Journal of Nursing Administration* 29(7-8):49-56, July-August 1999.

Pelfrey, S. "Financial Techniques for Evaluating Equipment Acquisitions," *Journal of Nursing Administration* 21(3):15-20, March 1991.

CHAPTER 12

Budgeting for operations

Pamela S. Hunt, RN, MSN

> "It's better to be prepared for an opportunity and not have one than to have an opportunity and not be prepared." — Whitney Young

Now that you've taken care of the staffing budget, the next challenge is the budget for operational supplies. You'll remember that the three functions of a budget are planning, management of ongoing expenses, and control of spending. Now let's examine the purpose of operational budgeting more closely.

Operational budgets

Budgeting starts with the facility's strategic plan, usually developed by the senior leadership and the board. Hopefully middle management and staff, as appropriate, can provide input as well.

   With the strategic plan in everyone's mind, smart financial planning occurs next. The goal of this type of planning is to achieve operating results that create sufficient excess capital. Adherence to board policies is at the forefront of every financial plan. Rate setting and debt or bond issuance are other components of the financial plan. The primary focus of bond issuance is the facility's ability to generate ongoing profits and cash flow from operations, proper management, and cash reserve levels. Facilities want to keep their financial state in a position that gives them an A+ bond rating. Those that have this rating have little trouble obtaining capital dollars for large-debt projects. With

251

strong financial planning, the facility builds a strong capital structure, which allows allocation of dollars for capital projects and day-to-day operations. In other words, your department should make enough revenue from the way it operates, the services it provides, the fees it charges, and the amount it actually gets paid to ensure that it has or can borrow the cash needed to provide necessary services.

Department budgets should be based on the department's goals and objectives. The need to manage expenditures to remain profitable should be on everyone's mind, but that doesn't mean cutting all expenses. Expenditures are necessary to generate revenue. The goal is to reduce expenses that don't generate revenue.

Operational supplies are also budgeted based on volume. No matter what department you're responsible for, it has a unit of service or volume measurement associated with it. For medical-surgical, it's number of patient days; for the laboratory, number of tests run; for dietary, number of meals served; for the emergency department, number of patient visits; and for the operating room, perhaps number of inpatients and outpatients. For your department, carefully look at what you do and how it's measured. (See *Factoring competition into revenue predictions.*)

Predicting revenue

Predicting revenue is important to guess how much money the facility might have available to buy supplies and equipment. Projects are approved based on projected revenue. Supply or operational budgets are predicted based on units of service multiplied by the projected reimbursement for the service.

Notice the term *reimbursement* instead of charge or cost. Facilities used to be reimbursed based on the fee for the service. Today, there are few places where the amount charged for a service is an indication of what the facility will be reimbursed for the service. The true revenue produced by that service is the dollar amount that the facility is reimbursed for the service.

What the service costs to provide remains important. Comparing the cost of a service to the reimbursement for that service gives a clear picture of the profit and loss margin for that service.

When talking about reimbursement, it's important for you as a nurse-manager to know what the payer mix is for your facility

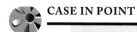

CASE IN POINT

Factoring competition into revenue predictions

The facility is looking to build a freestanding surgery center across the street. During the planning and building of the center, you predict that about 25% of your case volume will move across the street. Therefore, the operational budget and staff are reduced by 25% to account for the loss of cases. In the months to come, the low-risk outpatients do move across the street to the surgery center, and the number of cases decreases by 25%. However, the operating room in the facility is short staffed. Overtime increases to a new high, the call crew is working most of their call hours, and the staff is unhappy.

What's wrong? The cases at the center are minor cases that require minimum staffing, whereas the cases at the facility are inpatients and high-risk outpatients — that is, patients whose cases take longer in the operating room and require additional staff in the rooms.

What's the real unit of service? For the operating room, the unit that would explain this change isn't the number of cases but the number of operating room minutes. Comparison of operating room minutes before and after the opening of the surgery center show that the number of minutes has dropped only 13%. Therefore, know your units of service and make sure the unit of service you select projects the volume of work for the department.

and hopefully even your department. What is *payer mix?* It's used to describe your patient population in regard to how they're paying for their hospitalization. Common components of a payer mix for an acute care hospital are Medicare, Medicaid, commercial insurance, and self or charity care. The community your patient population comes from will dictate the percentage of the patient population that falls in each of these categories.

What can you assume about a facility in which its community's payer mix is 35% Medicare, 25% private insurance, 15% Blue Cross/Blue Shield, 10% Medicaid, 9% self-pay, and 6% charity care? Because of the large percentage of Medicare, this payer mix tells you that the facility is in a community with an aging population. The major employers in the community must carry Blue Cross/Blue Shield coverage. Medicaid, self-pay, and charity care totals 25%, which would lead you to assume the economy in this area is struggling.

If you're a facility that delivers care to a high percentage of Medicare patients, you should make it a point to read and keep up-to-date on the legislative acts that will affect your reimbursement for services. Let's say the major employer in your area happens to be an automotive plant. It's important for you, as a nursing leader, to pay attention to what's going on at that automotive plant, including contract negotiations, employee layoffs, and who the company is choosing to be their insurance carrier. All of these things can greatly impact your facility.

Expenses

Operational expenses are presented in detail to accumulate data and control costs. Each component is assigned a number for easy tracking. The first three digits of the number should represent the department cost center number; the last three digits, the component number where the supplies were used.

This detailed accounting and budgeting tool is normally distributed monthly and shows each component. In addition, the spreadsheet shows what is spent for that account in the current period (1 month) compared to budget and what was spent for the fiscal year compared to budget. The spreadsheet clearly shows the variances in dollars and in percentages. Some items naturally show variances on a monthly basis because those supplies or services aren't needed every day. This spreadsheet is one tool that the nurse-manager must look at and ask, "Do I understand? Can I account for what is occurring on this spreadsheet?"

When an account is over budget and the reason isn't obvious, look at the detailed listing of expenses for the period in question. This detailed listing is sometimes available within the facility's intranet, or you may have to call finance to run the report for you. Another list to look at for the variance is the accounts payable general ledger distribution list. This monthly report shows all external expenses charged to your department and indicates the vendor name and number with dollar amounts. Use all of these tools to manage the supply, minor equipment, and service expenses in your department.

Administration places special emphasis on variances over 5%. In response to administration inquiries, you may be asked to prepare an explanation of variances and submit suggested remedies.

Supplies or services can be considered variable, which means they're directly related to the volume fluctuations, or they can be considered fixed, which means they doesn't react to volume fluctuations. Some items that are expensed are even considered to be semivariable and semifixed.

Medical-surgical supplies, drugs, I.V. solutions, braces, oxygen, and X-ray film are all examples of variable expenses. The amount spent on each should directly reflect the number of patients served. Variable expense items are budgeted based on predicted volume and inflationary changes.

Physician and nonphysician fees are good examples of semivariable/semifixed expenses because they're sometimes related to the volume of a particular procedure performed or a fixed amount. Physician fees represent a payment made to the physician for professional services provided; nonphysician fees represent payment made to physicians and nonphysicians for administrative and consulting services. When budgeting for these services, calculate the estimates for the current year and future budget year according to the situation and contract period in effect.

Office supplies and other expenses include office supplies, minor equipment, dues, subscriptions, and travel and meeting costs. Some of these expenses may be considered fixed because the expense occurs regardless of volume fluctuations in the department.

There are three budget methods used for operational supplies: zero-based budgeting, unit-cost budgeting, and historical/trend budgeting.

Zero-based budgeting

Zero-based budgeting is used for fixed costs, such as travel expenses, meeting registration, memberships, and maintenance contracts. You start at zero and add the cost of each item based on your plan for the next year.

For example, in the travel budget for the unit, you want to send two staff members to your national conference and yourself to a management conference, all regional association meetings, and one other conference in whatever interest comes up during the year. You start with zero and based on what you know about where these predicted conferences are, how far you need to travel, how long the hotel stay is, and what meal and other travel expenses will be incurred, you build a predicted budget to support the goals of attendance. Hopefully you or one of your peers has data from previous years to help you in this planning.

Unit cost example

Medical supply: X-ray film
Fiscal year 2002 (6 months)

Actual expense	$27,400
MRI procedures	1,431
Unit cost	$19.15
Budgeted procedure	3,388
Budgeted expense	$64,880

Unit-cost budgeting

Unit-cost budgeting is used for variable costs, such as medical supplies, pacemakers, implants, and radiologic film. These items have variable costs but can be associated with a certain volume of procedures.

For this method, start with what you've actually spent for the current fiscal year. Divide that number by the number of procedures that you've done using this product in the same period. This number is an actual unit cost of the item. Next, predict how many of these same procedures will be performed in the coming year. Multiply the actual unit cost by the predicted number of procedures to find the budgeted expense. (See *Unit cost example.*)

Historical/trend budgeting

The method used for anything to which the other methods don't apply is the historical/trend budgeting. There are three different methods for historical/trend budgeting: prior year actual, projected, and annualized.

PRIOR YEAR ACTUAL METHOD To use the prior year actual method, you simply take the amount that was spent for the item in the prior fiscal year and add an inflation factor. This method is used if you predict the exact same volume, no new physicians performing the procedure or requiring the supply, and no new patient population needing the service. Current inflation factors

Inflation rates

Fiscal year 2002 budget

Expense classification	Inflation rate
Professional services	3.60%
Medical supplies	0.50%
Drugs and I.V. solutions	4.20%
Food	0.030%
Purchased services	4.00%
Rent/lease	0.00%
Plant and equipment maintenance	2.40%
Utilities	0.00%
Nonmedical supplies	2.20%
Leased property expenses	2.40%
Other expenses	2.20%

Source: December 1999, Rate Controls Publication.

usually come from finance or materials management and are based on the industry standard at the time. (See *Inflation rates.*)

Inflation factors may vary from product to product or service to service, depending on supply and demand. For example, orthopedic implant costs were being held to a very low inflation rate, with marginal increases given for about a 6-year period. After that 6-year period when the price increases were minimal, the inflation rate for the cost of implants took a turn and now companies are demanding — and usually receiving — above-average increases, compared to other medical supplies. Knowing the climate, networking with peers, and watching your monthly financial reports all help with predicting expenses.

PROJECTED METHOD In the projected method, you add the actual amount spent for the item in the last 6 months to the amount left in the budget for the next 6 months. This method is useful for items that may see fluctuations, according to the time of the year. Perhaps the first 6 months of the fiscal year showed a lower dollar amount spent, but because the winter months are in the

Historical and trend methods

➤ *Prior year actual:* Prior year plus inflation factor
➤ Projected: Actual 6 months of current fiscal year plus what's predicted to be spent in
   next 6 months
➤ *Annualized:* Most recent monthly figures, divided to get a monthly figure and multiplied
   by 12

last 6 months of the fiscal year, you expect more supplies to be needed because of increased volume. Another reason to use this method is for products that you purchase only quarterly or semi-annually.

ANNUALIZED METHOD The annualized method is the final historical/trend method. For the annualized figure, you take the most recent monthly dollar total spent for the item, divide by the number of months that figure covers, and multiply that number by 12 months to arrive at an annual prediction.

Take, for example, the opening of the surgery center earlier in this chapter. In the previous fiscal year, the nurse-manager had the total number of procedures, including those that went across the street, but she certainly didn't want to use this inflated number to predict expenses. At the time the budget was due, the surgery center had been open for about 9 months. In the last 5 months, the volume trends had leveled out, and most cases that were going to move to the surgery center had moved. Therefore, the nurse-manager took the last 5 months of current spending for the item and divided that by 5 to arrive at an average monthly spending. Then she took that monthly number and multiplied it by 12 months to arrive at a predicted amount to be spent in the coming fiscal year. (See *Historical and trend methods.*)

In the first fiscal year after the opening, the nurse-manager didn't want to use the last fiscal year's statistics to budget for the next year because the volume was obviously changing. Also, no one item was affected uniformly. For example, the implant component included orthopedic implants, which were used in the facility, and cosmetic surgery implants, which were used across the street. With these two items clumped together, budgeting accurately for the lost volume was difficult. Therefore, in trying to make the best guess, the nurse-manager took the most recent

5 months' worth of data, divided it by 5 to come up with a monthly number, then multiplied that number by 12 to arrive at a predicted annual figure.

When you don't make the budget

When budgeting for staffing, operational supplies, or capital equipment, the worst thing that can happen is to be way over budget or way under budget and not know why. Using critical thinking skills to justify, explain, and evaluate what caused the variance is vital. Here are factors you need to think of not only when explaining variance but also when budgeting for the next year.

New physicians. Are you expecting any new physicians to begin practicing at your facility? If the answer is yes, take note that it usually takes 6 to 9 months for a physician's practice to get built up to the point that it affects your volume. If possible, talk to the new physicians when they come on staff. Do they seem to practice similar to other staff physicians? Is there equipment that they used at other facilities that they're hoping to have you purchase here? What is their drug of choice for your most common diagnosis? Is that drug more or less expensive that what you currently see used? The answers to the questions may or may not affect what you're planning to spend in the next year.

New procedures are another factor to consider. Ask your physician group if they know of any new technology that may be implemented in the next year that could affect your budget. What supplies and disposables are necessary for these new procedures?

Pay attention to your *payer mix*. What's the local economy doing? If there are layoffs, you'll most likely see a drop in number of people accessing care, especially for elective procedures, such as cosmetic surgery and infertility treatments.

Payment contracts that materials management negotiates can affect your budget. Perhaps you noticed a variance in a particular expense, and no one let you know that materials management negotiated a 4% increase in the middle of the fiscal year. Similarly, if your facility is part of a buying group, prices and products can change in the middle of the fiscal year with little control from nursing. If you can't control it, why care? Remember: Being over or under budget isn't as critical as understanding why. Always make it your business to know why an account is showing a variance on the monthly report.

Change in a procedure or in regulations is another common reason for variance. An example of a regulatory change is the one involving latex sensitivity products. What a financial dent these products have made, but they're certainly a necessary compliance issue. The same thing happened in the 1980s, when nurses were required to wear gloves to start I.V.s, give patients a bath, or do a number of other patient-contact tasks.

Justifying variance

Don't forget to look at the budgeted volume for the department to justify a variance as well. Sometimes the reason that an item is over budget is because the volume of patients or procedures exceeds what was predicted as well. In the year the surgery center opened, the actual dollars spent in most of the operating room expenses were over budget. The budgeted volumes and operational supplies had been reduced by 25%, but the actual volume had only dropped by 13%. Comparing budgeted volumes to actual volumes can quickly give the answer to why supply expenses aren't in line with the dollars budgeted.

Justifying variances is seldom easy. The best practice is to look at these accounts on a monthly basis because it's easier to remember what happened last month to cause the variance as opposed to what happened last year. With everything that comes across your desk, looking at reports on a timely basis may not always be a top priority. However, being able to respond to the reports depends on your memory of what was going on clinically in the department when the expense occurred. Be disciplined enough to make notes throughout the month when you think of something that might cause a variance in the budget.

Budgeting for operational supplies can sometimes be overwhelming because the numbers are so large and the control of volume so minimal. Using accurate data to start with and building on what you know about your patient population and your community, you can make intelligent, informed projections of what you'll need for each item.

Capital equipment budgets

If you've been in health care for long, you may remember the times when a physician would request a piece of equipment, you would fill out a form, and the equipment would arrive. However, that's no longer the case. Extensive planning and complex justifications are now required to obtain the equipment you need.

Your facility may have its own definition of *capital equipment.* The most common definition is "a piece of equipment that costs more than $500 and has a life of more than 2 years." However, due to increased expenses, some facilities are revising this definition to "a piece of equipment that costs more than $2,000." This, of course, reduces paperwork for less-expensive items.

Although the paperwork is cumbersome, it's best to capitalize items that fit your facility's definition and not try to pass them through as noncapital items. When capitalized, the equipment will be tagged and added to the capital asset listing for your department. One of the main benefits of capitalizing equipment is that you can take advantage of the equipment's depreciation. The cost to be capitalized includes:

➤ the cost of the asset
➤ shipping and delivery costs
➤ taxes
➤ commissions
➤ installation costs
➤ financing costs
➤ other costs directly associated with acquiring the asset and putting it into use.

A 15-year plan is recommended when budgeting for capital equipment. How can you predict needs 15 years in advance at the rate health care is changing today? Any plan, especially 15 years, is just an educated guess. Most predictions past 5 years are based on predicted replacements.

Creating a map

In a spreadsheet such as this, there's a description, a quantity, and a coded indication for the status of the equipment — new, additional, or replacement (N = new, A = additional, and R = replacement).

New equipment is an item that the department doesn't currently own, rent, or lease and that isn't a replacement for existing equipment. Additional items are items that serve as supplemental to other like items in the department. For example, the department owns one per-

Capital budget 15-year plan

Asset Description	Qty.	Serial #	Acq. Date	Life	FY 2003	FY 2004	FY 2005	

Predicted replacements

Predicted replacements is the place to start in planning for capital equipment. You should have a current capital asset listing that indicates the original cost and purchase date of the equipment, the expected life of the equipment, and its depreciation value. Based on this, you can predict when equipment has outlived its predicted years. Many major expense items occur only once or twice in a 15-year period, but need to be anticipated so that smaller purchases during those years can be diverted.

For example, the year that new hard-wired monitoring equipment is needed would be a good year to avoid planning to purchase another large item. It's important to the facility for the department's budgeted totals per year to be somewhat level. Although narrowing it down to the exact dollar amount isn't possible, evening out expenses helps the facility to maintain control of dollars spent. Use a computerized spreadsheet to map out your 15-year plan, to help ensure that you're predicting replacement items on a routine basis. (See *Creating a map.*)

sonal computer and is requesting one additional personal computer, or the new equipment will function as backup for existing equipment. Replacement equipment items are items that replace existing equipment that will be traded in, sold, or discarded.

Listed next on the spreadsheet are the serial number from the current piece of equipment if available, the acquisition date, the expected life, and the year that the equipment needs to be replaced. A spreadsheet such as this clearly shows what equipment is budgeted, in what year, and the total dollar amount for the department.

FY 2006	FY 2007	FY 2008	FY 2009	FY 2010	FY 2011	FY 2012	FY 2013	FY 2014	FY 2015	FY 2016	FY 2017

New and additional needs

As with operational supplies, evaluate the current volume, new regulations, new physicians, and new procedures that may impact the department's capital equipment needs in the next year. Always ask physicians who admit the most patients to your department and staff who work in your department what their needs are. Physicians should help identify new procedures and products that they may be needing in the coming year. Likewise, who knows better than the staff who work with the equipment every day what needs to be replaced? Tap into these resources, and make physicians and staff members part of this planning process.

When evaluating a new service or product, you first want to assess whether the service or product produces good outcomes and is pertinent to your patient population. A good source for helping you assess whether new technology is clinically beneficial and appropriate for your needs is not only current literature but also other facilities that use the technology. (You may even be able to obtain a reference listing from the company.)

Use the group purchasing organizations that your facility belongs to as an information source. Call members and ask them what they have heard about the technology and if they're considering it as well. Here again, it's important to know your patient population and your community. Is this something that many patients will be accessing, or will it benefit only a few members of the community?

Prioritization

After replacement, new, and additional needs are identified, you need to prioritize. If you have a department with a significant amount of capital equipment, such as surgery, break your capital needs down into specialties. For example, under the total department capital asset request, there are the "subtitles": orthopedics; urology; obstetrics/gynecology; ear, eye, nose, and throat; and general. The department needs are capital items needed for the department in general, such as a medication refrigerator or copier. The other subtitles represent a clinical specialty, with the equipment needed listed underneath each. Subtotal the amounts in each clinical specialty or service line, and provide the department total at the end of the last page. These steps will make it easier to predict the budget and easier to manage it when the plan is made.

Justification

After the capital budget has been established and approved, every purchase request should be accompanied by a thorough justification. This justification should include the service provided, its necessity or importance, expected use, expected life, products evaluated, cost of equipment, and estimated savings or profits from the purchase of the equipment. Keep in mind, many facilities have their own justification formats to follow.

Necessity or importance

The service provided and the necessity or importance of the service should be self-explanatory. What will this equipment do? How will it benefit your patient care or physician practice? State how the equipment will help the facility continue to respond to its mission. If the equipment addresses safety or quality issues, address this in the opening statements of the justification. Also included in this section could be a statement that addresses whether your competitors are providing this service. If they are and if there's enough predicted patient volume for your facility to provide the service as well, then this could prove to be a great opportunity to gain more market share and provide a like service— only better! A word of caution: If your competitors are providing the service and there isn't a large market for it, then you first need to ask yourself if this is the right thing to do or if those dollars could be better used in another area.

Expected use

The expected use may be a bit more difficult to anticipate. It's expressed as a number pertinent to the product. For example, say the equipment is a noninvasive blood pressure module. The unit requesting this equipment is open 365 days/year. Based on the average daily census (ADC) of your unit, you predict the equipment will be used about 5 days/week. 52 weeks $\times$ 5 days = 260 days. 260 days divided by 365 total days leaves a use of 71%. There's no magical number of utilization percentage that instantly qualifies or disqualifies a piece of equipment for purchase. This logical step is a good critical thinking step to take when justifying purchases and prioritizing needs.

Expected life

The next area to address in a complete justification is the expected life of the equipment. The manufacturer of the equipment may provide this information, and it should be evaluated according to any history you have with like equipment. Keep in mind that companies commonly overestimate the useful life of a piece of equipment when you're purchasing it and underestimate the life of equipment after you own it.

Products evaluated

The justification should include products you've evaluated and their costs. Have you looked around, tested all products available, and selected the best choice based on clinical evaluation and price? This step in the justification process can be time-consuming, but it's essential in selecting the right product and proving responsible decision making.

On major purchases (over $25,000), you should always have quotes from at least three different vendors. Include in this section of the justification which vendors you tried, the dates the equipment was tested, the clinical evaluation, and the price of each. Just as with operational supplies, if you participate in a particular buying group, you may be hard-pressed to purchase only from the selected vendor. If no clinical difference is apparent, then selecting the group vendor is a good idea. Because cheaper isn't always better, the above process of evaluating products is important. You need to be able to prove that you evaluated various choices and then be able to explain why one is the best.

Cost

Next, you need to gather data on the cost of the equipment and the anticipated cost to your facility in using it and providing the associated service. This list should include the cost of the equipment as well as construction costs, the cost of disposables, the time the procedure would take, the number of staff it would take to perform the procedure, where the procedure would be performed, and any ancillary services that would be needed. The cost of the equipment and any construction cost is self-explanatory and was covered in the capital budgeting section.

You might want to investigate alternative companies at this time as well, but you may want to hold off testing those companies until you determine that you're going to move forward with this service in your facility.

The cost of disposables that are needed to do the procedure includes not only the cost of new disposables you must purchase but also any disposables that you may already have in stock. For example, if the procedure requires the patient to have an indwelling urinary catheter, then that cost should be added into the cost tally sheet.

One of the most expensive components of hospital costs is employees. How many staff members are needed to complete the procedure? If the procedure requires that conscious sedation standards be followed, you automatically need one nurse just to monitor the patient and possibly one other staff member if the physician needs an assistant during the procedure. Find out if the procedure can be done in a low-cost area, such as a medical-surgical room, or if it requires a high-cost area, such as an operating room. This will make a big difference in your cost tally sheet.

Finally, find out if ancillary services will be needed. Will the patient need laboratory work, radiology, or respiratory therapy, for example? When you begin assessing reimbursement for the procedure, revenue from ancillary services can be helpful.

Along with the true cost of the equipment, don't forget installation costs, which may need to be included in a capital construction budget. You, along with a representative from the equipment company, will want to contact your plant engineering department to discuss the installation of the equipment and the materials and manpower needed.

Remember also the warranty, maintenance agreements, and training expenses that may be associated with the equipment. These three factors can be very costly and aren't capital costs but costs that will show up on those subaccounts of the operational budget. During the capital budgeting period, you can negotiate and compare the warranty, maintenance agreements, and training costs, but realize that after the equipment is purchased, these expenses must be planned for in corresponding accounts of the operational budget. Also, don't forget that if you're purchasing a replacement piece of equipment, you must terminate the maintenance contract on the old equipment. This could save dollars for the first few years, when the new equipment is under warranty.

Reimbursement status

Speaking of reimbursement, now is the time to estimate how much the facility will get paid if they go forward to provide this service. The question isn't how much will be charged for the procedure, but how much will be reimbursed for the procedure. (You may want to check with your finance department.) In today's health care environment, few areas actually get paid what they charge. Therefore, a close look at what type of patients will be using this procedure and what kind of payment methods these patients use is necessary.

The answer to these questions may include private insurance payments, self-payment, and Medicare and Medicaid payments. With this information, you should be able to determine the average reimbursement rate for the procedure and additional charges for supplies associated with the procedure. Don't forget the ancillary services as well. Sometimes the payment for the procedure may not produce a good profit margin, but the ancillary services necessary to provide the procedure do.

Estimated savings or profits

The final point to be made on the justification is estimated savings or profits from purchasing the equipment or providing the service. To help you think in these terms, ask yourself, "Will the equipment decrease the patient's length of stay or time in the operating room? Most third-party insurance, Medicare, and Medicaid agencies compare length of stay and are constantly forcing them down lower and lower. Therefore, if this new equipment can decrease the length of stay by at least 1 day, this savings could be beneficial for the facility. Likewise, the average operating room minute costs $5.00 to $7.50. The math is easy. If the requested piece of equipment saves 20 operating room minutes, it could save $150/case. Let's say you do an average of 15 of those cases a month: That would equal an annual savings of $27,000!

$$20 \text{ minutes} \times \$7.50/\text{minute} = \$150.00 \times 15 \text{ cases/month} \times \$2,250 \times 12 \text{ months/year} = \$27,000$$

In addition, the saved operating room minutes would decrease anesthesia time and therefore lower the risk for the patient and improve room use.

Another area to think about in savings is proving a savings of staff time. Equipment, such as automatic blood pressure devices, can translate into time savings for nurses so that they can perform other essential functions.

Unexpected expenses

Sometimes things come up within the year that weren't budgeted—for example, equipment that didn't last as long as it was predicted to last, new technology that wasn't available when the budget was developed, or additional equipment needed to compensate for an unexpected increase in volume. If the item was budgeted for future years, mention that in your justification. Tell which year it was budgeted to be replaced and why it must be moved up to the current year. Make sure you adjust your 15-year plan accordingly when you complete your plan during the next budgeting period.

New technology and additional volume are two positive reasons for nonbudgeted equipment. Is there something in this year's budget that was included but now you don't think you'll need? If so, include in your justification that the item you want to purchase wasn't predicted to be needed; however, another item that was budgeted for (name the item and the budgeted dollar amount) is no longer needed. The approval may be better accepted if the committee knows that a switch of equipment is needed, not "extra" dollars. Even if no dollars are available to swap and the equipment wasn't budgeted, a strong, concise, but thorough justification can help you get the approval you need to make the purchase.

Submitting the capital justification

The capital justification should be concisely written and typed with bolded subtitles. Because these justifications are read and approved by the financial administrator and laypeople who serve on the governing board, you should use simple terms and clear language to explain the service provided and the need for the service. When writing the justification, choose your words carefully and put yourself in the place of the board member reading it. Answer the question, "What would make the board member think that it's necessary to approve this purchase?"

Justifications should include a summary with supporting documentation attached, if necessary. (See *Capital justification example,* pages 270 and 271.) There, the equipment has a high cost, so the justification requires well-defined comparison information for the board to review. Use this example and the information below to guide your justification for major purchases.

Drawing up a capital justification is a detailed process. To help ensure you include all the necessary elements, consider how each of the following can help bolster your case:

- ➤ introduction (objective)
- ➤ brief explanation of what equipment requested does in layman's terms (service provided)
- ➤ indication of whether equipment requested is new, replacement, or additional
- ➤ justification (explanation of why the equipment is needed)
- ➤ benefit for the facility (in layman's terms, as specific and concise as possible)
- ➤ additional usage/revenues
- ➤ specific new tests/procedures
- ➤ estimate of annual volume per test/procedure

(Text continues on page 272.)

Capital justification example

Surgery department
Objective
The surgery department is requesting the purchase of new surgical lights for two operating rooms.
Service provided
This equipment is used to illuminate the surgical field. These lights provide spotlight capabilities, are able to adjust field range, and have dimmer capabilities. Having adequate lighting is necessary to continue providing surgical care to the patient.
New, replacement, or additional
This is a replacement for the present equipment. On the asset listing, most of this equipment shows a useful life of 10 years. The present lights have been in use for over 15 years, and maintenance history shows frequent repairs in the last 2 years.
Justification
Why is the equipment needed?
The equipment is needed to perform surgical procedures to patients in the surrounding counties who come to the facility for surgery. The current equipment isn't providing the light needed.

Additional usage and revenues
Expected use
Use will be daily, or about 260 days/year. Room use is about 80% during scheduled hours. These rooms are also used for emergency cases, which are done 24 hours/day, 7 days/week. On average, 80 emergency cases are performed monthly.
Estimated savings or profits
We must have this equipment if we're to continue providing this service to our patients.

Additional usage
Not applicable.

Evaluation
1. **Conrad:** Conrad lights were brought into OR #7, installed on October 16, 2001, and left up for 6 weeks. During this time, the lights were used for actual surgical cases. Evaluation forms (attached) were handed out to all surgical staff and surgeons. The criteria for evaluation is listed on the form. The lights we're replacing are AMS, which is now Conrad. These lights have served us well over the past 15 to 20 years. These lights were the most favorable in the employee/surgeon evaluations.
2. **Tronics:** Tronics lights were brought into OR #5, installed on October 17, 2001, and left up for 6 weeks. During this time, the lights were used for actual surgical cases. Evaluation forms (attached) were handed out to all surgical staff and surgeons. The criteria for evaluation is listed on the form. These lights were the second favorite in the employee/surgeon evaluations. The sales staff and workmen with this light were outstanding in their customer service. The clinical evaluation of the lights, however, fell short compared to the Conrad light.
3. **Berch:** Berch lights were brought into OR #6, installed on October 15, 2001, and left up for 6 weeks. During this time, the lights were used for actual surgical cases. Evaluation forms (attached) were handed out to all surgical staff and surgeons. The criteria for evalua-

Capital justification example *(continued)*

tion is listed on the form. These lights were the least favorable in the employee/surgeon evaluations.

References
References were obtained from the following hospitals:

1. Conrad
Valley County Hospital, bed size 232.
Have had lights for 10 years. No problems with lights or service.
Tippecanoe Hospital, bed size 150.
Have had lights for 5 years. Very happy with lights and service.

2. Tronics
Community Hospital, bed size 250.
Have had lights for 7 years. No problems with lights or service.
Hancock Hospital, bed size 150.
Have had lights for 3 years. No problem.

3. Berch
Memorial Hospital, bed size 300.
Have had lights for 11 years. No problems with lights or service.
Happiness Hospital, bed size 162.
Have had lights for 5 years. Very happy with lights and service.

Evaluation summary
This trial was an effective way to evaluate these lights. Although somewhat time-consuming, it gave everyone a chance to use, move, focus, and adjust the lights in the actual setting that they'd be used. Both staff and surgeons evaluated them. References were a nonissue because all feedback was positive. As evidenced by the attached evaluations, the Tronics lights are preferred.

Price summary

Conrad		Tronics		Berch	
Cost:	$25,483.00	Cost:	$29,634.00	Cost:	$20,740.00
Less 41%:	$10,533.00	Less 40%:	$11,853.00	Less:	$ 1,865.80
Total Costs:	$14,950.00	Total Costs:	$17,781.00	Total Costs:	$18,874.20

Service contract summary

	Conrad	Tronics	Berch
Warranty period:	1 year	2 years	2 years
Cost of annual maintenance contract:	$370 labor only	$1,200 per room	$813 parts and labor

Service contract recommendation
Wouldn't recommend the extended service contract. Can opt for service contract at any time after purchase. These lights haven't required a great deal of outside service in the past.

Recommendation
Based upon all the information in Exhibit A, the recommendation is that the Conrad lights be purchased. These lights were the most favorable clinically and are the lowest priced.

➤ suggested patient charge
➤ projected annual revenue
➤ other enhanced usage (such as efficiency and productivity), if appropriate, even if additional revenue may not occur
➤ evaluation (listing information separately for each vendor)
➤ steps taken to evaluate equipment
➤ listing of references contracted with bed size (if it's a hospital) and key reference comments
➤ results of your evaluation (evaluation summary)
➤ conclusion statement for each vendor, including those not selected
➤ price summary for each vendor (separate column for each vendor with the vendor name in bold type and underlined at the top of each column)
➤ listing of the grand total cost for each vendor (separate column for each vendor, as under price summary); first item is a warranty period; next item, cost of annual maintenance contract, if applicable, and other maintenance factors pertinent to future cost
➤ service contract recommendation regarding maintenance alternative based on consultation with purchased services committee
➤ recommended vendor, including specific reasons for your recommendation (avoid repeating your reasons for justification) and criteria for decisions (which should be the lowest, best alternative).

Other capital expenses

In a facility, such as a hospital, there are several other major capital expenses besides equipment. These include building repair, land improvements, building additions, and automobiles. Although nurse-managers typically aren't asked to give detailed justifications and receive quotes for these types of major expenses, they are being asked to have more input in the identification, prediction, and decision making that goes into these expenses.

Your role as nurse-manager may be to make rounds in your departments and provide plant engineering with a list of repair and replacement expenses you're anticipating in these areas. Will your station need remodeling to improve efficiency? Is it in the plans to convert semiprivate rooms to private? Is there talk about installing patient showers in each room? These questions are examples of what you as the nurse-manager on the unit may know and need to communicate to plant engineering.

Making a decision

Now it's decision time. Based on your research and calculations, make an educated guess about how much the service will cost to provide and how much the facility will get actually paid. If the difference between the two is "in the black," then your decision is probably much easier. If the difference between the two "is in the red," then you'll need to decide whether it makes sense to go with something that's probably going to lose money for the facility.

Here are some more things to consider: Does it support your mission? Will it keep patients in town, or loyal to your facility and possibly be a means to establish a relationship with them so they use your facility for other health care needs? Can patients access this care somewhere else nearby? Is there another way to treat these patients without this equipment or new procedure?

Nurses, physicians, and finance people need to have a heart-to-heart discussion at this point. Remember, what is best for the facility may not be that it's going to lose substantial money from providing this procedure. On the other hand, those that make decisions based on their mission sometimes provide services that aren't profitable. Although the decision making can be tough, it's easier when you present a complete investigation of facts.

Total agreement isn't always possible among nurses, physicians, and finance people. However, completing the above process can help give everyone a more objective look at the possibilities. (See *Program evaluation example,* pages 274 and 275.)

Points to remember

The following points summarize the value of operational budgeting:

Program evaluation example

Service provided

Microwave therapy to treat benign prostate hyperplasia. Patient population is males, ages 50 to 80. The current surgical population is 45% Medicare.

Use

In a conversation with urologist Dr. Jones, who is requesting this new procedure, the estimate is 6 to 10 patients per month. This estimate is based on the patient population that he currently sees in his office.

Vendors used or evaluated

Information about the procedure have been with TNT technologies. This vendor is also talking to Durk, Community, and Chesterfield Hospitals, all in the VHA system. Another vendor who recently came into the market is Shields, Inc.; however, this group doesn't supply this state at this time.

Length of stay

This procedure can be done in a standard minor procedure room. The average procedure takes 90 minutes, with dismissal occurring 3 hours later. Total expected stay is 5 hours.

Cost of the service

There is no minimum number of patients per day. Each patient is billed for individually, according to the length of contract signed. (1 to 3 years). The following is a summary of the projected costs based on:

Per patient rental based on six procedures: $900
Supplies and drugs: $250
Nursing hours (2 × $22/hour): $44
Total estimated cost: $1,194

Reimbursement

Currently, reimbursement for this outpatient procedure is approved by Aetna and Blue Cross/Blue Shield at the contracted discounted rate, which would be $1,000. Medicare reimbursement for this procedure is $700. Based on the fact that 45% of the patient population is Medicare and that the target age for these patients is between 50 and 80, a high percentage of these patients should be Medicare eligible.
Cost/reimbursement estimates: Aetna and Blue Cross/Blue Shield patients = (−194); Medicare patients = (−494)

Ancillary services

On the average patient, no radiology or laboratory services are required.

Service satisfaction

It's difficult to determine service satisfaction at this time. Data are based on a small patient population. Although this procedure seems initially successful, long-term success can't yet be determined.

Program evaluation example *(continued)*

Summary
Based on the projected patient volume, high percentage of Medicare patient population, and the current Medicare reimbursement, this procedure wouldn't be financially beneficial for the hospital to provide. This patient population is currently being served with surgical intervention. With that in mind, the procedure, long-term outcomes, and evaluation of how many patients in our county are accessing this treatment elsewhere should be further investigated before moving to provide this service at this time.

➤ The functions of budgeting include planning, managing expenses, and controlling spending.

➤ Strong financial planning allows a facility to build a strong capital structure, allocating revenue for capital projects as well as daily operations.

➤ Awareness of reimbursement for a given service is necessary to calculate a profit and loss margin for that service.

➤ Variance in the budget requires critical thinking skills to justify and evaluate the cause of the variance.

➤ Purchase requests require justification of the equipment, including the service it will provide, the necessity of its use, and its expected life, cost, and profit. Supporting documentation should accompany all requests.

Selected readings

Blegen, M.A., et al. "Nurse Staffing and Patient Outcomes," *Nursing Research* 47(1):43-50, January-February 1998.

Cleland, V. *The Economics of Nursing.* Norwalk, Conn.: Appleton and Lang, 1990.

Finkler, S., and Kovner, C. *Financial Management for Nurse Managers and Executives,* 2nd ed. Philadelphia: W.B. Saunders Co., 2000.

Hunt, P. "Speaking the Language of Finance." *AORN Journal* 73(4):774-76, 779-82, 785-87, April, 2001.

Pelfrey, S. "Financial Techniques for Evaluating Equipment Acquisitions," *Journal of Nursing Administration* 21(3):15-20, March 1991.

Strasen, L. *Key Business Skills for Nurse Managers.* Philadelphia: Lippincott Williams & Wilkins, 1987.

Zimmerman, P.G. *Nursing Management Secrets.* Philadelphia: Hanley & Belfus, 2002.

13

Marketing your facility

Pamela S. Hunt, RN, MSN

"Far and away the best prize that life has to offer is the chance to work hard at work worth doing," — Theodore Roosevelt

Marketing has become a primary responsibility for many nurse leaders. Few nursing programs — whether they're associate's or bachelor's degree programs — include how to market a program or service. As a nurse leader, you certainly have the most knowledge about the services you provide, but how do you get this information to the public so that they can assess the care needed?

To answer this question, this chapter explores the goals of marketing, the process for developing a marketing plan, and the issues you need to consider when developing that plan.

Developing a marketing plan

The goals of marketing are to increase volume, maximize customer satisfaction, and improve the quality of life for your community by making them aware of the services you provide. All three are equally important.

Assessing the situation

The marketing plan begins with assessment, followed by the development of a plan, implementation, and evaluation — very much like the nursing process.

The assessment phase begins with knowing what your department has to offer. Make a list of the procedures and services you perform.

Next, assess the community your facility serves. This assessment should include, for example, the age of the population, services available to the community by all health care providers, teenage pregnancy rate, socioeconomic status, public transportation, and available social services. Answer the following questions: Who is our patient population? What services are they willing to access? (See *From cash cows to dogs*, page 278.)

Planning to get the word out

When you know which services you need to target and how much you're going to charge for them, you'll need to plan how you'll publicize them. Several promotional techniques are available. Simply choose the one that fits the service you're marketing.

- ➤ *Word of mouth.* Nothing is better than a personal recommendation. Word of mouth enables you to tell others about the services you're offering so that they can help spread the word. This marketing technique is quick and inexpensive and helps lend credibility to the service you're marketing.
- ➤ *Newspaper articles.* Another way to get the word out is to alert the media. If you live in a midsize or smaller community, the local newspaper may even feature the new services you're providing. However, don't sit back and wait for the newspaper to do the story. It may take a long time, or it may not happen. Instead, write an article to run the week your specialty is being recognized — for example, Critical Care Nurses Week or Perioperative Nurses Week. (Assistance and ideas for writing these articles can be found on the Web site for your specialty organization.) Make sure you also include the services that your department provides to the community on a regular basis.
- ➤ *Paid advertising.* Although paid advertising is another possibility, you may want to find out if your services qualify as public service announcements, which are free-of-charge and which many radio and television stations are required to offer.

From cash cows to dogs

Your marketing strategy should be directed toward programs and services that are profitable and that show a good growth potential, based on the needs of your community.

Services can be evaluated and placed into one of four categories: cash cows, rising stars, question marks, and dogs.

➤ *Cash cows.* Cash cows are services that are profitable but don't show a great deal of growth potential. Although you want to get the word out that you provide these services, you wouldn't want to spend most of your marketing dollars on these services because of the low growth potential.

➤ *Rising stars.* The rising stars are profitable and show good growth potential in your community, so this is where you want to concentrate your marketing efforts and dollars. An increase in volume of the rising stars is obviously going to result in an increase in revenue. Be aware that as time goes on, the rising stars usually become cash cows as the market becomes saturated and volume begins to decrease.

➤ *Question marks.* Question marks are services that don't have a good profit margin but can be moderate revenue producers if the volume is really boosted. Putting marketing dollars into question marks can be risky and tricky. Before investing in the question marks, thoroughly investigate the community to determine if there is sufficient growth potential in the population for these services. If there is, marketing efforts toward promoting these services may be justified.

➤ *Dogs.* Dogs are services that have little to no revenue-producing abilities and little to no growth potential. Dogs are services you provide because it's the "right thing to do" for the patients and the community, but they aren't services where you spend valuable marketing dollars. In the planning stage, determine what kind of promotional technique best fits the program or service you're marketing.

Coming up with a fee

Another planning factor is the price the patient pays for the service. When evaluating a new service, you should compare the cost of the equipment, cost of supplies, length of stay, and the number of staff hours necessary to care for the patient to the reimbursement for the service. When a service seems to be a money loser during this comparison, the facility must decide whether to provide the service because of its commitment to the community or to abort the program and use the dollars in another area.

When considering what the patient pays, money isn't the only factor to consider. Most patients today want little interruption in their activities of daily living; therefore, services should be evaluated as to how much time the targeted patient population would be willing to invest to obtain the service and how much they would be willing to pay for the service. However, before you set the price of the service, especially if it's one that people will pay for directly, check how much demand there is for this service. Some services tend to go in and out of style. For example, wellness services — such as yoga, massage therapy, exercise, and aromatherapy — are all currently in style. Many health care providers are offering these services and are paid directly by the patient. Before setting a price for a service, assess who else is providing these services, what they're charging, and how many people are accessing the service.

> *Community opportunities.* Go to health fairs and community screening programs. The county fair is always a big event and people are always interested in what's going on at the local hospital. Wear uniforms or scrubs, whichever you normally wear at work, and bring videos and props. The public will love it! Think like the patient who is going to access your service. If you're targeting a service that's going to be most valuable to senior citizens, ask to speak about the service to local senior citizen's groups and organizations. If the service is directed at young women and children, contact day care centers in the area or young women's groups. Ask yourself, "Where would I find the patients who need to know this information?"

> *Printed materials.* Printed materials are an important part of the marketing plan. Create pamphlets that are easy to read, have pictures, and tell how wonderful your facility is. Then get them into people's hands.

> *Introductory offers.* These offers are good ways to promote a number of services that the community has a choice and an opportunity to attend or obtain on a trial basis — for example, a cardiac rehabilitation program or a smoking-cessation class.

> *Traditional sales call.* These calls are well suited for occupational health services and health screenings — that is, services that are sold to other companies.

Planning the evaluation

When you've determined how, where, and when to promote your service, it's imperative that you write actual goals for the service with measurable outcomes. This step helps to guide your interventions and evaluate the effectiveness of the program.

 CASE IN POINT

A local hospital was in the process of developing a preadmission testing (PAT) program for surgical patients. It determined that its target population was all patients having scheduled surgery. One goal was to increase surgical PAT volume by 40% in the first 6 months. Interventions were then listed under the goal that would hopefully enable the facility to realize the 40% increase. Those interventions included meeting with the surgeon's office managers (who were going to hand out information about the PAT program), educating the surgeons, writing a feature in the hospital newspaper, and writing an article for the local newspaper. After implementing and evaluating these interventions, the hospital determined that it achieved 52% patient compliance in 6 months.

In continued evaluation, the facility brainstormed for ways to improve the percentage of compliance. Returning to the assessment phase, the staff realized that although the surgeons and office managers were doing a fair job of promoting the program, they wanted the program to be so well accepted that patients themselves would ask to go through the program when scheduled for surgery.

About this same time, two patients had written letters stating their appreciation of the PAT program and the anxiety that it removed from their surgical experience. Capitalizing on the positive feedback, the hospital produced a simple 60-second commercial for a local television station. It was filmed in the hospital cafeteria and featured one patient reading excerpts from the letter she had written telling how the PAT program had improved her surgical experience. Within a few weeks, the number of PAT patients began to increase. When scheduled for surgery, patients began asking their surgeons to refer them to "that nurse that talks with you before you have surgery." Within a few months, the program was seeing 97% of all scheduled surgical patients.

Further evaluation led to connecting the PAT nurse's home computer to the hospital network so that she could complete assessments during the evening for those patients who weren't at home during the day. ●

No matter how successful initial marketing interventions are, constant evaluation of the service, the goals, the patient population, and the pricing is necessary. As in the PAT example, the initial interventions were successful, but further evaluation and brainstorming lead to another intervention, using the patient's perspective, to increase compliance further and exceed the established goals. So remember the process you know best — assess, plan, implement, and evaluate. A program with thorough assessment, detailed planning, smooth implementation, and continuous evaluation will lead to successful marketing and goal achievement!

Writing the executive summary

Whether you're asking for additional employees, capital equipment, or operational supplies or outlining a marketing strategy, the information presented to the executive leadership should be concise and to the point. All critical, bottom-line information should be on the first page. Critical information includes the purpose of the request, how this request relates to the mission of the facility, and the final recommendation.

Attach supporting documentation and details behind the summary page for their information, including your work from the investigation and planning phase to come up with the recommendation. Depending on what you're asking for, the documentation may include calculations for additional staffing, predictions and methods for operational budgeting, thorough investigation and justification for the capital equipment, program evaluation steps, and complete marketing assessment, plan, and projected implementation. When able, use tables, pie charts, or line or bar graphs — any kind of visual aid to present or accentuate your point. Using colored charts and graphs as summaries can provide the impact that standard text simply doesn't have.

If you've done your homework well, by the time you get to the point where you're presenting it to administration, you'll feel confident in your recommendation and be able to speak the foreign language of finance.

The big picture

Now that you know a lot more about your department's financial needs and considerations, you need to take a look at some facilitywide issues, which may also impact what you're doing in your department. Remember, knowledge is power, and what impacts the bottom line of the facility impacts your passion as well.

Every facility has various spreadsheets to show financial status. These spreadsheets are designed in a way to clearly show the assets and the facility's liabilities. (See *Combined balance sheets,* page 282, *Combined statements of operations and changes in net assets,* page 283, and *Combined statements of cash flow,* page 284, to see examples of various statements used in most facilities.)

Review these spreadsheets to familiarize yourself with what's included. Then, if this information is available to you in your facility, make an appointment with someone in finance who can explain the spreadsheet. After all, it's better to be a nurse leader who goes to director meetings every month, reviews this infor-

Combined balance sheets

Assets	August 31, 2000	August 31, 1999
Current assets:		
Cash and cash equivalents		
Operating	$10,635,590	$16,351,137
Trustee-held funds	1,923,728	1,902,325
	12,559,318	18,253,462
Patient accounts receivable, less allowances for Doubtful accounts (2000 — $15,424,000; 1999 — $13,882,000)	53,686,982	47,110,045
Other receivables	869,853	1,048,370
Inventories, prepaid expenses, and other current assets	10,258,206	8,646,217
Total current assets	77,374,359	75,058,094
Investments limited as to use, less current portion:		
Construction and debt service funds held by trustee	3,240,636	4,315,000
Board designated capital and debt reserve funds	11,163,629	9,887,602
Temporarily restricted funds	1,378,266	1,322,717
Total investments limited as to use, less current portion	15,782,531	15,525,319
Property and equipment:		
Costs	154,167,866	146,231,766
Less allowances for depreciation	97,070,225	89,185,850
Total property and equipment	57,097,641	57,045,916
Other assets:		
Goodwill	1,420,464	1,564,874
Other	3,644,440	4,851,545
Total other assets	5,064,904	6,416,419
Total assets	$155,319,435	$154,045,748

Liabilities and net assets		
Current liabilities:		
Accounts payable and accrued liabilities	$9,545,359	$12,209,268
Salaries, wages, and related liabilities	6,558,650	5,715,997
Estimated payables to third-party payers	2,721,059	5,017,275
Current portion of long-term debt	1,157,124	2,861,725
Total current liabilities	19,982,192	25,804,265
Noncurrent liabilities:		
Deferred revenue	1,575,824	1,692,863
Accrued pension cost	3,620,023	3,422,975
Long-term debt, less current portion	39,128,529	40,264,997
	44,324,376	45,380,835
Net assets:		
Unrestricted	89,634,601	81,537,931
Temporarily restricted	1,378,266	1,322,717
	91,012,867	82,860,648
Total liabilities and net assets	$155,319,435	$154,045,748

Combined statements of operations and changes in net assets

	Year ended August 31, 2000	Year ended August 31, 2001
Unrestricted revenue and other support:		
Net patient service revenue	$226,009,321	$210,943,852
Premium revenue	12,605,477	17,242,802
Other revenue	7,424,125	9,070,442
Total unrestricted revenue and other support	246,038,923	237,257,096
Expenses:		
Salaries, wages, and benefits	101,873,002	96,867,314
Medical supplies and drugs	46,971,343	44,238,420
Contract and purchased services	31,762,478	32,493,277
Utilities, supplies, and other	32,009,262	29,476,285
Provision for doubtful accounts	14,639,719	16,462,942
Depreciation and amortization	9,102,050	8,501,404
Interest	2,152,632	2,493,246
Special charge for early retirement and employee separation	2,464,252	
Total expenses	238,510,486	232,997,140
Net income	7,528,437	4,259,956

mation, and understands the financial picture of the facility than one who doesn't.

Dealing with the changing reimbursement picture

With the "graying of America," most hospitals are serving a significant percentage of Medicare patients. Medicare regulations are like a living document—just when you think you understand them, they change. In 1965, Medicare reimbursement was based on the total percentage of Medicare patients served by the hospital and the total hospital expenses. Therefore, if the hospital's patient population was 40% Medicare, Medicare would pay 40% of the hospital's total expenses. As you can guess, this method of payment did nothing to control spending and expenses for the Medicare system.

In 1983, Medicare implemented the Diagnostic Related Group (DRG) method of payment for inpatients, which gives the hospital a predetermined amount of money based on the pa-

Combined statements of cash flows

	Year ended August 31, 2000	Year ended August 31, 1999
Cash flows from operating activities:		
Increase in net assets	$8,152,219	$5,607,113
Adjustments to reconcile increase in net assets to net cash		
Provided by operating activities:		
Depreciation and amortization	9,102,050	8,501,404
Equity in net income of joint venture and other	(715,830)	(1,593,508)
Net periodic pension cost	2,492,048	2,868,321
Net unrealized appreciation of investments	(245,128)	(888,662)
Changes in operating assets and liabilities:		
Patient accounts receivable, net	(6,576,937)	(4,015,945)
Other current assets	(1,433,472)	(527,268)
Accounts payable and accrued liabilities	(2,663,909)	(88,970)
Salaries, wages, and related liabilities	842,653	1,779,346
Estimated payables to third-party payers	(2,296,216)	1,500,737
Net cash provided by operating activities	6,657,478	13,142,568
Investing activities		
Purchases of property and equipment, net	(8,875,362)	(9,549,311)
Transfers from donor restricted funds for purchase of property		
and equipment	372,295	452,250
Net transfers into board designated funds	(1,061,756)	(1,401,994)
Purchase of trustee held investments	(7,231,744)	(7,211,621)
Release of trustee held funds for construction, debt service		
and other	8,267,148	7,138,952
Pension plan funding	(2,295,000)	(2,541,806)
Other investing activities, net	1,292,463	1,073,927
Net cash used in investing activities	(9,531,956)	(12,039,603)
Financing activities		
Repayments of long-term debt	(2,841,069)	(2,849,989)
Net cash used in financing activities	(2,841,069)	(2,849,989)
Decrease in cash and cash equivalents	(5,715,547)	(1,747,024)
Cash and cash equivalents at beginning of year	16,351,137	18,098,161
Cash and cash equivalents at end of year	$10,635,590	$16,351,137

tient's condition, regardless of how much it actually costs to complete the patient's care. With the DRG method of payment, more procedures, tests, and services doesn't equal more revenue and payment for the hospital.

It took until 1986 for Medicare to change the payment method for outpatients. That year, it began reimbursing selected outpatient services by a fee schedule (much like the DRG payments for inpatient care), although some were paid by a cost formula.

Continuing the desire to control Medicare costs, in August 2000, Medicare implemented Ambulatory Payment Classifications (APCs). APCs are the official DRGs of outpatient care. The facility receives one predetermined reimbursement for the patient's procedure. Seldom does the reimbursement for the service come near the charge for the service. As mentioned earlier, when you're doing a complete program evaluation, reimbursement versus the cost to provide the service becomes important in determining whether it's right to provide a service that you know is going to cost more than the reimbursement.

Medicare allows for additional reimbursement in outpatient care for supplies called the C codes of the Healthcare Common Procedural Coding Systems (HCPCS). HCPCS codes are pass-through codes for additional dollars on a limited number of supply items and devices. If a facility identifies and codes these allowable items properly, then it gets additional reimbursement, besides the procedure-coded APC; however, if it doesn't, then no additional reimbursement is made. What's more, large monetary fines exist if items are coded incorrectly. These regulations change so frequently that a detailed listing of what's currently on the pass-through list and what isn't would be out of date before the book was printed. There's a complete list in the *Federal Register,* which you can access on-line for more information.

Keeping current with health care reimbursement issues can be difficult and time-consuming, but it's necessary to understand potential revenue and resources for the facility. With limited resources, you must constantly make choices based on the priorities of the facility and the national and local economy and reimbursement issues that limit your choices.

Few professions have undergone the dramatic changes in role function, competency, and accountability as the bedside nurse and nurse-manager. Clinical competency isn't the only tool needed in an era where economics dominates the health care industry. As nurse leaders, you need to have the knowledge and foresight to ask the right questions, leading to the right answers, to give nursing the influence needed to plan for the future and protect patient care.

Points to remember

The following points summarize the value of fine-tuning the services your unit can provide to others:

➤ The goals of marketing are to increase volume, maximize customer satisfaction, and improve quality of life for your community.
➤ You can develop a marketing plan by following the steps included in the nursing process — assessment, planning, implementation, and evaluation.
➤ Keeping current with health care issues helps you identify potential revenue and resources for your facility.

Selected readings

American Organization of Nurse Executives. *Market-Driven Nursing: Developing and Marketing Patient Care Services.* Chicago: Health Forum, 1999.
Roederer, C. "Strategic Planning for Recruitment and Retention of Health Care Professionals," *Oncology Issues* 16(5):31-34, September 2001.

PART FOUR

Quality care skills

CHAPTER 14

Quality is key

Marie Brewer, RN, LNC

> "Customer and organizational perceptions of value may be out of sync because customer expectations are changing so quickly today. Organizations that are not tuned into their customers often miss these shifts — until someone else bursts onto the scene with more customer-responsive products or services." — Jim Clemmer, *Firing on All Cylinders*

Quality management, quality assurance, total quality management, and *continuous quality management* are all terms related to the same subject — improving what you do every day. It means learning from your mistakes, or "failing forward."

George Bernard Shaw coined the saying, "Success does not consist in never making mistakes but in never making the same one a second time." This is true when it comes to quality management and quality improvement processes. These processes prevent you from accepting that you've arrived and can do no better than you're doing right now.

Failing forward

Use mistakes as an opportunity to reexamine the process and rethink the goal. This is continual learning. Continuous improvement of quality has become a necessary and integral part of health care. The requirements for improving quality include a

It only takes a DIME!

The following four basic themes put quality management in simple terms. To be successful in your quality management programs, you must:
➤ *d*elight the customer
➤ *i*mprove the process
➤ *m*anage by facts
➤ *e*mpower the people.
It's simple; just remember the acronym DIME — delight, improve, manage, and empower.

common purpose and knowledge of concepts and methods so that changes result in improvement.

Measuring satisfaction

Responding to market changes and increased competition for patients, many health care facilities have shifted their focus to emphasize customer satisfaction and cost savings. The race is on to improve systems and to streamline care delivery, while continuing to improve quality of care.

To know that what you're doing is improving, you must have tools to measure your progress — and you can only have those tools after you identify your goals and objectives and then set policies, procedures, and protocols to define where you need to be and how you're going to get there. Total quality management is a business and life philosophy that embraces all activities through which the needs of the customer and the community and the objectives of the facility are satisfied in the most efficient and cost-effective way, by maximizing the potential of all employees in a continuing drive for improvement.[1] (See *It only takes a DIME!*)

Assessing quality

P.G. Martin defined *quality assessment* (quality management) as a formal, systematic program by which care rendered to patients is measured against established criteria.[2] Ongoing monitoring of systems is necessary to ensure that problems are identified early and appropriate intervention is initiated. Such inspection estab-

Total quality management

Three working premises emerge with the total quality management approach:
➤ Quality is important and can be measured.
➤ People are a critical part of the solution and not necessarily the problem.
➤ Change is fundamental and always present, but change can be managed to improve any organization.

lishes thresholds for acceptability and improves quality. This definition can be applied to any process, not just to patient care.

Replacing the traditional "search, blame, and punish" approach to quality assurance with the more positive approach of analyzing an entire event and looking for ways to improve the outcome of similar events invites all nurses and other staff to participate. This shift to emphasizing results or outcomes makes a lot of sense. Remember, though, that for any quality or improvement plan to work, it must have the involvement and support of all staff and a sincere commitment from management. According to the Joint Commission on Accreditation of Healthcare Organizations (JCAHO), any decision that affects the delivery of patient care in an attempt to improve the quality of the outcomes must have nursing input.[3]

The International Organization for Standardization (ISO) defines *quality management* as "a comprehensive and fundamental rule or belief for leading and operating an organization aimed at continually improving performance over the long term by focusing on customers while addressing the needs of all stakeholders."

Working toward improvement

All of the definitions and philosophies above boil down to one thing – doing what you do, whatever that may be, better and better. You benchmark first against yourself and then against your peers in your field of operation. The modern quality movement began with the work of W. Edward Deming, whose 85-15 rule states: "When something goes wrong, 85 percent of the problem is related to systems failure; 15 percent is the fault of the people involved." Quality management focuses on the system, not on the individual. Total quality management is a broad concept that includes the continuous quality improvement process. (See *Total quality management.*)

The face of quality

Quality in health care has many faces, definitions, and interpretations. Unfortunately, quality activities in health care are usually associated with what seems to be additional work, such as required measurements and tracking that seem to benefit the administration of the facility rather than patient care and services.

In this chapter, you'll review the different faces of quality and gain insight into what *quality* means in a health care setting. The continuous improvement of quality of care and services has become a necessary and integral part of health care. The requirements for improving quality are a common purpose and knowledge of concepts and methods so that change results in improvement. Improvement of quality is predicated on change. When you're thinking about quality management or quality improvement, remember the following humorous but true saying: "Insanity is doing the same thing over and over again but expecting a different outcome."

Unless you put a plan together and continually monitor and report feedback on results, you'll be doing the same thing and expecting something different to happen. You'll also not get the vital buy-in of all staff unless you have continual monitoring, support, and feedback.

Pioneers for quality

Three quality management pioneers whose styles should be recognized when considering the multitude of quality management programs are W. Edward Deming, Philip Crosby, and Joseph Juran. Each had his own model, with all having the goal of improving the quality of care and services. Although all three may not be relevant to your management style, all have merit in the challenging area of quality management in health care settings.

W. Edward Deming — points of quality

W. Edward Deming is considered a guru for quality in business. A physics major, he emphasized the concept of minimization of variation as an effective means toward quality management. Deming felt that management needed to be part of the solution and have active participation in quality programs. His points of quality are:

➤ Create consistency of purpose toward quality improvement.
➤ Adopt a philosophy that expects good products and service.
➤ Cease dependence on mass inspection and build quality into the product or service.
➤ Award business not solely based on price tag.
➤ Constantly improve the system of production and service.
➤ Institute on-the-job training, education, and self-improvement.
➤ Institute leadership; eliminate number quotas and management by objective.
➤ Drive out fear.
➤ Break down barriers between departments.
➤ Eliminate slogans, exhortations, and targets.
➤ Remove barriers to pride of workmanship.
➤ Take action to accomplish the transformation.

According to Deming: "Rational behavior requires theory. Reactive behavior only requires reflex action."

Philip Crosby — 14 essential components

Philip Crosby, philosopher and author, teaches that management can be more successful preventing problems rather than fixing them. "Do it right the first time!" is his credo. Crosby's 14 essential components to quality management are:

➤ Management commitment to quality improvement
➤ Quality improvement team to oversee action
➤ Quality measurement appropriate to the activities undergoing improvement
➤ Cost of quality evaluation using estimates as necessary
➤ Quality awareness promoted through various medical and supervisor involvement

➤ Corrective actions generated in response to the third and fourth points above
➤ Zero defect planning tailored to the company and its products
➤ Supervisory training at all management levels
➤ Zero Defects Day to celebrate a new performance standard
➤ Goal setting for individuals and groups
➤ Management's removal of the cause of the error after notification
➤ Recognition of goals met
➤ Quality councils' sharing of experiences, problems, and ideas
➤ Repetition (quality improvement is a never-ending process).

According to Crosby: "The new generation of management needs to understand their personal role in implanting quality and engaging the employees in the vision of the company."

Joseph Juran — Juran Trilogy

Joseph Juran — business executive, government administrator, lecturer, author, and consultant — was the first to incorporate the human aspect of quality management. The major points of Juran's quality management ideas include:

➤ Quality planning
– Determine customers.
– Determine customers' needs.
– Develop products or services for customers.
– Develop processes to produce products or services.
➤ Quality control
– Evaluate performance.
– Compare performance to goals.
– Act on differences.
➤ Quality improvement
– Establish infrastructure.
– Identify needs for improvements or projects.
– Establish project teams.
– Provide teams with resources, motivation, and training.

Says Juran: "It's your responsibility to school yourself and learn how to become a quality leader."

Quality management

With growing local, regional, national, and global competition, quality management is becoming increasingly important to the leadership and management of all facilities. This importance is related not only to the care you provide at the bedside but also to the basic administrative tasks you perform every day, for example, promoting your facility and handling billing, collection, staffing, recruitment, and retention issues.

Following principles

All quality initiatives have the goal of improving the quality of care or services to a customer at some level in the service chain. By applying the following eight Quality Management Principles from ISO, facilities can produce the benefit of improved quality for all customers (patients, owners, employees, suppliers, and the society at large).

Customer focus

Consider your customer, the most important person in any business. A customer is deserving of the most courteous, most attentive, and highest quality care and treatment that you can provide. A customer gives purpose to your work — and is the lifeblood of your business. All quality programs and processes should focus on improving the care and services rendered to your customers, regardless of who they are — patients, other nurses, vendors, physicians, or others. These programs should also be aimed as containing cost, preserving resources, and expediting care. (See *The disappearing customer.*)

Facilities depend on customers and therefore should understand current and future customer need, meet customer requirements, and strive to exceed customer expectations. A customer brings you his wants and needs, and it's your job to fill those needs and to provide the best care and service you can. It's your job to monitor the outcome of the care and service to determine how you performed and what you need to do better the next time. To meet and exceed customer expectation, you must continually measure satisfaction and act on improvements.

QUESTIONS & ANSWERS

The disappearing customer

Question: *Do you know the six reasons customers stop doing business with a facility?*
Answer:
➤ 1% die.
➤ 3% move out of the area.
➤ 5% do business with new acquaintances.
➤ 9% go to the competition.
➤ 14% are dissatisfied with a product or service.
➤ 68% have been mistreated by one of the staff.

Leadership

Leaders establish unity of purpose and direction within a facility. They provide vision, direction, and an understanding of shared values and then set challenging goals and objectives to achieve them. They coach, facilitate, and empower people to be successful. They create and maintain an internal environment in which people can become fully involved in achieving the facility's objectives. What's more, they empower and assign individuals to lead improvement initiatives by providing the time, resources, and support needed to make the individual successful and to promote the resulting improvement throughout the facility.

Involvement of people

The essence of any organization is people at every level — and their full involvement enables their abilities to be used for the organization's and the patients' benefit. Leaders establish competency levels and select, train, and qualify personnel. They provide clear authority and responsibility for employees. To have successful involvement of all employees, a facility must create personal ownership of its goals by maximizing employee knowledge and experience. Through education, it must encourage employees to become involved in operational decisions and the process as a whole.

Process approach

A desired result is achieved more efficiently by managing related resources and activities as a process. Continually monitoring, analyzing, and improving performance of clinical staff, services, and operational and administrative processes is the heart of performance improvement using a process approach.

System approach to management

Identifying, understanding, and managing a system of interrelated processes for a given objective improves the facility's effectiveness and efficiency. Leaders within the facility must explicitly identify internal and external customers and suppliers. They must focus on the planned use of resources in activities leading to effective use of people, equipment, methods, and materials.

Continual improvement

Continual improvement should be a permanent objective of the facility. Leaders must set realistic and challenging improvement goals, provide resources, and offer employees tools, opportunities, and encouragement to contribute to the continual improvement of processes and customer service.

Factual approach to decision making

Effective decisions and actions are based on the analysis of data and information. Effort is placed on minimizing cost, improving performance and market share, and improving customer service through the use of suitable tools and technology. Some of these tools and methods are discussed later in this chapter.

Mutually beneficial supplier relationships

Although most facilities are independent from their suppliers, a mutually beneficial relationship can enhance a facility's ability to create value, which improves the quality of patient care and services. You are, however, only as good as the employees or contractors that you employ.

Before using external contractors, you must adequately define and document all requirements. You must also review and evaluate performance to control the quality of products and services. When establishing strategic alliances or partnerships, ensure early involvement and participation by defining the requirements for joint development and improvement of products, processes, and systems. It might take valuable resources, but the time spent developing mutual trust, respect, and commitment to customer satisfaction and continuous quality improvement will be well worth the effort in the long term.

Following beliefs

Quality management is the process facilities use to improve their ability to satisfy customer expectations. A key to understanding this process is recognizing the central importance of the customer. In business, a customer buys services from a vendor and is free to buy — or not buy — from whomever he chooses. Patients — who are essentially customers of health care institutions — can select services that meet their expectations and reject those that don't. The following beliefs form the basis of the quality management approach and the measure of the health care facility's success for the future:

➤ Quality management is a positive strategy for growth and should be integrated into a facility's strategic plan.
➤ Top management must be committed to and actively involved in the quality management process.
➤ Quality management is a process, not a program.
➤ Quality improvement processes must be applied to all levels of a facility.
➤ Quality improvement benefits everyone, both internally and externally.[4]

Quality assurance

In traditional organizational structures, quality assurance activities are part of the organizational mandate to ensure that outcomes of work and services provided are as prescribed. Quality assurance has undergone many changes since its formal adoption into clinical nursing practice in the early 1970s. It was incorporated into all nursing organizations in the delivery of care and service to meet the requirements of the Joint Commission on Accreditation of Healthcare Organizations.

Quality assurance involves the monitoring of patient care activities, or other activities, to determine their degree of accuracy and excellence. Quality assurance in health care is comparable to

The manager's role in quality assurance

Quality assurance is a staff process. It relates directly to how the staff delivers the care and services required to meet patient needs. In nursing, the professional has an obligation to ensure that practice is consistent with the standards of the profession, the requirements of the patient, and the needs of the location or facility where the care is being provided.

Although you may strongly voice your concerns about the quality of care and services when others are performing the tasks, as a nurse-manager you must assume control of the decision and make the best choices by mastering the skill of delegation and directing the process. You must be assertive, not aggressive, in your pursuit of quality care and services to your patients. You must apply high standards of quality to every task.

The nurse-manager should develop methods at the unit or facility level to ensure that each nurse recognizes that quality assurance isn't a function separate from her role but a necessary component that should be incorporated into every aspect of work. If this is done effectively, quality activities should be written into the performance expectations of the job description.

quality control in the industrial setting. Its purpose is to set standards for care and service, to evaluate the care and services provided, and to initiate change in care or productivity when either doesn't meet the established or expected standards.

Many facilities don't focus directly on the quality assurance concept, because guaranteeing or ensuring that all quality standards are met can be quite a risk. The quality assurance component is a part of the entire quality management and continuous quality improvement program.

Following a program

A quality assurance program in a health care setting is designed to demonstrate and monitor the facility's actual performance against established standards or criteria. (See *The manager's role in quality assurance.*)

Any quality assurance program should encompass five general areas, including:

➤ monitoring and evaluating care and services
➤ identifying, hiring, and retaining the appropriate personnel to meet patient care and service need

Organizational tasks

In terms of quality assurance, the nursing organization has a responsibility to:
➤ develop the conceptual framework for nursing in the organization
➤ define standards of practice that can provide basic measurable criteria upon which to measure and validate performance
➤ develop a system that each nurse must follow that will identify her compliance with quality standards and identify any areas of needed improvements in the delivery of care
➤ develop a mechanism for continually monitoring the effectiveness of nursing care as both a collective and an individual professional activity.

➤ meeting rules, regulations, and standards set by the Center for Medicare and Medicaid Services, accrediting bodies, and professional organizations
➤ speaking to risk management issues
➤ addressing and resolving any identified problems or issues.[5]

The purpose, roles, scope, relationships, and effectiveness of a quality program can be assessed by addressing several questions as the program is being developed and used. Is there a clearly written plan that's based on the organizational mission, vision, and philosophy? Are goals clearly stated, and are they specific, realistic, measurable, and achievable with the resources that are available? Does the program meet all requirements of the various regulatory and accrediting bodies? Is the plan designed in a cycle that begins with clarification and problem identification and ends with sustained improvement? Are sufficient resources available to implement and maintain the plan? Are teams, committees, bedside staff, management, and other employees appropriately coordinated and integrated, and does the plan include all departments? Have both strengths and weaknesses been identified?[6] (See *Organizational tasks.*)

Continuous quality improvement

Continuous quality improvement (CQI) is a philosophy that encourages all members of a facility to identify new and better ways to do their job. CQI is sometimes referred to as total quality management (TQM). Both models are basically the same in their process and outcome.

For health care workers, the process requires cooperation among all departments and services to ultimately improve service and increase job satisfaction. For patients or other customers, on-going quality improvement saves time and reduces delays in service, reduces stress because patients know what to expect and when, avoids complications, and saves money and resources. With such outcomes, patients can recover more quickly and view their experience in the facility more positively.

According to Foster: "Quality is never an accident; it is always the result of high intention, sincere effort, intelligent direction, and skillful execution; it represents the wise choice of many alternatives."

Putting the customer first

In the CQI process, the customer, whether internal or external, always comes first. However, every employee is also important, and the CQI/TQM process encourages workers from every level to participate in improvement processes. Remember: Sometimes the best ideas come from the people who do the work.

CRUCIAL COMMUNICATION Internal and external customers need to talk and respond to one another. You need to ask how you did and find ways to streamline what you do. After all, the job of a good manager is to identify and remove speed bumps that may hinder employees. Simply remember to look at the process, not the person.

Ongoing improvement is crucial to CQI. Waiting for problems and dealing with them when they occur — also known as "fire fighting" — is a slow, costly, backward approach to quality improvement. Therefore, you must continuously find better ways of doing things. Finally, when you've made an improvement, you must sustain it. Nothing is worse than wasting valuable resources, not to mention the respect of the staff, when something that's finally working well is forgotten.

One of CQI's most important concepts is to celebrate your victories, no matter how minor. A leader spends a lot of time being a cheerleader for her staff and the facility. Tell people when they do well. Tell other people when someone does well. Celebrate the win!

Tools of the trade

Another important concept of CQI involves allocation of resources—specifically, not assigning a team to fix a simple problem. As Ross Perot said, "You don't need a committee to kill a snake!" So use your resources wisely, and pick the right tool to do the job.

Different tools can be used to analyze problems and improve performance. Again, some are complicated and some are easy. Most managers find that a simple graph tells a quality story much better than a written report.

The type of tool your facility selects isn't as important as the consistency of its use. It's impossible to get accurate data for making decisions if the tool keeps changing midstream. Consistent use of such tools is called "comparing apples to apples." Simply choose the tool that works best in your situation, and commit resources to it for at least a year, to obtain useful data.

FOCUS-PDCA One of the easiest and most used tools to improve quality in the CQI process is FOCUS-PDCA. It's a simple tool that can be used for any quality improvement undertaking.

The FOCUS-PDCA model works as follows:

F – Find a process to improve.

O – Organize a team that knows the process at hand.

C – Clarify current knowledge of the said process.

U – Understand all sources of variation.

S – Select the improvement.

P – Plan the improvement, and continue collecting data.

D – Implement the improvement, and collect and analyze the data.

C – Check and study the results.

A – Take steps to sustain any gains from the improvement, and continue improving.

FLOW CHARTS Flow charts show all steps in a process and give people a visual of the "big picture" so they see how each step is related to the next. Flow charts also help identify the most efficient way to complete a task or process.

PARETO CHARTS Pareto charts are bar graphs that show in descending order how often a situation occurs. They identify consistent or frequent problems, and they help the team decide where to begin the improvement process.

SCATTER DIAGRAMS Scatter diagrams show relationships between occurrences, situations, or actions. They allow the team to identify variables and the ways these variables affect the outcome.

FISHBONE DIAGRAMS Fishbone diagrams are visuals used to show cause and effect. They help people explore what, when, and why therapy went wrong (or right).

CONTROL CHARTS Control charts show the expected range of variation for a selected task or situation. They visually identify both trends and random variations in data. The standard requires at least seven points of data in order to see a true trend.

Setting priorities

As you read this chapter, think about all the areas that could be targeted for improvement in your facility, your city or town, and your home. Write these ideas down. If you're like most people, the list will be long and will cover many areas. Now, think of your resource pool. Few people, whether at work or at home, have a bottomless pocketbook. You have to pick and choose how to spend your time and money because you can't have or do it all. The same thing happens when a facility implements a quality improvement plan. All of a sudden, ideas for improvement seem to come out of the woodwork, with every one of them being just as important as the others in the eyes of those who proposed them. What do you do? You prioritize. One of the most common sets of prioritization criteria that health care facilities use determines rank (importance) by asking:

➤ Is it high risk clinically or financially?

➤ Is it a high-cost item?

➤ Is there a high incidence of occurrence?

Identified teams should measure each item on their list against these three areas to determine what they should work on first.

Most facilities have two tiers of performance improvement projects. The first are those that affect and involve the facility as a whole. The second are projects that are specific to a given area, such as wait time in an outpatient laboratory.

To measure or not to measure

You need to remember that you can't measure everything! If you do, you'll have huge—albeit interesting—collections of "so what" data. Some studies and data collection processes might be fun to do, but if the information being collected doesn't affect the bottom line clinically or financially, then most facilities simply don't have the resources to commit to the studies.

One recommendation commonly made to facilities embarking on a performance or quality improvement process is to conduct an inventory of all measures. Most people are amazed when they see that certain data are collected or certain studies are conducted simply because that's the way things have always been done. Going through this exercise with your facility is an eye-opening experience. People need permission to stop collecting data. They need a way to bring appropriate closure to something that has been done for years.

Giving feedback

People need both positive and negative feedback. They need to know what is expected of them, how much, when, and why. They then need to know whether they successfully accomplished what was expected and, if not, what they need to do differently next time. Giving feedback on these issues is all part of the performance improvement process. Think about watching an infant learn to walk. They have the objective of getting into and reaching more things, and they have an innate desire to learn and get better at what they do. Babies don't go from their bellies to their feet. They take many steps in between. They have to determine the best way to get up on their knees. When there, how do they move forward without falling on their noses? It's a progression of trial and error with a specific goal in mind that brings babies to their feet. Quality improvement is the same way. Set a goal and, through trail and error, find your way there. Celebrate the good, and rethink the areas that still need improvement.

Developing and using protocols

According to *Merriam Webster's Medical Dictionary*, a *protocol* is "a detailed plan or an official accounting of a procedure." Simply put, it's a road map of care that is developed using known history and variations in the outcomes of care of a particular diagnosis, treatment, surgery, or procedure. Clinical protocols are also known as care paths and clinical pathways. They're simply care and case management tools that organize expected patient care interventions and clinical outcomes for a specific category of patient across the various points of service in the continuum of care.

Protocols, guidelines, and pathways

In the medical domain, clinical practice protocols and guidelines build a commonly accepted way to improve patient health care and service delivery. The rationalization behind the development and use of clinical protocols is to increase productivity while simultaneously reducing cost of care without adversely affecting the quality of care. In fact, in many cases, the use of protocols improves care by increasing coordination and flow of services. One step toward this aim is the use of commonly accepted standardized health care procedures and protocols. Such treatment procedures are called *clinical practice guidelines* and protocols. In 1990, the Institute of Medicine defined *practice guidelines* as "systematically developed statements to assist professionals in making patient care decisions for appropriate health care intervention or specific clinical situations."[7] A clinical protocol is a more detailed version of a clinical practice guideline and refers to a specific class of therapeutic intervention. Protocols are used for utilization review, improving quality assurance, reducing variation in clinical practice, guiding data collection, ensuring better interpretation and management of the patient's status, activating alerts and reminders, and improving decision support.[8]

Not all protocols and pathways are set in stone. Many are kept flexible in order to meet the needs of all patients who fall within the same groups. The plan, just like a road map during a trip, may need to be modified based on patient condition, progress or regression, variations in need, and physician request. The clinical pathway or protocol should be developed by a multidisciplinary team in order to be most effective in predicting and improving patient care outcomes.

TAKING THE STEPS The steps involved in developing a protocol or pathway include:

➤ *Selecting the patient population.* Refer back in this chapter to the section on setting priorities. Most protocols are developed initially for high-cost, high-risk, or rarely done patient procedures.
➤ *Defining the boundaries.* Do you want the protocol to cover only the procedure itself, or do you want it to cover the continuum of care from the point of entry into your facility or the point of a particular service?
➤ *Collecting data.* What are the expected outcomes from the specified care paths or protocols? What has happened in the industry, and how does your facility compare? What is the cost? What is the length of stay? What do you want to improve?
➤ *Reviewing clinical practice.* This is probably the most important step in the development process. All aspects of care and disciplines involved in that care should be reviewed, with the final goal being to determine desired patient outcomes and to outline protocols that will support the desired outcome.
➤ *Drafting the protocol.* After all clinical practice has been reviewed and all data have been collected and analyzed, the protocol can be drafted.
➤ *Reviewing and revising.* After the appropriate team has reviewed and revised the selected protocol, the draft is shared with all others who will be involved in the implementation or who might have valuable input. When all input has been gleaned from other professionals, the protocol can be put in place.

TRACKING VARIANCE Part of developing a protocol includes determining early on what is to be improved through the use of the protocol. Based on this information, the next step is to track where and what variations may occur outside of the expected outcome. This will help determine whether the protocol is on track or needs adjustment and will also help leadership prioritize the variations to determine whether they're actually negative and whether they impact clinical or financial outcomes in a way that warrants changing the protocol.

EVALUATING THE OUTCOMES Evaluating the outcomes is the final step in the clinical protocol process. When you use a protocol, you want to look at what happens because of it. That involves measuring outcomes. Choose outcomes that the facility or the professionals providing the care have control over changing and that impact the facility. Using a few carefully selected measures that can be incorporated into routine care is the easiest way to accomplish this step. Outcomes need to focus on patient clinical status, customer satisfaction, and cost. The quality management plan in each facility is used to continuously analyze and improve patient care and service processes and outcomes.

JCAHO steps in the quality process

JCAHO performance improvement standards touch all chapters and functions of the JCAHO accreditation process. The overall goal of improving facility performance is to ensure that the facility designs processes well and systematically monitors, analyzes, and improves its performance to improve patient outcomes. Value in health care is the appropriate balance between good outcomes, excellent care and services, and cost. To add value to the care and services your facility provides, you need to understand the relationship between perception of care, outcomes, and cost and how these three issues are affected by processes that the facility carries out. (See *Organizational approach.*)

Most facilities identify more opportunities for improvement than they have time or resources to address. Consequently, they must design a way to prioritize the issues. Criteria for prioritizing the issues include:

Organizational approach

An organization's approach to performance improvement includes the following essential elements. These elements should be anchored in the everyday tasks and work of each employee.
➤ Designing processes
➤ Monitoring performances through data collection
➤ Analyzing current performance
➤ Improving and sustaining improved performance

➤ expected impact on performance
➤ degree to which the areas are high-risk, high-volume, or problem-prone areas
➤ relationship of the potential improvement to all other dimensions of performance in the facility
➤ available resources.

JCAHO focuses on "dimensions of performance." Performance is what is done and how well it's done; the characteristics of each are the dimensions of performance. Review the following information carefully, because it's the heart of why performance improvement programs are so important.

Doing the right thing

➤ The *efficacy* of the procedure or treatment in relation to the patient's condition (To what degree did the services or care accomplish the desired outcome?)
➤ The *appropriateness* of a specific test, procedure, or service to meet patient need (Was the care or treatment relevant to patient need as determined at the time?)

Doing the right thing well

➤ The *availability* of the needed test, procedure, treatment, or service to the patient who needs it
➤ The *timeliness* with which a needed test, procedure, treatment, or service is provided to the patient
➤ The *effectiveness* with which tests, procedures, treatments, and services are provided

➤ The *continuity* of the services provided to the patient with respect to other services, practitioners, and providers over time
➤ The *safety* of the patient and others to whom the service is provided
➤ The *efficiency* with which care and services are provided
➤ The *respect* and *caring* with which care and services are provided.

Tips for transitioning

For a successful quality management program, managers and staff must think in a new way. They must know their boundaries and be allowed to move within those boundaries. Here are 10 tips to use as you begin your quality management transition.

➤ *Instead of making lists to assess a problem, use lateral or creative thinking.* Problem solving requires vertical thinking. For example, people usually make a list of things to do, often prioritizing the items on the list. Most facilities have a hierarchy, a structure with someone in charge of a group of people. However, work doesn't flow linearly. Working from a mental model of the workflow rather than relying on the management hierarchy can be more helpful in producing innovative solutions to problems. Lateral, or creative, thinking emphasizes rearranging ideas in new ways. Instead of listing consequences, map essential concepts; the object is to identify relationships between issues being discussed. Let people know how important they and their jobs are to the whole. Quality is every person's responsibility every day. It isn't something that's done once to make a business better.
➤ *Develop a culture that loves questions.* Learn to love the questions that arise from delivering care and services. Use provocative questions to open up and guide discussions. Stress to all staff that no question is silly; every question is worth asking.
➤ *Become comfortable having your thoughts challenged.* Questioning is both a process and an attitude. Most people feel uncomfortable and become defensive when others ask for an explanation of how they arrived at a decision. Instead, you should welcome any chance to examine your own thinking. Answer questions with enthusiasm. Also, remember that most adults don't want

to look uninformed or foolish, so if they ask a question, they deserve a thorough answer.

➤ *When discussing potential solutions to problems, suspend personal judgment.* Creative thinking is about exploring alternatives and picking the best one. Entertain a variety of options. The point is to reach a consensus and arrive at the best solution.

➤ *Consider all aspects and approaches to an issue.* Issues can be discussed from three main directions: the feeling associated with the issue, the vision or overall facts associated with it, and the associated patterns or actions. You can't view every problem purely from a factual standpoint. There are always feelings involved, especially when you're dealing with change.

➤ *Describe any situation from various perspectives.* There are four types of speech: framing, advocating, illustrating, and inquiring. There may be a variety of ways to approach a situation.

➤ *Constantly reflect on boundaries and the way new regulations affect the boundaries of practice.* The world of health care is mired in regulations, and no matter how good an idea might be, it still must fall within the boundaries of those regulations. Your quality management team and process must be constantly alert to changes and the way they affect care and services.

➤ *Be prepared to be wrong.* Learn to examine your own thinking; when you find gaps or errors, admit it. Revisit each point where you made key decisions and try to understand how you came to your conclusion. Think aloud. Intellectual humility is an important characteristic of good managers.

➤ *Be a lifetime learner.* Be inquisitive. Explore all options. Listen to your customer.

➤ *See the humor in situations.* Celebrate wins no matter how minor they seem. Rather than reacting in anger to a problem, look for the irony in the situation. Don't take life too seriously.

Points to remember

The following points summarize how to monitor quality:

➤ CQI is an integral part of health care. It includes identifying goals and forming objectives to establish policies, procedures, and protocols.

➤ TQM is a philosophy that strives to meet the needs of the customer and community and the objectives of the facility as well as maximize the potential of all employees.

➤ The success of any quality or improvement plan is dependent on the involvement, support, and commitment of the staff and management.

➤ Quality assurance involves monitoring activities for accuracy and excellence in order to set standards for care and service that ultimately improve patient outcomes.

References

1. St. Clair, G. *Total Quality Management in Information Services.* New Providence, N.J.: Bowker-Saur, 1997.
2. Martin, P.G. American Society for Healthcare Risk Management. *Risk Management Handbook for Health Care Organizations.* Chicago: American Hospital Pub., 1990.
3. Hansten, R., and Washburn, M. *Clinical Delegation Skills: A Handbook for Professional Practice,* 2nd ed. Gaithersburg, Md.: Aspen Pubs., 1998.
4. Moen, R.D. *Quality Improvement Through Planned Experimentation,* 2nd ed. New York: McGraw-Hill Book Co., 1999.
5. Kavaler, F., and Spiegel, A. Risk *Management in Health Care Institutions – A Strategic Approach.* Sudbury, Mass.: Jones and Bartlett Publishers, 1997.
6. Meisenheimer, C. *Quality Assurance for Home Health Care.* Rockville, Md.: Aspen Pubs., 1989.
7. Field, M., and Lohr, K. *Clinical Practice Guidelines: Directions for a New Program.* Washington, D.C.: National Academy Press, 1990.
8. Pattison-Gordon, E. *Requirements of a Sharable Guideline Representation for Computer Applications.* Technical Report #SMI-96-0628. Stanford: Stanford University, 1996.

Selected readings

Becher, E., and Chassin, M. "Improving the Quality of Health Care: Who Will Lead?" *Health Affairs* 20(5):164-69, May 2001.
Walldal, E., et al. "Quality of Care and Development of a Critical Pathway," *Journal of Nursing Management* 10(2):115-22, March 2002.

CHAPTER 15

Quality in nursing practice

Marie Brewer, RN, LNC

> "Quality is never an accident; it is always the result
> of high intention, sincere effort, intelligent
> direction, and skillful execution; it presents the wise
> choice of many alternatives." — William A. Foster

Defining nursing practice

What is a nurse? How do you describe nursing practice? How
have others described it over the years? The word *nurse* means to
nurture, nourish, and protect. The word *practice* means to do or
perform and to become proficient and excellent in a particular
area or skill. Therefore, *nursing practice* implies proficiency in the
skill of nurturing and protecting others.

The successful nurse-manager is viewed as the "mother" of the
unit and should be aware of how the nursing profession is defined and regulated. With that said, this chapter begins by taking
you on a journey through the definitions of *nursing practice* over
the past century and a half.

In 1859, in *Notes on Nursing*, Florence Nightingale defined
nursing in the following way.

> The following notes are by no means intended as a rule of
> thought by which nurses can reach themselves to nurse, still
> less as a manual to teach nurses to nurse. They are meant sim-
> ply to give hints for thought to women who have personal

311

charge of the health of others. Every woman or at least almost every woman in England has, at one time or another during life, charge of the personal health of somebody, whether child or invalid — in other words, every woman is a nurse. Everyday sanitary knowledge, or the knowledge of nursing, or in other words, of how to put the constitution in such a state as that it will have no disease, or that it can recover from disease, takes a higher place. It is recognized as the knowledge that everyone ought to have — distinct from medical knowledge, which only a profession can have.

If then, every woman must, at some time or other of her life become a nurse, i.e., have charge of somebody's health, how immense and how valuable would be the produce of her united experience if every woman would think how to nurse.

I do not pretend to teach her how, I ask her to teach herself, and for this purpose I venture to give her some hints.[1]

In 1917, *Goodnow's First Year Nursing* described the nursing profession as follows:

The young nurse will do well to bear in mind that the accepted principles of nursing ethics have not only been carefully thought out, but tested over and over again in actual life; so that her attitude should be that of a child that obeys at first because it must and later because it has seen the reasons of obedience.

It is pretty generally conceded that nursing is a profession, and the nurse should bear in mind that her work is therefore upon a higher plane than that of an ordinary occupation. More is, and ought to be, expected of her, and if she is not willing to attempt to carry out the program which is set before her, she would better choose some other work.

The actual work done by a nurse can be learned by a person of ordinary intelligence, but the fine art of nursing is a thing that requires special fitness, special and long training, and determined application. We hear of the "born" nurse. There is no such person, though we may by courtesy apply the term to her by her interest, enthusiasm, faithfulness, diligence and loving spirit, puts the work of caring for the sick among the professions. She may have talent for nursing, as a painter or musician has a talent for art or music, but she must, as they do, possess the determination which makes her go through years of training in the technique and spirit of her art.[2]

Some 50 years later in 1967, *Fundamentals of Patient Care: The Emergence of Nursing,* by Kozier and DuGas, defined *nursing practice* in the following way.

Nursing is a service in which people are helped to meet needs related to their general health. From its earliest inception nursing has had a nurturing quality, and today this quality is incorporated into practices that are designed to assist patients physically, psychologically and sociologically.

Generally, nursing practices are adjunctive to medical practice but nurses have varying degrees of autonomy in their functions. Nursing has been described as a helping art in which the nurse helps a person to meet certain needs he has at a particular time.

The nurse has the following functions: to teach patients and personnel, to assist in the curative process, to provide nursing care, to coordinate the activities of personnel, and to participate in research.

The nurse should no longer regard herself merely the "'handmaiden of the physician'" but rather as a competent member of the health care team. She works cooperatively with the patient and his physician to help the patient overcome health problems. She has a technical and scientific background which gives her a foundation for her professional function as well as communication skills which enable her to offer her patient the guidance he requires.[3]

The final, most current definition comes from the National Council on State Boards of Nursing. As you read and compare these definitions, you'll find that no matter how the definition is worded and how comprehensive nurses' education is, nurses are still first and foremost caregivers of the human body and spirit.

> The practice of nursing means assisting individuals or groups to maintain or attain optimal health, implementing a strategy of care to accomplish defined goals and evaluating responses to care and treatment. This practice includes, but is not limited to, initiating and maintaining comfort measure, promoting and supporting human functions and responses, establishing an environment conducive to well-being, providing health counseling and teaching, and collaborating on certain aspects of the health regimen. This practice is based on understanding the human condition across the life span and the relationship of the individual within the environment.[4]

Now that we've explored the various definitions of nursing practice, you may be wondering how you're expected to conduct yourself as a nurse in today's world. In 1995, the American Nurses Association (ANA) published the Nursing Social Policy Statement. In brief, it states: "The authority for the practice of nursing is based on a social contact that acknowledges professional rights and responsibilities as well as mechanisms for public accountability." This statement is based on the assumption that humans possess an essential unity of mind, body, and spirit and that the human experience is contextually and culturally defined. Health and illness are human experiences; the presence of illness doesn't preclude health, nor does optimal health preclude illness. (See *ANA definition of nursing.*)

The ANA goes further to specify and define the four areas that are required as a knowledge base for nursing practice. These areas are:

> ➤ *phenomena of concern.* Nurses must focus on human experiences and responses to birth, health, illness, and death within the context of individuals, families, groups, and communities.
> ➤ *diagnosis.* Nurses must facilitate communication among health care providers and the recipients of care and provide for initial direction in choice of treatments and subsequent evaluation of the outcomes of care.

ANA definition of nursing

The American Nurses Association (ANA) defines nursing as:
➤ attention to the full range of human experiences and responses to health and illness without restriction to a problem-focused orientation
➤ integration of objective data with knowledge gained from an understanding of the patient or group's subjective experience
➤ application of scientific knowledge to the processes of diagnosis and treatment
➤ provision of a caring relationship that facilitates health and healing.

➤ *interventions.* Direct or indirect, nursing interventions involve both physical and emotional intimacy. Nurses provide physical care, emotional support, and health teaching or counseling. They assist with recovery or a peaceful death.

➤ *outcomes.* Nurses must evaluate the effectiveness of their interventions in relation to identified outcomes. They must continually revise their diagnoses, outcomes, and plans of care.

As first and foremost caregivers of the human mind, body, and spirit, nurses have an obligation to respond to health and illness without restriction, to integrate what they objectively know with the patient's subjective response and, finally, to continuously make an effort to learn and apply this knowledge to the diagnosis and treatment of their patients.

Standards of care

What are the standards of care for the practice of nursing? These are the rules or definition for what it means to provide competent care as a registered nurse. The registered professional nurse is required by law to carry out care in accordance with what other reasonably prudent nurses would do in the same or similar circumstances. Thus, providing high-quality care consistent with established standards is critical.

ANA

The ANA provides guidelines for nursing performance and nursing standards. Other sources for standards of care are statutes

ANA standards of nursing

As defined by the American Nurses Association (ANA), *standards of nursing* consist of three components:
➤ Professional standards of care define diagnostic, intervention, and evaluation competencies.
➤ Professional performance standards identify role functions in direct care, consultation, and quality assurance.
➤ Specialty practice guidelines are protocols of care for specific populations.

and regulations, authoritative textbooks and journals, state practice acts, state practice guidelines, job descriptions, critical pathways and clinical guidelines, administrative codes relative to certain settings, court decisions and administrative rulings, the Joint Commission on Accreditation of Healthcare Organizations (JCAHO) and, finally, facility and unit policies and procedures. (See *ANA standards of nursing.*)

Clinical nursing practice can vary considerably, depending on the setting in which the nurse is employed and the patients cared for in that setting. The ANA has developed and published standards for clinical nursing practice and 18 other specialty areas of nursing practice, including community health nursing.

JCAHO

JCAHO defines *practice guidelines,* or *standards of care,* as descriptive tools or standardized specifications for care of the typical individual in the typical situation, developed through a formal process that incorporates the best scientific evidence of effectiveness with expert opinion. Synonyms include *clinical criteria, parameter, practice parameter, protocol, algorithm, review criteria, preferred practice pattern,* and *guideline.*

AACN

The *Standards for Acute and Critical Care Nursing Practice* describe the practice of the nurse who cares for an acutely or critically ill patient no matter where that patient is cared for within the health care environment. In 1998, the American Association of Critical-Care Nurses (AACN) Board of Directors formed a

Practice Standards Task Force to evaluate and revise the current standards. In support of the ANA position that specialty standards should be framed from the general clinical nursing practice standards, the AACN Practice Standards Task Force used the latest edition of the *ANA Standards of Clinical Nursing Practice* as a template for its work. The task force evaluated each Standard of Care and Standard of Professional Performance for its relevance to and inclusion of acute and critical care nursing competencies. The original standards statements were either left unchanged or revised to better articulate the professional expectations of competent acute and critical care nursing practice. The measurement criteria, which detail how nurses meet each standard, were evaluated and revised as necessary to reflect the unique aspects of acute and critical care nursing.

There are six standards of care for acute and critical care nursing. Even though these were written specifically for acute and critical care nursing, they're the same standards that should be used in any nursing care situation because they follow the nursing process.[5]

STANDARD OF CARE I: ASSESSMENT Nurses collect relevant patient health data. They recognize that data collection involves the patient, family, and other health care providers, as appropriate, to develop a holistic picture of the patient's needs. The priority of data collection activities is driven by the patient's immediate condition and anticipated needs.

Pertinent data are collected using appropriate assessment techniques and instruments. These data are documented in a retrievable form, and the data collection process is systematic and ongoing.

STANDARD OF CARE II: DIAGNOSIS The nurse analyzes the assessment data to determine diagnosis. The nurse recognizes that the diagnoses are derived from the assessment data and that identified diagnoses are validated throughout the nursing process by interacting with the patient, family, and other health care providers involved in the care. All identified diagnoses are prioritized and documented in a manner that facilitates determining expected outcomes and developing a care plan.

STANDARD OF CARE III: OUTCOME IDENTIFICATION The nurse identifies individualized, expected outcomes for the patient. Outcomes are derived from actual or potential diagnoses. These outcomes are mutually formulated with the patient, family, and other health care providers when possible and appropriate. The outcomes are individualized in that they are culturally appropriate and realistic in relation to the patient's age and present and potential capabilities. Outcomes should always be attainable in relation to resources available to the patient and in time frames that meet patient need. Outcomes provide direction for continuity of care so that the nurse's competencies are matched with the patient's needs.

STANDARD OF CARE IV: PLANNING The nurse develops a care plan that prescribes interventions to attain the desired and expected outcomes. The care plan is individualized to reflect the patient's characteristics and needs and is developed collaboratively with a team consisting of the patient, family, and health care providers, in a way that promotes each member's contribution toward achieving expected outcomes and reflects current acute and critical care nursing practice. Priorities for care are established, and the plan provides for continuity across the care continuum.

STANDARD OF CARE V: IMPLEMENTATION The nurse implements interventions identified in the care plan. These interventions are delivered in a manner that minimizes complications and life-threatening situations. The patient and family participate in implementing the care plan, based on their ability to participate in and make decisions about care.

STANDARD OF CARE VI: EVALUATION The nurse evaluates the patient's progress toward attaining expected outcomes. Evaluation is systematic and ongoing, based on certain criteria, and is the collaborative effort of the patient, family, and health care providers involved in the evaluation process, as appropriate. Evaluation occurs within an appropriate time frame after interventions are initiated. Ongoing assessment data are used to revise the diagnoses, outcomes, and care plan as needed. All revisions in diagnoses, outcomes, and the care plan are documented, along with the effectiveness of interventions in relation to outcomes.

Explaining APIE

The planning method that goes by the acronym *APIE* is defined as "a systematic, rational method of planning and providing nursing care."

➤ *Assess and analyze.* Collect and organize data and form a statement of the actual or potential needs.
➤ *Plan and prioritize.* Formulate your plan. This involves devising goals and expected outcomes, setting priorities, and identifying interventions to help reach the goals.
➤ *Implement and intervene.* Put your plan into action.
➤ *Evaluate.* Assess your outcomes and see how they measure against the goals.

And remember: All of the above steps in the standard of care process should be documented accurately and completely in the medical record.

APIE

In the April 2002 edition of *Nursing Spectrum* magazine, Judith Brumm, RN, writes about the "APIE" method to guide nursing practice.[6] The process is simple to remember and easy to implement. (See *Explaining APIE.*)

Standard of care is a term used to designate what is accepted as "reasonable" under the circumstances. It's a measuring scale. The standard of care is the degree of skill, care, and judgment that a care provider uses under similar circumstances. The accepted standard of care may vary based on the circumstance and on the clinician's level of professional education.

Standards of professional performance

Standards of professional performance are described in terms of competency, not in terms of reasonable care. These are authoritative statements that describe a competent level of behavior in the professional role, including activities related to quality of practice, performance appraisal, education, collegiality, ethics, collaboration, and resource management. Technological advancement provides new and better aids and equipment to treat patients. The criteria used to measure compliance with the use of such new technology also change. Criteria to determine the standards of practice are continuously being developed by specialty areas of medicine and nursing.[7]

Regulations

Nursing practice, and the corresponding standards for professional performance, are regulated by individual state practice laws, the ANA, and other such organizations. The standards and regulations define the practice base, provide for research and the development of that practice base, establish a system for nursing education, establish the structures through which nursing services will be delivered, and provide quality review mechanisms for the following:

➤ *Code of ethics.* This area includes standards of practice, structures for peer review, and system of credentialing.
➤ *Certification.* This area encompasses the judgment of competence made by nurses who are themselves practicing in nursing or in an area of specialization, the successful completion of an examination, the content of course work, and the amount of supervised practice that's required.
➤ *Legal regulations.* All nurses are legally accountable for actions taken in the course of nursing practice as well as actions delegated by nurses to others assisting in the delivery of nursing care. The regulations also delegate accountability that might arise from licensure criminal and civil statutes.
➤ *Statutory definitions.* These must be compatible with the profession's definition of its practice base but general enough to provide for the dynamic nature of an evolving scope of nursing practice. There should be a goal for both professional and legal regulatory mechanisms with consistent definitions and criteria.
➤ *Self-regulation.* The nurse is accountable for the knowledge base of practice, formal, and continuing education. Mechanisms that hold nurses accountable for practice based on the profession's code of ethical behavior should be in place. Peer review certification is an important component of self-regulation.

The ANA published the *Nursings' Social Policy Statement* in 1995. This statement describes the scope and definition of nursing practice in the United States, including:

➤ the values and social responsibility of the profession
➤ nursing definition and scope of practice
➤ nursing knowledge base
➤ the methods by which nursing is regulated.

The statement is both an accounting of nursing professional stewardship and an expression of the continuing commitment to the society nurses serve.

Professional levels of nursing

Several established professional levels guide the scope of performance and nursing practice in the United States. The first, which covers basic nursing and the generally accepted requirements for a nurse who completes nurse's training and education, includes the following:

➤ graduates from an approved school of nursing
➤ qualifies by the national exam to be a registered nurse
➤ cares for patients and families
➤ selects interventions based on desired outcomes
➤ teaches caregivers
➤ coordinates care
➤ integrates patient service delivery
➤ prepares patients for tests and procedures
➤ monitors responses to interventions.

Nurses in advanced practice acquire specialized skills and knowledge through study and supervised practice at the master's or doctoral level in nursing. The term *advanced practice* is used exclusively to refer to advanced clinical practice.

Advanced practice registered nurses (APRNs) are distinguished by the autonomy to practice at the edges of the expanding boundaries of the nursing scope of practice; the ability to work toward self-initiated treatment regimens, as opposed to dependent functions and complexity of clinical decision making; and the skill to manage organizations and environments. They assess health needs; diagnose; plan, implement, and manage care; evaluate outcomes of care plans; advocate care; promote health; prevent diseases and disability; direct care or manage systems of care for complex populations; manage acute and chronic illness;

Expectations for the APRN

What distinguishes advanced practice registered nurses (APRNs) from other nurses is their specialized skills and knowledge. These include:
➤ a knowledge base that concentrates one's focus on one specialized area of nursing
➤ practice experiences (Expansion refers to the acquisition of new practice knowledge and skills, including those legitimizing the role autonomy within areas of practice that overlap traditional boundaries of medical practice.)
➤ integration of specialized theoretical, research-based, and practical knowledge that occurs as a part of graduate education in nursing.

assist with childbirth; and so on. In many cases, they can also prescribe, administer, and evaluate drug treatment; serve as a consultant in practice; educate; conduct research to expand the knowledge base; provide leadership for practical changes; and contribute to the advancement of the profession. (See *Expectations for the APRN.*)

Cultural diversity

Another area that directly affects standards of professional performance is cultural diversity issues in nursing.[8] Knowledge and skills related to cultural diversity can strengthen and broaden health care delivery systems. Other cultures can provide examples of a range of alternatives in services, delivery systems, conceptualization of illness, and treatment modalities. Knowledge about cultures and their impact on interactions with health care is essential for nurses, whether they're practicing in clinical, education, research, or administrative settings. Cultural diversity addresses racial and ethnic differences; however, these concepts or features of the human experience aren't synonymous.

Knowledge of cultural diversity is vital at all levels of nursing practice. Concepts of illness, wellness, and treatment modalities evolve from a cultural perspective. Concepts of illness, health, and wellness are part of the total cultural belief system. Because culture is one of the organizing concepts upon which nursing is based and defined, nurses need to understand:

➤ how cultural groups understand life processes
➤ how cultural groups define *health* and *illness*
➤ what cultural groups do to maintain wellness

MANAGER'S TIP

Supporting cultural diversity

Nurse-managers need to foster policies and procedures that help ensure access to care that accommodates varying cultural beliefs. They must be knowledgeable about and sensitive to the cultural diversity among providers and consumers. They also must be aware that nurse-researchers are attempting to use the cross-cultural body of knowledge to ask pertinent research questions.

Through exploration of other cultures, nurse-researchers and practitioners have found that although cultures differ, many similarities exist among the groups. The good news is that nurses are in a position to influence professional policies and practice in response to cultural diversity. The nurse-manager simply needs to encourage such behavior from her staff and continually emphasize the importance of cultural awareness.

➤ what cultural groups believe to be the causes of illness
➤ how healers cure and care for members of cultural groups
➤ how the cultural backgrounds of nurses influence the way care is delivered.

It's important that nurses consider specific cultural factors affecting individual clients and recognize that cultural variation means that each client mut be assessed and respected for individual cultural differences. This is especially true in the home health care arena because the nurse sees patients in their own homes, their cultural environment.

Nurses in clinical practice must use their knowledge of cultural diversity to develop and implement culturally sensitive nursing care. Nurses take pride in their role as client advocates. Recognizing cultural diversity, integrating cultural knowledge, and acting, when possible, in a culturally appropriate manner enables nurses to be more effective in initiating nursing assessments and serving as client advocates.

All nursing curricula should include pertinent information about diverse health care beliefs, values, and practices. Such educational programs would demonstrate to nursing students that cultural beliefs and practices are as integral to the nursing process as physical and psychosocial factors. (See *Supporting cultural diversity*.)

National Center for Health Services Research

The modern roots of the research movement go back to 1968, when the National Center for Health Services Research was established within the U.S. Department of Health, Education, and Welfare. In 1989, this center became the Agency for Health Policy and Research, which was reauthorized by Congress in 1999 as AHRQ (Agency for Health Policy and Research). The reauthorization affirms the agency's existing goals and research priorities:

➤ to support improvement in health outcomes

➤ to strengthen quality measurement and improvement

➤ to identify strategies to improve access, foster appropriate use, and reduce unnecessary expenditures.

Research-based care

The word *research* is defined as careful, systematic study and investigation in a field of knowledge that's undertaken with the intent to establish facts or principles. The very heart of the nursing process lends itself to "research" that uses outcomes to predict and direct better care. Assessment of the effectiveness of patient outcomes and treatment cost and accessibility—as opposed to assessment of treatment efficacy alone—isn't a new field of research. (See *National Center for Health Services Research.*)

Nurses have a key role in the research agenda of the Agency for Healthcare Policy and Research, especially in the areas of primary care, outcomes research, translation of research into practice, and quality of care.[9] Research-based nursing practice is absolutely vital for nursing today. In accordance with their requirement for accountability and responsibility, nurses must use research in all areas of practice. Research findings offer opportunities to enhance patient care while expanding the body of nursing knowledge. The widespread introduction and use of research will be one of the most important factors in the new era for nursing.

As professionals, nurses need to continually update their knowledge to ensure effective, safe, high-quality care. This is a professional obligation. They must be able to justify and be accountable for the care they give and be confident that it's the best care, based on current information. Nurse-managers now have a clear responsibility to raise research awareness and appreciation in their staff, helping them create an environment conducive to the critical examination of current practice. A culture of "valuing

Explaining evidence-based practice

Question: *What is evidence-based practice?*

Answer: Evidence-based practice is the process by which nurses make clinical decisions using the best available research evidence, and clinical expertise. Three areas of research competence are interpreting and using research, evaluating practice, and conducting research. These three competencies are important to evidence-based nursing and research-based care. To carry out this process, the following factors must be considered:

➤ Sufficient research must have been published on the specific topic.

➤ The nurse must have skill in accessing and critically analyzing research.

➤ The nurse's practice must allow her to implement changes based on the evidence from the research.

The knowledge generated through nursing research is used to develop evidence-based practice, improve the quality of care, and maximize health outcomes and cost-effectiveness of nursing interventions.

research" is vital when applying research to practice. Management and education practice should also be based on valid research findings. The introduction of a purchaser-provider split in health care provision means that health care professionals must demonstrate that care is clinically sound and cost-effective. Evidence-based practice, which is based on research, demands that nurses examine their practices in all spheres, evaluate care, and ensure that the best possible evidence related to nursing practice is disseminated as widely as possible.[10] (See *Explaining evidence-based practice.*)

Participating in research

Nurses must be clinically accountable for the care they provide to patients, and their clinical decisions must be based on as much scientifically documented evidence as possible. Nurses are central to research-based care because they're the ones who are in the best position to articulate and evaluate the interventions they use. The continuing quest for quality and cost-effective health care has brought evidence-based practice and nursing research into the foreground.

A systematic process that seeks to add new nursing knowledge to benefit patients, families, and communities, nursing research and research-based care encompass all aspects of health related to nursing, including promotion of health, prevention of illness, and care of people of all ages during illness and recovery or toward a peaceful, dignified death. Nursing research applies the scientific approach in an effort to gain knowledge, answer questions, or solve problems.

One area in which nurses might be active participants in research-based care is the clinical trial process. Medicare, known now as the Centers for Medicare and Medicaid Services (CMS), defines *clinical trials* as research studies designed to evaluate the safety and efficacy of medical care. They're key to understanding the appropriate use of medical interventions of all types and informing payers about which services to cover. In the past, Medicare didn't pay for items and services related to clinical trials because of their experimental nature. As a result, only a small percentage of elderly people participated in clinical trials, although seniors bear a disproportionate burden of disease in the country.

On June 7, 2000, the President of the United States issued an executive memorandum directing the Secretary of Health and Human Services to "explicitly authorize [Medicare] payment for routine patient care costs...and costs due to medical complications associated with participation in clinical trials." In keeping with the President's directive, CMS is engaged in defining the routine costs of clinical trials and identifying the clinical trials for which payment for such routine costs should be made.

Understanding the ethical issues

Regardless of the setting or the situation, ethical issues are commonly involved in research-based care or clinical trials. The Association of Clinical Research Professionals published a written Code of Ethics on April 10, 2001, to state and affirm commitment to upholding the highest standards of personal and professional behavior in the field of clinical research. Through this Code of Ethics, they commit to:

➤ hold the safety and welfare of human subjects as their highest goal

➤ execute their work according to scientific standards of objectivity, accuracy, and integrity
➤ continue to advance their knowledge and understanding of their profession through education and training
➤ safeguard the quality and credibility of their professional judgment from inappropriate influence
➤ ensure that the principles of informed consent are honored both in spirit and in practice
➤ observe both in spirit and in working practice all legal, ethical, and regulatory requirements for the conduct of clinical research, including the confidentiality of all relevant records and communications
➤ avoid conflicts of interest in their own affairs and make full disclosure in advance of undertaking any matter that may be perceived as a conflict of interest
➤ be prepared to draw attention to, or challenge, practices of others that may be detrimental to good clinical practice or in breach of relevant legal, ethical, or regulatory standards.

Nurses play a key role in research-based care, especially in the areas of primary care, outcomes research, translation of research into practice, and quality of care. You know your patients, where they are, what they need, and what outcomes you can expect. As a nurse, you need to use your holistic approach in patient care as a means to predict and improve care in common patient groups. You learn from what you do and apply it to the next case. Nurses and other clinicians use a wide range of judgment, decisions, actions, and recommendations, including:

➤ clinical expertise — everything you know from past experience and good observation skills
➤ patient perspective — empathy, compassion, and respect
➤ context of care — patterns within the community
➤ human biology — understanding of how things work
➤ clinical care research — ability to spot fair comparisons as well as understand how numbers can be applied to the clinical setting.

Defining satisfaction

The Joint Commission on Accreditation of Healthcare Organizations[11] defines *satisfaction* as measures that address the extent to which patients (or enrollees, practitioners, or purchasers) perceive their needs to be met. Satisfaction measures that focus on the delivery of clinical care from the patient's, family's and caregiver's perspective include, but aren't limited to, the following aspects of care: patient education, medication use, pain management, communication regarding plans and outcomes of care, prevention and illness, improvement in health status, and so forth. A satisfaction measure may address one or more aspects of care.

Patient satisfaction

As health care is becoming more consumer driven, health care organizations are finding that patient satisfaction data are necessary for communicating with current and potential patients and for improving the quality of care they bring to their communities. More sophisticated than in the past, today's health care consumers now demand more accurate and valid evidence of health plan quality. Patient-centered outcomes have taken center stage as the primary means of measuring the effectiveness of health care delivery. It's commonly acknowledged that patients' reports of their health and quality of life, as well as their satisfaction with the quality of care and services, are as important as many clinical health measures. Patient satisfaction with care is an important outcome measurement for health care providers as the competition for a consistent customer base intensifies in the communities. (See *Defining satisfaction*.)

Quality of care

Quality of care, which is directly linked to patient satisfaction, is the degree to which health services for individuals and populations increase the likelihood of desired health outcomes and are consistent with current professional knowledge. Dimensions of performance that affect satisfaction include patient perspective issues, safety of the care environment, accessibility to care, appropriateness of care and treatment, continuity, effectiveness, efficacy, efficiency, and timeliness of care.[12]

Measuring patient satisfaction

Over time, the measurement of patient satisfaction has become less of a luxury and more of a necessity for health care organizations. It's increasingly important that a patient-satisfaction program be done well, using sound protocol and methods. Numerous ways to process and analyze patient-satisfaction data exist. Statistical analysis can range from simple counts or frequencies of patient responses to more complex procedures, such as correlational analysis or quality-control charting that highlights relationships and variations in the data. In addition, technologies for tabulating and analyzing survey data range from relatively simple spreadsheets to more sophisticated statistical analysis programs.

The main thing to remember is the importance of objectivity in satisfaction measurement. Many accrediting agencies require that patient satisfaction data used for accreditation purposes be collected by an outside survey vendor. This has a twofold benefit for the organization. First, the outside vendor can be totally objective and, second, there's comparative data to benchmark. Getting valid results begins with understanding what you want evaluated, whom you're going to ask, what you're going to ask, and how often you're going to ask the questions. It's also necessary to determine at what point you want to assess patient satisfaction. Do you want to determine satisfaction with the entire episode of care or just with one point of care? In general, however, consumer data are collected to achieve the following goals:

➤ to identify and prevent problems
➤ to evaluate organizational performance
➤ to plan staff education
➤ to improve public image and reputation
➤ to identify and plan new services
➤ to give meaningful feedback to patients, payers, regulators, accrediting bodies, and others.

According to H. James Harrington: "Measurement is the first step that leads to control and eventually to improvement. If you can't measure something, you can't understand it. If you can't understand it, you can't control it. If you can't control it, you can't improve it."

Assessing patient satisfaction

In assessing patient satisfaction, you open yourself to the potential for patient complaints. Not everyone will always be satisfied with the care they receive, and there are as many reasons for this as there are complaints. As a health care provider, you need always to remember that the greatest opportunities for improvement of care and services can come from the consumer who isn't satisfied on some level. By giving you the message that something is wrong, that patient is giving you the opportunity to fix the problem for the next customer.

Patient satisfaction is a personal thing. Satisfaction with care begins with communication of expectations and plans, respect for differences in people and their needs or perceived needs, courtesy, timeliness, and other "soft" skills that go above and beyond the technical and professional skills that you use as registered nurses. As was stated in the beginning of this chapter, nurses are first and foremost caregivers of the human mind, body, and spirit and have an obligation to respond to health and illness without restriction; to integrate what they know objectively with the patient's subjective response; and to continuously make an effort to learn and apply this knowledge to the diagnosis and treatment of their patient.

Health care education

JCAHO states that the goal of patient education is to improve patient health outcomes by promoting recovery, speeding return to function, promoting healthy behaviors, and appropriately involving the patient in decisions about care. Through the process of patient education, nurses can influence patients to gain the knowledge, attitudes, and skills needed to maintain and improve health. The desired outcome of any education process is to change a behavior.

The nurse's role in education

Nurses are also teachers and are key to providing effective education. Patient teaching hasn't always been a top priority for the health care professional — or the patient, for that matter. Patients

Documenting teaching

One of the most compelling reasons for clear, complete documentation of patient teaching is that it can keep you out of court. The courts recognize the patient's right to informed consent — that is, to have appropriate information when making decisions about health care. This puts the burden of decision on the patient, but it also makes you responsible for helping that patient make an intelligent choice.

Nurse practice acts in many states now make nurses responsible for patient teaching. The Joint Commission on Accreditation of Healthcare Organizations also has set national standards for documentation that the courts use as guidelines. So if a patient claims he was harmed by inadequate teaching and your documentation falls short of these standards, the courts may decide that you provided substandard nursing care — even if the patient teaching you provided was thorough.

Delegate wisely

Of course, dietitians, physical therapists, and others also do patient teaching. However, nurses do the referring to ancillary staff members, making nurses ultimately responsible for the teaching outcomes. For this reason, document each referral and the specific material you expect that person to teach, and delegate only to those qualified to teach. Remember: Licensed practical nurses aren't taught the fundamentals of patient teaching — it's beyond the scope of their practice. But they can reinforce what you've already taught the patient, as long as you follow up, evaluate, and document what the patient learned.

Document what you don't teach

Keep in mind that documenting what you didn't teach is just as important as documenting what you did teach. For example, you'll have to postpone or redirect your teaching if it causes the patient too much stress or if he decides that he'd rather have you teach a family member instead. Just make sure you record his response to your teaching attempts.

One last caution

As health care agencies and consumer groups become more sophisticated about patients' rights to information, careless patient teaching may become a common ground for lawsuits against nurses. To avoid litigation, document and delegate responsibly.

haven't always asked questions and been involved in their care at the level that are today. In these times of staffing, resource, and time shortages, it's usually easier to do something ourselves rather than take the time to teach someone else to do it. A good nurse promotes independence and self-reliance in patients. Patient education is one of the most crucial roles in nursing practice. Nurses who fail to provide or document adequate patient education increase their risk of liability should something happen to the patient when the patient is no longer under the care of the nurse or facility. (See *Documenting teaching.*)

The traditional view of patient information didn't require the dissemination of valuable and vital information to patients. Gradually, under the impetus of professional and legal demands for nursing accountability, nursing philosophy on the patient's right to know has changed. The nursing process now stipulates patient and family education as a major responsibility of the registered nurse.[13] JCAHO looks for evidence of three major processes when they evaluate patient education in an organization: evidence of the organization's internal focus on education, the way education itself is accomplished, and the way the organization evaluates and determines that both overall and individual education goals have been set and reached.

The nursing goal must be to give patients and caregivers the best and most accurate information available to help them achieve an optimal level of health and safety. To tend only to the physical needs of patients without teaching them to obtain, retain, or regain health is a job half done. Lavinia Dock (1858–1956), a nursing pioneer in public health, emphasized the nurse's role in preventive health through teaching. Although the primary responsibility of nurses is to teach patients what they need to know to recover from the present illness or procedure, they also need to inform and support the patients and others involved in their care as to what to expect when they leave the care setting.

This area of education is even more important than ever with short-term stays, same-day surgery, and diagnosis-related group or managed care–based models. Patients simply don't stay in a facility long enough for traditional education, so the nurse must develop ways to assess need, readiness, and ability to learn; identify others to teach; teach what is relevant to the patient; and evaluate the response. Patients and their families or other caregivers must know enough about their illness or condition to be able to safely return home with self-care and to know when and why to call for assistance. The education process can, and should be, a combination of face-to-face time, literature or some type of visual, and questions and answers to determine whether goals have been met. All of this should be carefully documented. As a nurse-manager, you need to promote and support the teaching efforts of your staff. Guide them in the priorities of teaching and the value of documentation. (See *Prioritizing teaching*.)

Prioritizing teaching

Sometimes, teaching patients what they need to know seems time-consuming — there's too much to cover and not enough time to do it. If you're hard-pressed to find time for teaching, try this method:
➤ List the patient's learning needs.
➤ Rank these needs in order of importance.
➤ Write your "teaching to be done" list based on this ranking.

This method helps you distinguish the patient's *learning* needs from his *nursing care* needs. It also helps you organize your time and quickly redirect your actions after an interruption.

Of course, the hardest part is ranking the patient's learning needs. To simplify this task, classify each learning need as:
➤ *immediate* (one that must be met promptly, such as teaching the patient who's being discharged in 2 hours) or *long range*
➤ *survival* (life dependent such as teaching the warning signs of adrenal crisis) or *related to well-being* (nice to know but nonessential such as describing the effects of stress in cardiovascular disease)
➤ *specific* (related to the patient's disorder or treatment such as preparing him for upcoming coronary artery bypass) or *general* (teaching that's done for every patient such as explaining hospital visiting hours).

After you've classified the patient's learning needs, establish priorities. An immediate survival need, for example, would be the top priority.

Culture's effect on education

As you approach the education of a patient, you must always be cognizant of patients' own values about health and illness. What is their cultural background, and how does it affect their acceptance of teaching? Cultural awareness is a learning process by which the nurse becomes aware of, appreciates, and becomes sensitive to the values, beliefs, practices, and problem-solving strategies of other cultures. For the nurse, this also means examining and addressing any personal biases she may have that could affect the care and education of a patient. This awareness and acceptance of cultural diversity is never more important than in the home setting, when the home health nurse goes into the heart of a patient's home and culture to provide care. In all care and education, you're expected to assess and treat each patient as an individual. This individuality begins with the patient's cultural and ethnic background.

Using the nursing process

Teaching is a collaborative process that involves intimate communication between the nurse, the patient, and possibly multiple caregivers. The goal of education is to add something to the patient's knowledge base that will improve his ability to care for himself. The learning that results causes a permanent change in behavior that the patient chooses, or doesn't choose, to accept. The process of patient teaching can be modeled after the nursing process.

Before any educational interventions can be planned, assessment of knowledge must occur and goals (both short and long term) must be set. The nurse must assess the patient in his current environment; in cooperation with the patient, identify needs; together write educational objectives; establish and implement an education plan; and continually assess and evaluate results. The education process must also be interdisciplinary. In most cases, because the nurse is the consistent team player in the care of a patient, the nurse should facilitate and coordinate the education process, acting as the point person to ensure that the patient and family are well prepared with the information and skills they require. (See *Early steps in teaching*.)

The more nurses teach, the more they learn. There's no best way to teach all patients. The best technique is the one that works for each individual nurse and patient. All professionals should be familiar with the four generally accepted assumptions about adult learning that follow:

➤ *Adults value self-direction.* Adults want the information necessary to assist them in making their own decisions and taking responsibility for their own choices. They need to know why they're being asked to change a behavior and what will or could happen if they don't make the change.
➤ *Adults bring various life experiences to every learning situation.* As an educator, you must take time to assess that experience and build on it as you introduce new information.
➤ *Adults are strongly influenced by social roles and developmental tasks.* You must be careful that as you provide education and training, you consider and respect the role and abilities of the patient outside of the facility.

Early steps in teaching

Before teaching, take the following steps. First, set teaching outcomes for your patient. Then collect and evaluate data. Last, form a statement of the patient's readiness, willingness, and ability to achieve those outcomes — your "teaching diagnosis." You may discover more areas for teaching based on what your patient and his family want to learn. If so, reassess the patient or modify your outcomes to create a workable teaching plan.

1. Set teaching outcomes
➤ What must the patient learn?
➤ What does the health care team want him to learn?
➤ When should teaching occur?

2. Collect data
➤ What do patient and family interviews tell you about learning needs, outcomes, and response?
➤ What does the patient's chart reveal?
➤ What information can the health care team give?

3. Evaluate data
➤ What does the patient want to learn?
➤ Do his goals conflict with his family's or the health care team's goals?
➤ What learning barriers exist?
➤ What factors can promote learning?

4. Establish a teaching diagnosis
➤ What is the patient ready, willing, and able to learn?
➤ Do the patient, family, and health care team confirm your findings?
➤ Do you need to set new teaching outcomes?

➤ *Adults are oriented to the present.* They need to be able to immediately apply new knowledge or skills to their current condition and needs.

Dealing with change

Learning means changing a behavior — and change is frightening to most adults. Also, in many cases, the patient is in pain or is fatigued, anxious, or afraid, which also affects the ability to learn. Recognizing this in a patient will help you choose the time and amount of teaching to be done in one sitting. Begin the education process by asking the patient about himself and his work, family, and hobbies. Move from that point to the patient's immediate and future concerns and needs. What goals has he set for himself relative to his illness or condition? What is he most interested in learning about? What does he already know?

The next step is to identify how this person best learns. Does he like to read, listen, or watch videos? Is there a time of day when he is more alert? Is he aware of anything that may prevent

Assessing learning readiness

To help you determine the patient's readiness, willingness, and ability to learn, assess his:

☐ developmental level
☐ emotional maturity
☐ emotional state
☐ health beliefs
☐ intellectual status
☐ learning goals (and his family's, too)
☐ learning style
☐ life experiences

☐ physical condition
☐ religious beliefs
☐ self-esteem
☐ sociocultural background
☐ socioeconomic status
☐ stage of adaptation
☐ support system, including family and other groups.

him from learning? Is there someone else who needs to be with him during this time? Finally, based on the information gleaned from the above questions, mutually determine reachable and quantifiable goals — both short and long term — for the patient. Using this information, select the education materials or methods that best suit this patient and put together and implement the education plan. (See *Assessing learning readiness.*)

Barriers to learning

Nurses and other health care professionals must do more than merely pass on information to the patient and his family. They must also take the time to identify any potential or real barriers to the patient's learning and putting this new information to practical use. The nurse facilitates the learning process and clarifies issues or misunderstandings between what is being taught and what is being relayed back by the patient. The responsibility of the health care professional is to give patients the tools and knowledge to act on their own behalf, to carry out recommendations from the care plan, to be aware of and able to choose alternatives, and to apply this new knowledge in their everyday life.

Complying with learning

Compliance with instructions and education is a huge issue in health care. Simply informing patients as to what they need to do isn't educating them and doesn't guarantee compliance. A patient is usually considered compliant when he or she agrees to

Deciding learning outcomes

How can you express learning outcomes clearly? First, focus on specific behaviors you want to influence. The patient's learning behaviors and the learning outcomes that you develop fall into three domains: cognitive, psychomotor, and affective. For example, understanding dietary changes falls into the cognitive domain, whereas complying with these changes falls into the affective domain and taking the patient's blood pressure falls into the psychomotor domain.

With these domains in mind and with input from the patient, you can write clear, concise learning outcomes. They should explain what you're going to teach, indicate the behavior you expect to see, and set clear criteria for evaluating what the patient has learned.

Review the two sets of sample learning outcomes below for a patient with chronic renal failure. Notice that the outcomes in the well-phrased set start with a precise action verb, confine themselves to one task, and describe measurable and observable learning. In contrast, the poorly phrased goals may encompass many tasks and describe learning that's difficult or even impossible to measure.

Well-phrased learning outcomes

Cognitive domain
The patient with chronic renal failure will be able to:
➤ state when to take each prescribed drug
➤ describe symptoms of elevated blood pressure
➤ list allowed and prohibited foods on his diet.

Psychomotor domain
The patient with chronic renal failure will be able to:
➤ take his blood pressure accurately, using a stethoscope and a sphygmomanometer
➤ read a thermometer correctly
➤ collect a urine sample, using sterile technique.

Affective domain
The patient with chronic renal failure will be able to:
➤ comply with dietary restrictions to maintain normal electrolyte levels
➤ verbalize his feelings about adjustments to be made in the home environment
➤ keep scheduled appointments with his health care provider.

Poorly phrased learning outcomes

Cognitive domain
➤ know his medication schedule
➤ know when his blood pressure is elevated
➤ realize his dietary restrictions.

Psychomotor domain
➤ take his blood pressure
➤ use a thermometer
➤ bring in a urine sample for laboratory studies.

Affective domain
➤ appreciate the relationship of diet to renal failure
➤ adjust successfully to limitations that chronic renal failure has imposed
➤ realize the importance of seeing his health care provider regularly.

and follows the recommendations for care. The extent to which a patient chooses to follow and to be compliant with instructions must be addressed. This is one reason why it's so important to carefully assess and choose the best method to teach each patient and then to evaluate and document the outcome of each education session. (See *Deciding learning outcomes*.)

Identify the necessary tools. Mutually set the goals that the patient is expected to reach. Have the patient or family sign or initial the education record as they verbalize understanding or reach the desired outcome. One thing to remember when teaching patients new information is that just because a patient nods his head or verbalizes understanding, learning hasn't necessarily occurred. The nurse must ask for specific feedback, recall, and practical application of the new information and skills.

Teaching is an art that takes time and practice. In health care, it's the art of transferring usable and practical knowledge from one person to another in order to improve the quality of life. Nurses need to always remember that even with all of the highly skilled and technical requirements that come with profession, they're first and always teachers and caregivers. They have an obligation to their patients to help them rise to the highest possible level of self-care and independence as possible.

Teaching the teacher

Now that the importance of teaching patients is clear, it's the extended responsibility of the nurse-manager to ensure that the nurses under her direction also participate in learning as well as teaching. The manager can apply some of the same goals and techniques used for teaching patients to teach nurses. Although the manager may not be the person directly teaching the nurses on her unit, she needs to promote and support continuing education for her staff. Most institutions offer continuing education through the staff development department. These programs should be posted in an area highly visible to the staff. Classes or seminars pertinent to a particular unit should be highlighted. Required education, such as Basic Life Support or Advanced Life Support, should be monitored and attendance arranged on a timely basis. Nurses engaged in personal continuing education, such as college courses or certification classes, should be encouraged and supported. Remember: With all the continual change that occurs in health care, the nurse may not have time or energy to learn without management support.

Referring to the "Nursing Philosophy" from the University of Kentucky seems a good way to end this chapter. Their philosophy ties together all of the components covered in this chapter.

Nursing is a professional discipline concerned with meeting the health needs of a diverse and changing society. Nursing is concerned with diagnosing, treating, and evaluating human responses to actual or potential health problems across the life span. Clients may be individuals, families, groups, or communities. Nurses assist clients to achieve their human potential by promoting or restoring health or by supporting them to achieve a peaceful death....

Nurses must analyze, synthesize, apply, and evaluate knowledge from nursing and other disciplines in order to provide high-quality care. They must demonstrate caring, commitment, and respect for the dignity of all people. Excellence in nursing is exhibited through adherence to professional standards and through contributions to changes in professional standards as the role of the professional nurse changes....

Health is a dynamic state reflecting a client's ability to adapt to changes in the environment. The environment consists of internal and external forces that influence biopsychosocial and spiritual functioning. Nurses support and enhance clients' capacities for health by fostering care and personal growth in an increasingly complex health care system. Nursing is a dynamic discipline and nurses provide care through cooperation, collaboration, and consultation with healthcare professionals of other disciplines.[14]

Points to remember

The following points summarize the role of quality in nursing practice:

➤ Nursing practice has been redefined over time. However, its general implication pertains to how nurses perform in their role to protect and nurture others by following the best established standards of care.
➤ Standards of care provide guidelines for nursing performance that incorporate the best evidence of effective nursing practice.

➤ Standards of professional performance describe a competent level of behavior in the professional role and are regulated by individual state practice laws, the ANA, and other such organizations.

➤ The use of research in the nursing profession offers opportunity to expand the body of nursing knowledge and enhance patient care.

➤ Improving patient satisfaction and education are key goals of the health care professional. Such improvement promotes positive attitudes, independence, and self-reliance in patients regarding their health outcomes.

References

1. Nightingale, F. *Notes on Nursing: What It Is and What It Is Not.* Commemorative ed. Philadelphia: J.B. Lippincott Co., 1992.
2. Goodnow, M. *Goodnow's First Year Nursing: Text-Book for Pupils During Their First Year* of Hospital Work, 2nd ed. Philadelphia: W.B Saunders Co., 1916.
3. Kozier, B., and DuGas, B. *Fundamentals of Patient Care: A Comprehensive Approach to Nursing.* Philadelphia: Philadelphia: W.B. Saunders Co., 1967.
4. Model Nursing Practice Act. National Council of State Boards of Nursing, 1994.
5. Brent, N. *Nurses and the Law: A Guide to Principles and Applications,* 2nd ed. Philadelphia: W.B. Saunders Co., 2001.
6. Brumm, J. "Put Time on Your Side: Part 2," *Nursing Spectrum* 3(4):26SE, April 2002.
7. Bogart, J.B. *Legal Nurse Consulting: Principles and Practice.* Boca Raton, Fla.: CRC Press, 1998.
8. Cultural Diversity in Nursing Practice. Position Statement Originated by: Council on Cultural Diversity in Nursing Practice, Congress of Nursing Practice Adopted by: American Nurses Association Board of Directors. Effective Date: October 22, 1991. *www.nursingworld.org/readroom/position/ethics/etcldv.htm.*
9. Burstin, H., et al. "Future Directions in Primary Care Research: Special Issues for Nurses," *Policy, Politics, & Nursing Practice* 2(2):103-7, May 2001.
10. Greenwood, J. "Nursing Research: A Position Paper," *Journal of Advanced Nursing* 9(1):77-82, January 1984.
11. Joint Commission on Accreditation of Healthcare Organizations. Comprehensive Accreditation Manual for Hospitals (CAMH): The Official Handbook *Update* 4:GL21, 2002.
12. Joint Commission on Accreditation of Healthcare Organizations. Op. cit.

13. Lorig, K. *Patient Education: A Practical Approach*, 3rd ed. Thousand Oaks, Calif.: Sage Publications, 2001.

14. University of Kentucky School of Nursing philosophy statement. *www.uky.edu/nursing/intro/phil.htm.*

Selected readings

Nativio, D. "Guidelines for Evidence-based Clinical Practice," *Nursing Outlook* 48(2):58-59, March-April 2000.

Rodham, K., and Bell, J. "Work Stress: An Exploratory Study of the Practices and Perceptions of Female Junior Healthcare Managers," *Journal of Nursing Management* 10(1):5-13, January 2002.

Sleep, J., et al. "Achieving Clinical Excellence Through Evidence-based Practice: Report of an Educational Initiative," *Journal of Nursing Management* 10(3): 139-144, May 2002.

CHAPTER 16

Managing risk

Sally Austin, JD, ADN, BGS

> "Deliberate with caution but act with decision and promptness." — Charles Caleb Colton

A nurse-manager needs to be aware of the various aspects of her unit that may cause legal problems, such as an inadequately trained staff, flawed equipment, or standards of care that aren't adequately upheld. Although many facilities employ risk managers, an effective nurse-manager is aware of the different aspects of risk management that will assist in the successful outcomes of her unit. The nurse-manager should also be aware of the role of the risk manager.

Overview of risk prevention

With the explosive increase in malpractice litigation arising in the late 1970s, health care facilities were forced to find ways to prevent lawsuits and to control costs associated with lawsuits. Initially, physicians and hospitals were the target of malpractice lawsuits. Hospital liability was based on either corporate negligence or *respondeat superior,* the legal principle that holds an employer responsible for an employee's wrongful acts. Nursing practice continued to evolve into more specialized roles with greater autonomy and accountability. Subsequently, nurses found themselves named as codefendants to lawsuits.

Not only did the explosion of malpractice actions become commonplace, but the passage of government regulation to control the cost and quality of health care also increased. In addition, the Joint Commission on Accreditation of Healthcare Organizations set out specific requirements, not only for the risk management program but also for the quality improvement program, necessary in order to receive accreditation standing. In response to these forces, health care facilities scrambled to implement risk management programs to protect their facilities' financial interests both by controlling insurance premium costs and other liability exposure costs and by reducing the frequency and severity of incidents while ultimately improving patient care. In general, most definitions of *risk management* recognize that it's an internal systematic program aimed at reducing preventable injuries to patients, employees, and visitors; procuring cost-effective and adequate liability insurance coverage; improving patient care; and reducing financial losses of the facility through risk identification and evaluation processes, risk analysis, and risk control measures.[1] Stated another way: "*Managing* risks means taking immediate steps to control the possibility that a patient, an employee, or a regulatory entity will complain of the quality of care delivered. It means taking steps to minimize risk before complaints are lodged and lawsuits filed."[2]

Managing risks isn't just the responsibility of the risk manager but is also implemented through a team effort under the leadership of the risk manager. The risk manager works very closely with legal and human resources. In addition, the team approach includes the incorporation of committees, such as a risk management committee, a morbidity and mortality committee, an infection control committee, and a surgical committee. The importance of the risk management committee can't be overstated. The membership should consist of representatives of the facility's governing body, administration, operations, and medical staff and the risk manager. Risk information reviewed or analyzed by other committees should be referred to the risk management committee for its evaluation as to appropriate action.[3] If the facility has an in-house legal counsel, this person should serve as legal counsel to the committee. If external legal counsel provides the facility's legal services, the law firm should provide guidance and direction to the committee. The coordination of risk management and risk prevention principles is also a component of compliance programs. Many, if not most, health care entities have incorporated a compliance program. One of the first steps taken to establish the compliance program is to do a risk identification analysis. It isn't unusual for the risk manager to serve as a committee member on a corporate compliance committee.

Components of risk management

An effective risk management program incorporates the following components:

➤ identification of risks through the incorporation of incident reporting and audits
➤ use of a grievance or complaint mechanism to process and resolve grievances of patients or their representatives
➤ collection of data regarding negative health care outcomes
➤ identification of the cause of each injury
➤ early intervention and sympathetic care after accidental injury
➤ creation and maintenance of a database of risk information
➤ analysis of risk information collected (number of losses, frequency, and overall effect of losses on health care delivery) through the use of trending reports
➤ development of corrective action plans to reduce liability exposure and address issues identified
➤ development of training programs to reduce liability exposure
➤ creation of an effective patient advocacy program.[4]

Risk management programs are generally considered to be reactive in nature. However, an effective program incorporates proactive components by establishing active decision-making processes that the health care team uses in responding to potential liability claims. After the causes of an incident are determined through risk management efforts, quality improvement principles are incorporated to define steps to be taken to establish, improve, refine, or revise processes in order to prevent the same type of incident from occurring again.

Risky business

Both risk management and quality assurance identify high-volume, high-risk health care; analyze data to determine areas of noncompliance with regulations or standards of care; analyze the frequency and severity of an incident; and implement corrective actions. Quality assurance continually looks at delivery processes and seeks ways to streamline and improve the process, with the ultimate goal of becoming a more efficient delivery system with fewer errors. Both programs determine root causes of a particular incident and develop means to prevent the incident from occurring in the future. Risk management processes identify ways to diminish financial liability exposure. Quality assurance principles monitor the effectiveness of any corrective actions enacted.

Depending on the culture and structure of the health care entity, the risk manager's role incorporates varying responsibilities. The basic responsibilities include risk identification and evaluation as well as education. Some facilities expand the role to include the procurement of risk insurance and claims management.

Basic elements of a risk management program

Risk management programs are established to minimize exposure to legal risks and liability, collect and analyze data to decrease risk to staff and patients, and improve and maintain quality patient care — all of which require collaboration among staff members.

Identifying risk

The first element of both an effective risk management program and a corporate compliance program is risk identification. The goal of risk identification in the risk management process is to identify and evaluate liability exposures, such as professional negligence, corporate negligence, general negligence, employee-related claims in workers' compensation, and claims based on employment law. The goal of risk identification in the corporate compliance process is even broader and looks at risks in all areas of operation, including regulatory requirements and billing practices.

Risk identification can be characterized as reactive, internal, or proactive.

Unexpected outcomes

One cause of malpractice litigation is "unexpected outcomes" — that is, things that occur as a result of a procedure but that neither the patient nor the patient's family anticipates. When a procedure is performed and a particular adverse outcome isn't discussed as a possibility when informed consent is provided to the patient, the patient or patient's family may have questions or anxieties about the adverse outcome. If these questions remain unanswered or the anxiety continues, the patient or his family may look to place blame on the health care provider as a way to displace any unresolved or unexpressed anger or guilt.

What can a nurse do to prevent unexpected outcomes? Make sure the patient and his family are aware of all possible effects that the procedure can have. The more complete your patient teaching is, the more likely you are to avert malpractice litigation.

➤ *Reactive* identifiers include external communications, such as lawsuits, medical record requests, patient complaints, and billing disputes.
➤ *Internal* identifiers include internal communications, such as incident reports and audits.
➤ *Proactive* identifiers include the use of peer review committees, social services, patient advocate programs, and quality assurance programs.

When risk exposures are identified, steps are taken to find ways to improve processes and reduce the likelihood of the incidents occurring or recurring.

Although incident reporting will be discussed in greater detail later, it's important to note here that a policy or procedure should define when the incident report is created, the type of incident identified, and the specific information required on the form. This information is then reviewed and trended. Audits should also be developed to randomly review medical record documentation using defined criteria or generic indicators, such as unexpected hospital deaths, unplanned post discharge readmissions to hospital within a certain time frame, unexpected infections, and return trips to the emergency department within a defined time frame. Audits should also be performed and results trended on reports completed as the result of work-related injuries.

To help define risk exposure, the manager should be aware of specific incidents that tend to result in malpractice actions or other types of legal actions, such as general liability (for example, slips, falls, or other injuries to visitors), or employee claims (for example, workers' compensation or employment law–related claims). Recognized causes of malpractice litigation can then be categorized as can employee injuries. (See *Unexpected outcomes.*)

Medical errors

A common cause of professional exposure is medical error, such as surgical mishaps, misdiagnosis, incorrect treatment, medication errors, obstetrical mishaps, informed consent, and futile medical care (care withheld or withdrawn). Of these, medication errors are extremely common. Another indicator may be an injured patient where a weak health care provider–patient relationship exists or where the individual has an uncertain financial future — for example, a disgruntled patient or family member who has a previous financial status and is looking for a way to gain financial income through a legal claim.

Breach of confidentiality

Breach of confidentiality is a category that's receiving a great deal of attention in today's health care environment. With the use of electronic records and the electronic transmittal of health care information, the risk of patient-specific health care information getting into the hands of someone who doesn't have a "need to know" increases. It's also imperative that protections are in place when vendors have access to a computer database that contains patient information. Therefore, facilities must take steps to protect this information, including developing policies and procedures that address the handling of patient information, implementing password protection, providing access to patient information only on a need-to-know basis, and strategically placing computer screens so they aren't in open view. Staff must also use great care not to discuss a patient where someone in the general public can overhear, such as in an elevator or at a party. More on this topic is discussed later in this chapter.

Elevated standards of care

Another category of potential risk is clinical practice guidelines. When such guidelines are developed, they should be drafted in such a way that they don't elevate the required standard of care. Any elevation of the standard created in the guideline can increase the risk of medical malpractice.

MANAGER'S TIP

Equipment risks

Health care facilities are responsible for selecting, providing, and maintaining the medical equipment and supplies necessary to provide safe patient care. Nurse-managers assume some of that responsibility by identifying risks associated with the use and maintenance of such equipment, including incorporating routine checks and keeping a maintenance log. In addition, the manager must ensure that health care staff members receive the appropriate training on the use of new equipment and supplies.

Equipment failure can result from improper maintenance, improper repair, or a defect in the manufacture, design, or warnings associated with the use of the equipment. Equipment failures and any injuries associated with them should be reported to the risk manager or to the institution representative legally responsible for reporting such incidents to the appropriate government agency.

Corporate negligence

Numerous duties apply to the health care facility as the result of patient care being rendered within the facility. Failure to properly perform these duties can increase the risk of liability. These duties include but aren't limited to:

➤ duty to properly maintain the facility and equipment
➤ duty to have necessary equipment and supplies (see *Equipment risks*)
➤ duty to hire, supervise, and retain competent and adequate staff
➤ duty to develop and implement policies and procedures that promote quality of care
➤ duty to properly train and orient staff.

Workers' compensation

To this point, this discussion of the risk identification process has focused on patient care. However, the manager must also consider the work environment. Enacted to protect the employer from being sued, workers' compensation laws are regulated by state statutes that vary from state to state. However, some principles are consistent among the states. In all states, the employee's only recourse is to file a workers' compensation claim. Dollar amounts for recovery for injuries and lost wages is defined by law. The fa-

Providing a safe environment

To minimize liability risks and ensure appropriate patient care, health care facilities must provide a safe environment. Ways of ensuring a safe environment include providing protective equipment, vaccines or medications for infectious diseases to which a health care worker has been exposed, routine tuberculosis testing, appropriate in-services on safety techniques, and education on the proper and safe use of equipment and supplies.

Not only must the facility provide a safe haven for the patient to receive care and a safe workplace for its employees, but it must also ensure a safe environment for visitors, including vendors, consultants, family and friends of patients, and others. This includes clearly defining hazardous areas — for example, posting a sign indicating that the floor is wet in a particular area, as a means to help prevent falls.

cility is responsible for providing a safe environment for health care staff. (See *Providing a safe environment.*)

To qualify as workers' compensation, the employee's injury must meet two criteria: It must arise out of the employer's business and be within the scope of carrying out that business. The first criterion is easily met if the injury occurs while the employee is either on the premises or on an errand for the employer (such as transporting a patient to another facility). If an employee is injured while on the job but either failed to meet safety requirements (for example, by not wearing gloves and goggles) or performed tasks that weren't for the employer's benefit (not within the scope of the employer's business), the second criterion wouldn't be met.

The risk manager may be asked to investigate employee-related injuries. In general, most states require an employee injury to be reported to the employer within a specific time frame. The employer is required to report employee injuries to a specified state agency. The required form must be completed within a time frame defined by law. Ultimately, however, the employee is responsible for notifying the employer about the injury.

Analyzing risk

Identified risks must be analyzed to determine probability of a loss. This process takes into effect the number and frequency of losses experienced and the overall effect of the losses on the facility, using statistical or mathematical evaluation.[5]

Risk control functions

Nurse-managers and staff nurses alike work together to control risks and make their health care environment a safer place. Essential risk control functions include:
➤ ensuring good medical record documentation
➤ effectively drafting policies and procedures
➤ adhering to adopted policies and procedures
➤ establishing education and training programs on use of medical supplies and equipment and current medical practices
➤ ensuring appropriate informed consent
➤ ensuring accurate and complete nursing assessments
➤ ensuring that patients' rights are recognized
➤ developing effective patient advocate programs
➤ using incident reporting and occurrences screening.

When risks have been identified and the probability and frequency of loss established, the risks must be prioritized. Prioritization focuses on the degree of frequency and severity of the risk in terms of safe patient care and financial exposure to the facility. This process involves assessing proper response to the identified risk and either allocating appropriate resources to prevent the risk from occurring or diminishing the extent and exposure of the risk incurred. Those risks that carry a high degree of frequency and severity to the organization should be high priority for reactive or proactive action. Good patient advocate programs can help reduce financial exposures.

Controlling risk

The next element of the risk management program is risk control, with loss prevention and reduction as key components. Educating the staff about the importance of risk management and individual responsibility in risk identification, prevention, and correction is an important aspect in any risk control program. (See *Risk control functions.*)

Basic steps

As soon as an incident occurs, information that can be used to potentially reduce financial obligations is gathered and documented according to the facility's risk control program. The following are sample steps.

Elements of professional negligence

The elements of professional negligence include a duty, a breach of duty, damage to the patient, and a direct connection between the breach of duty and the damage to the patient. Standards of care represent the identified duty applicable to the health care provided to the patient. For a duty to exist, a health care provider–patient relationship must also exist. Determining whether any injury to the patient is the direct result of a failure to follow the standards of care is also imperative.

Step 1. The incident undergoes initial investigation. The incident is first reported to the nurse-manager and then to the risk manager — for example, through an incident report, a patient complaint, or a letter from the patient's attorney.

Step 2. The risk manager obtains and reviews the patient's medical record. This review can help the risk manager determine whether health care staff carried out the appropriate standard of care. To make this determination, the risk manager must have a working knowledge of the elements of professional negligence and then keep these elements in mind while reviewing the medical record. (See *Elements of professional negligence.*)

The risk manager should note what a plaintiff's attorney looks for in the medical record, because these tips help the risk manager identify problems. The plaintiff's attorney will typically look for charting inconsistencies, substandard or inappropriate care, time delays in initiating care, lack of treatment, chart battles between health care professionals, errors in medication administration, late entries (not documents as such), and evidence of an incident report.

Step 3. The risk manager should identify the individuals involved in the incident and interview these individuals as soon as possible after the incident, while memories are still fresh. The risk manager will want to document the interview, either in writing or through taping of the interview. If the facility has an in-house legal department, it's wise to seek direction from them on conducting the interviews. In this manner, the documentation can be either protected under attorney-client work product or prepared in anticipation of litigation.

Step 4. If the organization has no in-house legal counsel, the risk manager may want to seek direction from an outside counsel in order to obtain whatever legal protections apply. After interviewing those individuals involved in the incident, the risk manager will interview any witnesses to the incident who may know of applicable information. The types of questions include open-ended questions that allow the interviewee to tell the story. The interviewer wants to know what happened, when it happened, where it happened, why it happened, how it happened, and who observed it. Again, it's best to let the witness tell the story, as long as the defined questions are answered.

Step 5. The risk manager must identify, document, and secure physical evidence that may be relevant and has the potential for becoming lost. Such evidence includes electrocardiogram strips, fetal monitoring strips, X-rays, magnetic resonance images, computed tomography scans, and laboratory specimens such as slides. Last, the risk manager will collect all medical bills and request that billing is held.

More steps

Another aspect of risk control incorporates steps used and adopted to avoid lawsuits. The risk manager can play a major role in this effort but must have the cooperation of all health care staff. Specific efforts include:

➤ creating realistic policies and procedures
➤ creating realistic expectations
➤ ensuring that questions are answered completely
➤ alleviating a patient's anxiety
➤ allowing the patient to express anger
➤ developing a strong relationship with the patient and his family
➤ recognizing most common signs of malpractice
➤ minimizing consequences
➤ establishing good recordkeeping
➤ handling patient complaints effectively.

Risk management tools

Nurse-managers use some or all of the following tools to identify and manage risk.

Aspects of the incident report

The incident report should be in an easy-to-use format to capture required information. The process for filling out the report should be set out in a written policy and procedure document that includes:
➤ the definition of an incident
➤ the purpose of completing the report
➤ the circumstances that require completion of the report — for example, cardiac arrest, unexplained death, return admission to the intensive care unit, medication errors, break in sterile technique, transfusion reaction, infections following surgical procedures, falls, and malfunctioning of equipment
➤ the process for filling out the report
➤ follow-up efforts initiated as the result of a reportable incident
➤ the responsible party required to review the incident report
➤ the time frame in which the report should be filled out following an incident.[6]
Keep in mind that any information captured on the form should be objective and should include:
➤ patient-identifying information
➤ a description of the incident that occurred
➤ any injuries sustained
➤ any care rendered to maintain the patient's, employee's, or visitor's status while awaiting medical examination
➤ medical treatment required as a result of the incident.

Incident report

One of the most beneficial tools at the risk manager's disposal is the incident report. This report serves as a communication tool to provide information about an adverse patient incident that could lead to a potential claim. The incident report serves a multifold purpose. If completed promptly after an incident occurs, the report can help establish a means for resolution to a potential claim before a lawsuit is filed. Besides signaling a potential patient claim, the report provides a mechanism for determining the need to revise a policy or procedure. The incident report can also help provide a means for monitoring the performance of individual health care professionals — for example, incident reports may indicate numerous medication errors committed by one registered nurse. By identifying this concern, the facility is then able to provide appropriate remedial measures related to the nurse in question. (See *Aspects of the incident report*.)

Many, but not all, states have laws that protect the disclosure of incident reports in the event of medical negligence litigation.

The rationale for this protection is to establish a means for facilities to identify problems and take corrective actions to improve patient care. To claim the privilege, legal counsel should review those incident reports that document breaches in the standard of care or injury to a patient or visitor. Incident reports shouldn't be filed in the medical record — and no reference to an incident report being drafted should appear as documentation in the medical record. Rather, the chart entry should objectively state how the patient was found, what happened and any medical intervention provided including assessment, and treatment.

When the incident report is directed to the risk manager's attention, the form should be reviewed and categorized as to degree of priority depending on incident; degree of risk, including financial and the potential for legal action against the facility; the patient's medical status; and anxiety of the patient or the patient's family. The risk management committee reviews the information on the incident report. The data on incident reports is trended into selected categories, and appropriate actions are taken to address any identified concerns. (See *Using the incident report.*)

Keep in mind the following principles when drafting policies and procedures on how an incident report should be completed:

➤ Use consistent writing style.
➤ Be accurate and concise.
➤ Document interventions.
➤ Avoid pointing fingers.
➤ Be honest.
➤ Sign the report, and include the date and time.

Risk financing

At some facilities, the risk manager may be responsible for risk financing — that is, shopping for insurance or helping to set up self-insurance programs. Some facilities elect to retain risk. Under this scheme, the facility pays for any losses with internal funds. The facility may be required to set aside in a trust fund the anticipated amount of liability exposure for each identified exposure.

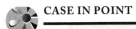
CASE IN POINT

Using the incident report

You, as an operating room manager, have received an incident report indicating that Patient Wilson was readmitted to the hospital after a recent abdominal surgery. At the time of readmission, Patient Wilson was experiencing severe abdominal pain, high temperature, and chills. She was taken back to surgery, at which time a lap pad was found. Patient Wilson underwent a colostomy as a result of the retained sponge. The family knows of the incident and is extremely angry. As manager, you set out to investigate this incident. After reviewing the incident report and Patient Wilson's medical record, you request that Nurse Brown (the operating room nurse assigned to the first surgical case) come in so you can take her statement. Your intent is to tape the statement to maintain the information in case of litigation.

You need to develop an outline of the facts that are important to document, relative to what happened in this incident. How would you begin the session? What questions need to be answered?

The risk manager is the optimal person to take charge of incident reports. If your facility doesn't employ a risk manager, follow these recommendations to decrease risk.

1. Develop good listening and investigative skills to participate in the interview and recorded statement process. While performing the interview or taking a recorded statement, seek answers to such questions as:

➤ What happened?
➤ Who was involved?
➤ When did it happen?
➤ Where did it happen?
➤ How did the incident occur?
➤ Why did it happen?
➤ What was the immediate outcome?
➤ What steps were taken to maintain the patient's condition while awaiting medical examination?
➤ What care was rendered to the patient as a result of the incident?
➤ Were there any witnesses?
➤ Was the incident discussed with anyone, including the physician, the patient's family, and the patient?

It's advisable to let the interviewee tell the story and to ask specific questions if the information isn't provided.

2. When documenting the interview or recorded statement, the manager should document the date and time of the interview or statement, the identity of the individual conducting the interview or statement, and the identity of the individual giving the interview or statement. If the statement is recorded, the risk manager needs to obtain permission from the interviewee. The best practice is to capture the permission on tape. Also, it's important to document that the interviewee is older than age 18.

This model is effective when the health care facility has adequate cash flow and the capacity to satisfy funding requirements. The facility also must be sophisticated enough to set aside appropriate reserves, which include the anticipated cost to resolve the claim, including damages and attorney fees. Any losses incurred are covered with operational funds.

Alerting the insurance company

Other facilities elect to transfer risk by acquiring commercial insurance coverage (primary and excess). Insurance policies are written as "occurrence based" or "claims made." Under occurrence-based policies, the date the incident occurred is the important criterion for determining applicable coverage. If the incident occurred during the policy period, it's covered. It doesn't matter if it was reported when the policy expired. Under claims-made policies, the incident is covered if the claim is reported during the policy period. When the event occurred has no bearing on applicable coverage. Tail coverage should be purchased at the end of a claims-made policy to cover potential negligent acts that may be reported after the policy lapses. Tail coverage is usually purchased for as long as the statute of limitations is applicable. If the facility continues to procure claims-made insurance in the year after the current policy period has ended, tail coverage is unnecessary. Generally, facilities have "claims-made" coverage.

The risk manager must follow specific reporting criteria to alert the insurance company, especially if the facility has a claims-made policy. If a claim arising under the claims made policy isn't reported in a timely fashion, the insurance company can deny coverage. Generally, insurance companies set the time frame and the types of claims that must be reported.

Scope of coverage

In addition to the type of insurance coverage elected, the risk manager must also be informed as to the limits of coverage. This is generally defined in terms of total amount of coverage per occurrence and in the aggregate. *Per occurrence* is the maximum amount covered per incident during the policy period. *In the aggregate* is the total amount the insurance company will pay out on all claims during a policy period.

The risk manager must also be concerned with the scope of coverage of the insurance policy, which is normally set out in the policy language. The policy creates a contract between the insured and the insurer. Normally, intentional actions and criminal actions aren't covered. If an intentional claim is raised, the insurer may be required to provide defense counsel during the legal process. Should the defendant be found liable for an intentional action, the defendant likely would be required to repay the insurer for legal fees as well as make individual payment for any damages awarded to the injured party. An additional exclusion to most insurance policies is punitive damages — that is, damages awarded that are punishing in nature. Other damages awarded to an injured party are compensatory in nature — that is, damages awarded that attempt to make the injured party whole — and are generally covered by insurance up to a specified dollar amount per incident.

As an additional safety protection, some facilities require medical staff members or those who are part of a network to maintain minimum levels of insurance.

Overview of the litigation process

As a manager, you need to have some knowledge of the stages and elements of the litigation process related to medical malpractice suits.

For a plaintiff to bring a cause of action in negligence against someone (a defendant) or some entity, the plaintiff's case must meet certain elements: a duty by the defendant to the plaintiff, a breach of the duty (or failure to perform a required action because of the duty required by the relationship), a damage to the plaintiff (either physical or financial), and a direct relationship (casual connection) between the breach of the specific duty that resulted in the specific injury the plaintiff suffered.

Statute of limitations

The plaintiff has a specific period of time to bring a lawsuit against the defendant. This period of time is known as the statute of limitations. This time frame varies from state to state and varies with the type of action. Some jurisdictions require that the plaintiff present the case to a panel for review before permitting the compliant to be filed in a court of law.

Filing of the lawsuit

The cause of action is brought when the plaintiff files a lawsuit against the defendant in the appropriate court. After the lawsuit is filed, it must be served upon the defendant according to statutory requirements. The defendant then has a specific time frame to file an answer. If the answer isn't filed within the time frame, the defendant is considered in default. If the default can't be remedied, then the plaintiff prevails on the liability portion of the claim; only the damages need to be determined by the jury. The defendant's answer specifically addresses each allegation that the plaintiff raised. Any allegation not specifically denied is considered admitted. The defendant must also raise in the answer any affirmative defenses the defendant has against the plaintiff. Some affirmative defenses must be raised in the answer or are forever waived. If the defendant believes that the plaintiff didn't set out the required elements in the complaint, the defendant could raise the affirmative defense of failure to state a cause of action upon which relief can be granted. At this point, the defendant could seek a motion to dismiss.

Discovery

After the answer is filed with the court and served upon the plaintiff, the discovery process begins, provided the defendant doesn't prevail on a motion to dismiss. During this phase, the parties have the use of specific tools to gain documentation and information to support or defend the party's position. These tools include:

➤ interrogatories
➤ depositions
➤ request for production of documents
➤ independent medical examination.

Interrogatories are questions set out from one party to another. These questions must be answered and the truth of their accuracy certified. Deposition is testimony taken before a court reporter that records the questions asked and the responses given. Depositions can normally be taken of anyone who has information relevant to the facts of the case.

During the discovery phase, the defendant could determine that the plaintiff hasn't met the elements of his claim. At this time, the defendant can seek a summary judgment motion. If the defendant prevails at this stage, then the suit would be resolved at this point.

Additional efforts to seek resolution

If the lawsuit continues, additional efforts can be used to seek resolution. Some jurisdictions require that a medical negligence action be presented to a panel as a prerequisite to trial. The parties could decide to reach a settlement following this proceeding or at any other time during the phases of the legal process. The parties could agree to mediation, during which a third party works with the two parties to try to resolve the matter amicably.

Some jurisdictions require arbitration. In arbitration, a third party listens to the evidence that each party presents, asks questions of the parties, and then makes a decision based on the facts and the law applied. Arbitration can be binding or nonbinding. With binding arbitration, the parties must accept the arbitrator's decision; with nonbinding arbitration, the parties can proceed to trial.

Come to order

During the trial phase, both parties present testimony and introduce evidence in the courtroom. In medical negligence cases, expert testimony is required to establish the standards of care and any breach. Normally, these actions are brought before a jury, which makes the final decision. Until the jury returns with its verdict, the parties can agree to reach a settlement. If the matter is left to the jury, the jury will determine whether the plaintiff or the defendant prevails. If the plaintiff prevails, the jury will determine the damages due the plaintiff.

Product liability

In addition to assisting with medical negligence cases, the risk manager also may assist legal counsel in actions involving product liability. These types of actions can involve liability exposure to a manufacturer, seller, or supplier of medical equipment for any injuries sustained by a third party because of a defect in the product. This liability applies not only to medical equipment but also to drug products. Product liability actions can be brought as negligence actions. If the cause of action is based on negligence, the elements previously addressed under medical negligence apply.

A second theory for product liability actions includes breach of an expressed or implied warranty. In an expressed warranty, the manufacturer specifically promises or guarantees a certain action. In some instances, the courts may find that a warranty is implied as a matter of public policy for the protection of the public.

Manufacturers of medical equipment or drugs are required to publish appropriate instructions regarding safe use as well as any warnings. With drugs, any adverse effects must be disclosed. Should the manufacturer fail to provide such warnings, the manufacturer has breached a duty.

Blood isn't subject to product liability actions. Courts have held that blood is a service that hospitals provide, rather than a product.

Claims management and coordination with legal counsel

Your facility should have in place an effective claims management process. The purpose of the process is to follow the status of potential claims, actual claims, and litigated matters. Potential claims can be identified through incident reporting, communications from the patient or patient's family, and communication from the patient's attorney requesting the medical record. The facility could be alerted to an actual claim through communication from the patient's attorney, whereby the attorney indicates that the patient intends to file suit against the facility.

The medical review and the interview of appropriate staff and witnesses make up an important part of the claims management process. They help the risk manager determine whether the facility risks liability exposure. As mentioned previously, it's important to conduct interviews with the staff, the patient, the patient's family, and any witnesses as soon as possible after the incident to document the findings.

Claims management process

During the claims management process, the risk manager monitors the developments of any claim and the progress of potential claims to actual claims or lawsuits. Because an injured patient must bring a lawsuit within the time specified in the statute of limitations, a claims management database should monitor a potential claim for the statute of limitations period. As well as monitoring a potential claim and an actual claim, the stages of a lawsuit to its resolution should also be recorded.

The risk manager should track the following data as part of the claims management database:

- the date of the incident
- the patient or party involved (an employee claim or a visitor claim)
- any civil action file number (for those claims that are at a lawsuit stage)
- insurance company, policy number, and policy period
- the statute of limitations time period
- a summary of the events
- the current status of the matter
- potential for liability exposure
- any reserves assigned to the matter.

Keeping reserves

Setting aside reserves that represent the likely cost for resolving the matter, including legal costs and any damages the injured party is likely to be awarded, is important. However, the risk

Sample claims management case

The following example shows a form that can be used to maintain the claims management database and sample entries:

Claimant:	**Doris Jones**
Patient:	Doris Jones
Nurse:	Bonnie Bell
Surgeon:	Ron Wells, MD
DOI:	8/10/00
SOL:	8/10/02
Civil Action File #:	00-00983
Insurance Info:	AON, 1/00/00-12/31/00
	#1789833
Incident:	Retained sponge left during abdominal surgery on 56-year-old patient. Resulted in two additional surgeries and a total colostomy.
Status:	Suit filed 2/15/01. Answer filed 3/10/01. Early discovery phase. Interrogatories responded to on 6/30/01. Currently depositions being taken of hospital staff and surgeon. Depositions taken of patient and patient's family members.
Exposure:	Substantial
Reserves:	$150,000.00

manager may need assistance in determining reserves. If the matter is being coordinated through a commercial insurer, the insurance company will set the reserves and advise the risk manager. If the suit or claim is being handled by outside counsel retained by the facility, the outside counsel can help the risk manager determine appropriate reserves.

Factors to consider when assigning reserves include the likelihood that the injured party will prevail in a legal action; the financial injury to the patient, including any medical costs affiliated with treating the injury; any lost wages that the patient incurs from being unable to work because of the injury; and other damages, such as damages to family members that are dependents to the injured party and legal fees and costs incurred to defend the action. (See *Sample claims management case.*)

Malpractice insurance

If the facility has malpractice insurance through a commercial carrier, then the carrier will typically select outside counsel to represent the interests of the facility in case of legal proceedings.

If a substantial deductible (whereby the facility is self-insured up to a stated dollar amount) must be met, the facility might have some say in the use of outside legal counsel. If the facility is self-insured, then the selection of legal counsel will rest with the facility. The risk manager may be asked to help select the appropriate legal representation. Price shouldn't be a determining factor, although it does play a part. The most important factor is the expertise of the firm selected to assist with professional malpractice, general liability issues, and employment matters.

If a commercial insurer selects counsel, the insurer will probably establish expectations of legal counsel at the outset. In these instances, the insurer is likely to set the limits of authority that the outside attorney would have in resolving the legal claim or lawsuit. Although the facility may have some input, the final decision commonly rests with the insurer. If the facility selects legal counsel and directs the activities, then the facility should establish expectations related to billing practices, coordination of investigation, and reporting requirements, through either the risk manager or in-house legal counsel, or both. When self-insured or insured with a large deductible, the facility would be responsible for setting limits of authority for outside counsel for settlement purposes.

The role of counsel

When a claim or lawsuit is assigned by the insurer or the facility, a primary attorney should take responsibility for overseeing the case. The risk manager is likely to be called upon to provide the assigned counsel with a summary of the pertinent factors involved in the incident that have been revealed to date. This consists of a review of the medical record findings and both the contents and a summary of determinations made as a result of any interviews of parties or witnesses to the incident. At this point, areas requiring additional research and investigation are identified and assigned.

The risk manager will likely be asked to provide the assigned attorney with copies of the medical record and related documents, such as monitor strips and X-rays; all medical billing information and a copy of the incident report; any written statements; and a summary of any interviews or actual tapes of interviews, if available. The risk manager may be asked to assist outside counsel in gathering additional information.

Outside counsel then conducts a review of the medical record and any other information provided by the risk manager. The attorney develops a plan of action. If the facility is self-insured, the risk manager can request that the assigned attorney provide the facility with an action plan setting out the financial costs at each stage of the litigation process. Regardless of whether counsel is assigned by the commercial insurer or retained by the facility, the risk manager may well play an active role in assisting the assigned counsel with preparing and resolving the claim or lawsuit. Thus, it's appropriate for the risk manager to request such a plan, even if outside counsel is assigned by the insurer.

Providing information

At various points during the discovery and the claim or lawsuit preparation process, the assigned attorney should provide the risk manager with periodic reports setting out significant discovery findings to date, legal exposures the facility faces, likelihood of success at time of trial, likelihood of success on a summary judgment motion (to be discussed in greater detail below), and any affirmative defenses the facility has available to raise.

As the discovery phase of the claim or litigation process proceeds, the risk manager plays an integral role in assisting counsel in responding to such discovery requests as interrogatories and request for production of documents. The risk manager may be asked to help set up interviews with appropriate staff or help identify and retain expert witnesses in support of the facility's position. If the lawsuit proceeds to trial, the risk manager may play an active role during the trial phase.

Effective policies and procedures

The risk manager can play a crucial role in making sure that policies and procedures are drafted in such a way that they protect the facility. This is why the risk manager should be on any committee that establishes policies and procedures and should have a strong command of the principles for effectively drafting policies and procedures. (See *Defining policy and procedure.*)

Defining policy and procedure

A *policy* typically defines the minimum standard at the facility and creates the boundaries of acceptability. A *procedure* defines how a task or function should be performed. Procedures standardize and establish parameters of care. They should be drafted to provide for discretion to be exercised by health care providers.

Using appropriate terminology

When drafting policies and procedures, consistent terminology should be used throughout. Any abbreviations should be standard and recognized and should be defined in the document. The policy or procedure should be realistic and should reflect current and accurate national standards. Terms such as *responsible for* and *highest standard of care* should be avoided. When the term *responsible for* is used, the ability to delegate a task, even when permissible, could unnecessarily be hampered. A better practice is to incorporate the wording *or a designee.* This allows for the nurse's discretion when determining when a task is appropriate to assign to another person who assumes responsibility for carrying it out.[7]

Health care facilities are required to provide safe patient care. The use of the term *highest standard of care* actually elevates the standard that's required. When referring to standards of nursing care, reference should be made to the appropriate standard of care consistent with current nursing standards. The purpose of the procedure helps determine how specific the final product should be. A good practice is to minimize step-by-step procedures and, instead, to set guidelines to reach an end result.[8]

Policies and procedures shouldn't be drafted in a way that unnecessarily "boxes in" or "confines" the facility or the health care professional. Such terms as *shall* and *must* and terms that specify a time frame, such as *every 4 hours,* should be avoided. These terms create absolutes — that is, standards of care that are breached if the specific task isn't carried out within the established time frame, which could result in medical negligence if the patient is injured because the specific task wasn't performed within that time frame. The better practice is to use such terms as *when warranted, as conditions indicate, in the registered nurse's discretion,* and *within every ___ hours.*

Keeping policies and procedures current

When a policy or procedure is drafted, it should be dated to reflect when it became effective. All policies and procedures require periodic review and updating to ensure that they represent current health care practice and that terminology is consistent. All revisions should be dated and documented. The risk manager should maintain a copy of the policy or procedure not only in the form in which it became effective but also in each revised form, in case a cause of action is brought against the facility.

Keep in mind that if a policy or procedure were revised after an incident, that revised form wouldn't necessarily reflect the established practice at the time of the incident. It's important to ensure that the policies and procedures in place at the time of the incident are used to help establish the current standard of care at the time in question.

The role of education

Education and training programs play an important role in risk management. Programs include general orientation about the components of a risk management program and staff responsibilities to further risk management efforts. General information includes the definition of *risk management,* the functions of the risk manager, and an overview of professional liability programs that outlines who is insured, describes the insurance coverage, details the steps for reporting incidents, and explains why individual coverage of professional liability insurance is recommended or required. Other general topics include reasons why risk management practice is critical to the survival of the facility, and the health care staff's obligations to support risk management, including the significance of early reporting of potentially compensable events, criteria to be used to identify a claim, and the way trending data are used in the facility's loss control efforts.

Using in-service

Focused in-service education is required on a routine basis to address such areas as patient safety efforts, medical injury prevention, legal aspects of patient care, use of new equipment, intro-

Typical allegations

The following are examples of typical allegations in lawsuits involving nurses:
- Failure to adequately document patient care
- Failure to monitor the patient
- Failure to initiate treatment in an appropriate and timely fashion
- Failure to follow physician orders
- Failure to notify the physician
- Failure to identify abnormal signs and symptoms and to respond appropriately
- Failure to identify and rule out potential problems
- Failure to identify high-risk patients
- Failure to convey discharge instructions
- Failure to follow facility procedure
- Failure to report questionable care or substandard medical practices
- Failure to ensure patient safety
- Failure to use medical equipment and supplies safely
- Failure to administer medication correctly
- Failure to provide adequately trained staff and adequate supervision.

duction of new clinical practices, and ways to develop rapport and communicate with patients and their family members. These programs provide a means for the risk manager to advise staff of new risk control techniques and to provide an overview of any newly enacted regulatory requirements.

Education programs can also provide information related to recently identified loss trends. Data collected from analysis of trending reports is important in identifying weaknesses and determining whether the weaknesses are systemic, individual, or related to a specific clinical area.

Know the allegations

Managers should be aware of the allegations typically made against nursing staff in medical malpractice actions. Knowledge of these allegations assists managers in initiating proactive steps. These allegations become evident in trial cases. (See *Typical allegations*.)

The following section reviews allegations commonly raised in lawsuits. Some case law is also provided to demonstrate the prin-

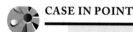

CASE IN POINT

Failure to inform

In a Nebraska case,[9] the nursing staff practiced good documentation but failed to keep the physician informed of the patient's condition.

Patient Critchfield gave birth to twins by cesarean delivery. The admitting assessment on one twin, whose birth weight was 4 pounds 10 ounces, revealed that he was having difficulty breathing as evidenced by retractions during attempts to breathe, cyanosis, pallor, a weak cry, and flaccid muscle tone. He was admitted to the neonatal intensive care unit. About 12 1/2 hours after birth, the nurse noted that the baby was lethargic. About 4 hours later, the nurse documented that the baby demonstrated poor muscle tone, shallow respirations, and little movement, but she didn't alert the treating physician of her findings. About 3 hours later, the nurse noted chest retractions, which continued over the next 3 hours. Once again, she made appropriate documentation of her findings but didn't notify the attending physician.

Ultimately, the baby suffered brain damage, and a lawsuit was filed. Expert testimony at trial indicated that had the nursing staff advised the attending physician of the baby's deteriorating condition, the brain damage potentially could have been alleviated with the administration of oxygen. Therefore, the attending nurse was found to have breached the standard of care. The court found in favor of the plaintiff. The lesson here? Good documentation is good nursing practice, but it won't protect the nurse if the physician isn't kept informed.

ciples presented. Case law is a good resource for the risk manager in providing proactive educational programs.

Medical documentation

Much has been written about the importance of medical documentation. Documentation records information that tells the story of the patient's condition and treatment while receiving care at the facility. Documentation should be objective, factual, accurate, and complete. The best practice is to document as the care is being given. Documentation must be legible. Something should be documented subjectively only when it's a direct quote from a patient or the patient's family. Only approved abbreviations should be used. If a note is indecipherable, then it can be misinterpreted, and faulty care can result. The reader shouldn't have to guess what the writer intends. (See *Failure to inform.*)

Each facility should develop policies and procedures on how corrections and late entries are to be made in a medical record.

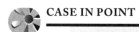

Altered nurse's notes

The principle of late entry is demonstrated in a Louisiana case[10] in which nurse's notes were found to be altered and missing.

Patient Gordon was transported by ambulance to the hospital with shortness of breath and chest pain. While en route, she received oxygen. According to emergency medical service documentation, she arrived at the hospital emergency department at 7:49 p.m. The emergency department record indicated that she arrived at 7:50 p.m. The 7:50 p.m. time element was altered such that no one could determine what was originally documented.

At some point, the emergency department nurse removed Ms. Gordon's oxygen. Shortly after Ms. Gordon's admission, her son came to the hospital and was advised that she wasn't in the emergency department. He frantically searched for her and eventually found her alone in the emergency department. Ms. Gordon collapsed as her son tried to help her to the bathroom. The son called for help. A code was called. All resuscitation efforts failed, and Ms. Gordon was pronounced dead. A wrongful death suit was filed.

At the time of trial, expert testimony indicated that Ms. Gordon could have survived had she received oxygen and been treated immediately. During the trial, evidence was introduced indicting that the medical records had been improperly altered. Rather than marking through the incorrect time, recording the correct time, and initialing the entry — which would have been proper procedure for altering a nurse's notes — the nurse wrote over the original time. The court found for the plaintiff.

The general practice for correcting an entry is to draw a line through the misstatement and to initial and date the correction. Any late entry should indicate the patient care date in question and the pertinent information, and it should be initialed and dated. Although it's advisable to have a record of what happened during patient care, it's inadvisable to make a late entry after an attorney has requested the patient's medical record or the facility has received some other communication from the patient's attorney. (See *Altered nurse's notes*.)

Medication errors

Medication errors generally involve one of the five rights of medication administration: the dose, route, patient, medication, or time. The person administering medication is responsible for having a basic knowledge of the medication's actions, the normal

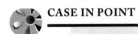 CASE IN POINT

Medication documentation error

The importance of indicating the site and mode of administration in the medication documentation was the issue in another case.[11]

Patient Pellerin was admitted to the emergency department with chest pain. The emergency department physician examined Ms. Pellerin and placed an order for an injection of 50 mg of meperidine (Demerol) and 25 mg of hydroxyzine (Vistaril). After the medication was administered, Ms. Pellerin felt a sharp pain and burning sensation in her hip. These symptoms continued to extend in her hip area and progressively worsened over the next several weeks.

Ms. Pellerin brought suit. The nurse had failed to indicate the site and mode of administration in her documentation in the patient's medical record. Expert testimony revealed that the patient's injury could have been caused if Vistaril wasn't injected into the muscle; however, the injury more likely resulted because of improper mechanics of injecting the needle. The jury found in favor of the plaintiff.

dose, and any adverse effects or contraindications related to the drug. (See *Medication documentation error*.)

Patient condition issues

The importance of accurate and appropriate monitoring of the patient's condition goes without saying. The patient care plan is developed incorporating the status of each patient's initial condition and modified to meet the needs of the patient's ongoing condition. Liability exposure becomes an issue when the patient's condition isn't monitored or when the health care staff fails to notify the patient's physician of any change in the patient's condition. The nurse's responsibility doesn't end with placing a call to the physician. The responsibility requires actual communication of the patient's change of condition. Of course, it's then important that this communication be appropriately documented to include the reported change in condition, the time it was reported, the name of the physician who received the report, and any orders that the physician gave. All attempts to reach the physician, including times and when the physician responded, should be documented.

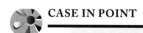
CASE IN POINT

Inconsistent orders

A Massachusetts case[12] demonstrates the nurse's responsibility to spot inconsistent physician orders.

Mr. St. Germain underwent lumbar surgery, during which he had fixation hooks and rods inserted. The surgery was performed by an orthopedic surgeon and a neurosurgeon. After surgery, the orthopedic surgeon ordered the patient to be on bed rest for 4 to 5 days. However, 2 days after the surgery, a first-year orthopedic resident wrote an order for Mr. St. Germain to receive a soft orthopedic support and to be moved out of bed to a chair. The resident wrote these orders in the physician order section of the chart, in the physician progress note section, but the resident made note only of the order for the bandage and failed to note the order to get the patient up.

The orthopedic surgeon visited the patient and acknowledged the resident's progress note. The surgeon added to the progress note that Mr. St. Germain was to receive an X-ray the next day and, if OK, was to be moved out of bed to a "tilt table." The surgeon failed to cosign the orders written by the resident.

The charge nurse noted the orders of the surgeon and the resident. The next morning, the assigned nurse encouraged Mr. St. Germain to get out of bed and walk. However, as Mr. St. Germain tried to stand up, a large snapping sound from his back was noted, and he fell backward back onto the bed. The orthopedic surgeon was called. Mr. St. Germain was returned to surgery at which time it was noted that the rods and hooks had shifted position. The corrective surgery was unsuccessful.

Mr. St. Germain brought suit of medical negligence. The court found against the hospital, citing that the hospital nursing staff had breached the standard of care to spot inconsistencies in the orders of the surgeon and those of the resident.

Transcription of orders

Not only must nursing staff ensure that medical orders are correctly transcribed, they must also ensure that the order is appropriate for the patient. This includes making sure that no inconsistencies between orders and no contraindications exist. (See *Inconsistent orders.*)

Falls

Interestingly enough, patient falls are responsible for more negligence lawsuits against hospitals and hospital staff than any other causes.[13] In addition, the use of restraints has caused much attention in light of recent patient rights efforts. Therefore, the use of restraints to help prevent falls has limited application. Nursing

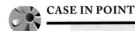

Result of a fall

Mr. Lamarca was admitted to the intensive care unit with shortness of breath, dizziness, and a history of heart disease and arthritis. He was placed on several medications, some having a sedative effect.

The next day, Mr. Lamarca's wife found him unconscious. The nursing staff advised her that Mr. Lamarca had been injured in an accident. The incident report indicated that the patient had fallen out of bed. As a result of the fall, Mr. Lamarca suffered a broken hip. He remained hospitalized and suffered complications, which ultimately resulted in his death.

Trial testimony revealed that the nurse hadn't placed the patient on appropriate fall risk prevention. The court held that the hospital was responsible for Mr. Lamarca's fractured hip, which ultimately resulted in his death.[14]

staff can help alleviate falls by performing adequate and appropriate assessments, assuring that the patient is provided with the appropriate support necessary to safely ambulate, and making sure the environment is uncluttered. (See *Result of a fall*.)

Transfer of care

If a patient requires transfer to another facility where necessary care is available, appropriate steps must be taken to ensure a successful and safe patient transfer. Such steps include stabilizing the patient before transfer, adequately communicating the patient's condition and needs to the receiving facility and to the staff transporting the patient, and providing appropriately trained staff to care for the patient during transport. (See *Patient transfer*.)

Standards of care

Policies and procedures establish standards of care. When adopted policies and procedures aren't followed and injury results to the patient, the nurse and the facility can be held liable. (See *A crash cart incident*, page 374.)

Health care staff using medical equipment must be in-serviced on its appropriate and safe use. Liability exposure may be demonstrated for failing to meet this standard. In one case, the plaintiff died during surgery when certain medical apparatus was used inappropriately.[15] Testimony at trial found that two nurses were unfamiliar with the use of the equipment in question and

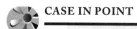

CASE IN POINT

Patient transfer

The Romo case[16] represents legal and ethical issues that can arise from a patient transfer.

Mr. Romo was admitted to Union Memorial Hospital with complaints of vomiting and abdominal pain. He was diagnosed with gastroenteritis, discharged, and given discharge instructions. Two days later, he came to the hospital with right-sided abdominal pain, chills, and nausea. Mr. Romo was assessed, and orders were written that he was to be monitored. However, the nurses' notes indicated that his vital signs weren't monitored during two periods of extended time.

A second physician examined Mr. Romo and determined that he needed to be closely monitored in the intensive care unit. Because no beds were available at Union Memorial Hospital, arrangements were made to transfer Mr. Romo to another hospital. After transfer, he was diagnosed with probable perforated appendix with sepsis. Before he could be taken to surgery, Mr. Romo suffered a cardiac arrest. Following resuscitation, he underwent surgery, during which he died.

His wife brought suit. The issue before the court was whether the transferring hospital had stabilized Mr. Romo's condition, as required by the Emergency Medical Treatment and Active Labor Act, before the transfer. The court found against Union Memorial Hospital, citing that the hospital had breached the standard of care required by not adequately stabilizing Mr. Romo's condition.

had never received in-servicing on its use. The equipment in question used a clip on a piece of tubing. At the time of the surgery, the clip wasn't in place, which left the tubing hanging. The court found that the clip was in place when the equipment left the manufacturer. This tube was inadvertently attached to an outflow port during surgery, resulting in the patient's death. The court held that the nursing staff breached a standard by not being trained on the equipment before using it. The court also found that the supervisory nurse should have been aware of the lack of experience of the operating room staff related to this piece of equipment. (See *Medical negligence,* page 375.)

As mentioned previously, health care facilities are required to provide adequate medical equipment and supplies to provide safe patient care. The Citron case resulted in an adverse decision against the hospital for failure to have sufficient blood products available.[17] In this case, the decedent who was 26 weeks pregnant was experiencing back pain, cramps, and nausea. Her physi-

CASE IN POINT

A crash cart incident

A North Carolina case[18] demonstrates the failure to follow a policy and procedure requiring the checking and restocking of the crash cart after use.

In this case, Mrs. Dixon was intubated when she went into respiratory failure early one morning. Throughout the day, her condition improved to the point that she was able to be weaned from the ventilator and extubated. However, shortly after extubation, her condition deteriorated.

Mrs. Dixon arrested before she could be reintubated. A code was called. The crash cart, which was located outside of Mrs. Dixon's room, was brought into the room. The respiratory therapist responding to the code attempted to intubate Mrs. Dixon but didn't have the appropriate size endotracheal blade because the one from the crash cart had been used earlier in the day to intubate Mrs. Dixon.

After several attempts to intubate Mrs. Dixon failed, one nurse secured the requested endotracheal blade and gave it to Dr. Taylor, who then easily and successfully intubated Mrs. Dixon. However, Mrs. Dixon never recovered consciousness, and she ultimately died.

Suit was brought against the hospital. The court found against the hospital, stating that the hospital's policy and procedure required that the crash cart be checked and restocked after each use. The court determined that less time might have passed securing a fully stocked crash cart than trying to intubate Mrs. Dixon with the wrong size blade — and damage to the patient might have been avoided. The court also noted the ease in which Mrs. Dixon was intubated when the appropriate size blade was provided.

cian directed her to go to the emergency department. By the time she reached the hospital, she had no vital signs. Following resuscitation and stabilization for an intra-abdominal bleed, she was taken to the operating room. During surgery, it was noted that she had lost at least half of her blood supply. The hospital didn't have sufficient whole blood or platelets to treat this patient. She died about 4 hours after surgery. Her surviving spouse brought suit against the hospital. The court found for the plaintiff, citing failure to have or secure sufficient blood products to meet the patient's needs.

Staff issues

Another concern for corporate exposure involves allegations for failing to have adequately trained staff and adequate supervision. Nursing shortages have occurred to varying degrees for the past

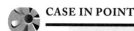

Medical negligence

The following case[19] demonstrates how the plaintiffs were unable to prove that the four elements of medical negligence were met.

In this case, Patient Beilke was admitted to the hospital in labor. It was noted that she was allergic to latex. At the time of admission, her blood pressure was elevated. Mrs. Beilke was given an epidural, after which the nurse decided to catheterize the patient with a rubber catheter. After catheterization, the patient experienced a warm and itchy feeling along with shortness of breath. Subsequently, the unborn baby's heart rate dropped. An emergency delivery was carried out with the use of forceps. At the time of birth, the baby wasn't breathing. The baby was resuscitated but was eventually diagnosed with cerebral palsy (CP).

The plaintiff brought suit against the nurse, alleging that she caused the baby's CP by inserting a rubber catheter. The court found in favor of the hospital, holding that the CP wasn't proximately caused by the insertion of the rubber catheter. This decision was based on the expert testimony provided at the time of trial.

---

several decades. In light of the shortages, unlicensed assistive personnel are hired to assist in performing tasks that can be delegated. (See *Inadequate training,* page 376.)

Product liability

In addition to being sued for patient care provided or required, efforts have been made to sue hospitals under a products liability theory. However, to prevail, the plaintiff must show that the health care facility is the seller or manufacturer of a medical product. For example, the plaintiff in an Indiana case[20] failed to provide testimony to prevail on a product liability cause of action brought against the hospital.

Patient Casko was admitted to St. Mary's to have a pacemaker inserted. Allegedly, the pacemaker failed, and the patient died. Suit was brought against the hospital, the physicians, and the medical company that allegedly manufactured, sold, and distributed the pacemaker. Indiana's product liability law required that the injured party prove the seller distributed a defective product unreasonably dangerous to a consumer and that the defective product reached the consumer in the same defective condition without substantial alteration. The hospital argued—and the

Inadequate training

The following case[21] represents allegations of breach of the duty to have adequately trained staff.

Mrs. Merritt fell and broke her hip after trying to crawl out of bed while the attending nurse was responding to a code in another room. The patient had tried getting out of bed on several occasions, despite the fact that the side rails were documented as being up and that she was cautioned to seek assistance from the nursing staff when trying to get out of bed.

The patient underwent surgery for repair of the hip fracture. Several months later, she died as a result of complications allegedly related to the fall. The surviving family brought suit.

Testimony at the time of trial indicated that the patient was the nurse's only patient; however, following facility policy, the nurse left the patient to respond to the code. The court found for the surviving family.

court found — that the hospital wasn't a seller of a product but rather a provider of services.

Disability

The Americans with Disabilities Act (ADA) generally applies to the treatment of the disabled workforce. However, the Act was applied in a California case involving patient care.[22] Mr. Aikins collapsed at home. His wife, who was deaf, sought the assistance of a neighbor in calling 911 to have Mr. Aikins transported to the hospital.

Upon arrival to the hospital, the emergency department (ED) physician examined the patient. The ED physician was under the mistaken belief that Mr. Aikins had been without oxygen for only 4 minutes before the emergency medical services team arrived. The ED physician decided to perform an angioplasty but wasn't able to communicate with Mrs. Aikins to get permission because of her deafness. Mrs. Aikins requested an interpreter on a couple occasions. However, the hospital failed to grant her request. Ultimately, Mrs. Aikins learned though a written note that her husband wouldn't survive without life support.

The day after Mr. Aikins was admitted to the hospital, the attending physician learned that 15 minutes had lapsed between the time Mr. Aikins collapsed and the time cardiopulmonary resuscitation was initiated. An EEG was ordered; it showed no brain activity. The following day, Mr. Aikins's daughter arrived and learned of her father's condition. This was reportedly the first time Mrs. Aikins received answers to her questions. The decision was made to withdraw life support, and Mr. Aikins died. Mrs. Aikins brought suit against the hospital, alleging that the hospital failed to provide interpreters in violation of the ADA. The court found that the hospital violated the Act when it failed to show that an undue burden was placed on the hospital to provide an interpreter to communicate with Mrs. Aikins.

Liability prevention

Following are liability prevention tips specific to common allegations. These tips can assist the risk manager in developing proactive efforts.

Failure to maintain patient safety

➤ Follow the care plan established by physician orders (unless there's a question about the appropriateness of the order).

➤ Provide for proper assistance for bed, bath, shower, and tub.

➤ Provide for proper use of physical restraints as indicated and ordered.

➤ Appropriately document steps taken to ensure patient safety.

Failure to follow policies and procedures

➤ Draft policies and procedures to reflect actual practice.

➤ Beware of such words as *shall* and *must*.

➤ Avoid the term *responsibility for* because it prevents delegation.

➤ Avoid the term *highest quality* because it increases the required standard of care.

➤ Use words that provide for discretion.

➤ State as little as possible.

➤ Draft policies and procedures in the form of guidelines.

➤ Establish a system to seek approval for any deviations, and document reasons for the deviations.

➤ Provide for accessibility of policy and procedure manuals.

Failure to maintain equipment

➤ Keep equipment in working order.

➤ Keep appropriate maintenance logs.

➤ Remove dangerous or malfunctioning equipment.

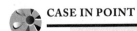

CASE IN POINT

Violence in the workplace

In a Louisiana case,[23] one of the hospital's nursing staff was stabbed in the hospital elevator. On the evening of the alleged incident, Nurse Mundy maintained that no security guards were present at the elevator she usually used when coming on duty. She testified that normally guards were present. As Nurse Mundy entered the elevator, someone jumped into the elevator and stabbed her with a knife. She suffered knife wounds to her back, neck, chest, and hand.

Nurse Mundy brought suit against the employer for failing to provide a safe work environment. The court held that the facility has a duty to exercise reasonable care for the safety of persons on its premises. Employees and other guests of the facility shouldn't be subjected to unreasonable risk of harm. This court found, however, that the duty doesn't extend to "unforeseen or unanticipated" criminal acts of a third party.

➤ Make sure necessary equipment is available.
➤ Keep clutter to a minimum.

Environmental safety

In addition to liability issues related to patient care, the facility must provide a safe environment for the staff. The safety of the environment includes not only the physical plant but also actions of other employees or visitors. (See *Violence in the workplace.*)

Workers' compensation

Another exposure area for which the risk manager may have responsibility is monitoring and overseeing workers' compensation cases. This could include helping to determine whether the injury "arose out of and in the scope of employment," ensuring that medical expenses are appropriate and paid in a timely fashion, and ensuring that the injured employee appropriately receives disability payments for time off from work. The goal is to help the injured worker return to work as soon as possible after an injury.

Workers' compensation generally doesn't cover injuries incurred commuting to or from worka, although there are exceptions to this rule. In the Deland case, the court found in favor of the injured employee.[24] Ms. Deland had completed her normally assigned shift. When her replacement called in sick, she had to continue to cover the unit for an additional shift. As a result, she worked 28 of 40 hours. On her way home, she fell asleep at the wheel and crashed into a pole, suffering facial and leg injuries. She filed for workers' compensation, which her employer denied. She then filed suit. The court found that there was a nexus between her injury and the schedule she was required to work.

Points to remember

The following points summarize the importance of risk prevention and management:

> ➤ A comprehensive risk prevention program can be truly effective only when the staff isn't expected to resolve difficult risk management issues alone but, rather, incorporates a team effort. Such a program requires the inclusion of quality assurance principles and compliance programs, a proactive approach to preventing injuries arising as a result of an unsafe environment or resulting from substandard care, and specific, careful, and defined responses to complaints as they arise.
> ➤ Given the major role the staff has in controlling exposure to liability in the health care environment (by following appropriately drafted polices and procedures and established, realistic standards of care), there's no substitute for a risk management program that provides the hospital staff with immediate problem-solving support.

References

1. Brent, N.J. *Nurses and the Law — A Guide to Principles and Applications,* 2nd ed. Philadelphia: W.B. Saunders Co., 2001; Pozgar, G. "Tort Reform and Reducing the Risks of Malpractice," in *Legal Aspects of Healthcare Administration,* 8th ed. Gaithersburg, Md.: Aspen Pubs., 2002; and Dzingleski, L. "The Basic Principles of Managing Risk," *Provider* 13(3):8, 10, 12, March 1987.
2. Brill, J.M. "Risk Management is Team Effort," *American Nurse* 22(3):34, March 1990.

3. Pozgar, G. Op. cit.

4. Pozgar, G. Op. cit.

5. Hagg, S. "Elements of a Risk Management Program," in *Risk Management Handbook for Health Care Organizations*, 2nd ed. Edited by R. Carroll. Chicago: American Hospital Publishing Co., 1997.

6. Johson, V.P. "Taming the Scourge of Incident Report Analysis," *Perspectives in Healthcare Risk* Management 10(2):9-12, Spring 1990.

7. Feutz-Harter, S.A. *Nursing and the Law*, 6th ed. Eau Claire, Wis.: Professional Educational Systems, 1999.

8. Feutz-Harter, S.A. Op. cit.

9. *Critchfield v. McNamara*, 532 N.W.2d 287 (Neb. 1995).

10. *Gordon v. Willis Knighton Medical Center*, 661 So.2d 991 (La. App. 1995).

11. *Pellerin v. Humedicenters, Inc.*, 697 So.2d. 590 (1997).

12. *St. Germain v. Pfeifer*, N.E.2d 848 (MA 1994).

13. Feutz-Harter, S.A. Op. cit.

14. *Lamarca v. U.S.*, 31 F. Supp. 2d 110 (NY 1998).

15. *Chin v. St. Barnabas Medical Center*, 711 A.2d 352 (NJ Super. 1998).

16. *Romo v. Union Memorial Hospital, Inc.*, 878 F. Supp. 837 (NC 1995)

17. *Citron v. Northern Dutchess Hospital*, 603 N.Y.S.2d 639 (NY 1993).

18. *Dixon v. Taylor*, 431 S.E.2d 778 (NC 1993).

19. *Beilke by Beilke v. Coryell*, 524 N.W.2d 607 (ND 1994)

20. *St. Mary Medical Center, Inc. v. Casko*, 639 N.E.2d 312 (Ind. 1994).

21. *Merritt v. Karcioglu*, 687 So.2d 469 (LA 1996).

22. *Aikins v. St. Helena Hospital*, 843 F. Supp. 1329 (CA 1994).

23. *Mundy v. Department of Health and Human Resources*, 620 So.2d 811 (LA 1993).

24. *Deland v. Hutchings Psychiatric Center*, 611 N.Y.S. 2d 44 (1994).

Selected readings

Aiken, T.D. (ed.) *Legal and Ethical Issues in Health Occupations.* Philadelphia: W.B. Saunders Co., 2002.

Carroll, R. *Risk Management Handbook for Health Care Organizations*, 3rd ed. San Francisco: Jossey-Bass, 2001.

Lee, N.G. *Legal Concepts and Issues in Emergency Care.* Philadelphia: W.B. Saunders Co., 2001.

Levine, M.L. (ed.) *The Elderly : Legal and Ethical Issues in Health Care Policy.* London: Ashgate Publishing Co., 2002.

Youngberg, B.J., ed. "Integrating Quality Assurance and Risk Management," *The Risk Manager's Desk Reference*, 2nd ed. Gaithersburg, Md.: Aspen Pubs., 1998.

CHAPTER 17

Performance appraisal

Marie Brewer, RN, LNC

> "Leaders recognize the hidden qualities that bring about success, and focus on the 'specialness' of their people." — Art Williams, *Pushing Up People*[1]

Managers in health care must do more than manage day-to-day operations in their facilities. They must also coach the professional growth of the people who choose to work with them in the joint endeavor of patient care. After all, if your employees are successful, then you're successful.

Although to be successful in a job, a person needs to know what's expected of him. It's the manager's job to communicate the job requirements and remove the barriers that prevent an employee from being successful. Consider the role of manager at the beginning of the performance continuum, starting with an excerpt from *The Sales Coaching Playbook.*

"In working with managers from banking to health care to real estate to technology, I've concluded that there are three main reasons for [a] manager's failure. They:

➤ don't know what the job involves.
➤ don't know how to do the job.
➤ don't have the tools to get the job done."[2]

Managers wear two main hats — that of an administrator and that of a coach. Administrators focus on the management core, such as oversight of policy, procedures, employee compensation,

Benefits of coaching

Coaching employees has many benefits. It:
➤ improves professionalism
➤ improves communication within the team
➤ improves employee commitment, ownership, and involvement
➤ reduces turnover
➤ improves relationships and increases confidence and competence of the team
➤ increases performance and productivity

and strategic development. Coaching involves administration, but it also focuses on helping a person develop in a way that he attains his maximum potential. It's about communicating with him and tapping into his internal influences and energy. (See *Benefits of coaching.*)

Value of one-on-one talks

The most significant benefit of the performance appraisal process is that, in the hectic pace of daily working life, it offers a manager and an employee the rare chance for a one-on-one discussion of important work issues that might not otherwise be addressed. For many employees, the performance appraisal interview may be the only time they have exclusive, uninterrupted access to their manager.

When the performance appraisal process is conducted properly, most managers and employees report the experience as beneficial and positive. This time offers a valuable opportunity for a manager and an employee to focus on work activities and goals, to identify and correct existing problems, and to encourage better performance that will enhance the performance of the entire facility. The value of this intense and purposeful interaction shouldn't be underestimated by either party or by the facility. It's vital to the professional growth of the employee, manager, and facility.

Origins of performance appraisal

Performance appraisal is a method of evaluating an employee's job performance by comparing actual results to expected outcomes — although its history is quite brief.

Frederick Taylor and Henry Ford

The modern origin of performance appraisal can be traced to 1907 to 1914, Frederick Taylor's time-and-motion studies, and Henry Ford. Ford realized he would need a more efficient way to produce cars in order to lower the price. He and his team looked at other industries and found four principles that would further their goal — interchangeable parts, continuous flow, division of labor, and less wasted effort.

Ford divided the labor by breaking the assembly of the Model T into 84 distinct steps. Each worker was trained to do just one step. Ford called in Frederick Taylor, the creator of *scientific management,* to do time and motion studies to determine the exact speed at which the work should proceed and the exact motions workers should use to accomplish their tasks.[3]

Saul Sells

As a management tool, formal evaluation of work performance dates back to World War II and a man named Saul Sells. Throughout his career, Sells stressed the significance of organism and environment interactions in understanding and predicting behavior; he also emphasized the need to study behavior in its natural setting. The first project he conducted was adaptability screening of Air Force pilots, which later became a prototype for research in pilot selection and validation design. It involved a worldwide program for testing pilots in training, and later assessed their performance in combat during the Korean War. Sells later studied similar issues confronted by the National Aeronautics and Space Administration as they began planning long-duration space missions.[4]

Salary justification

Performance appraisal systems started as a way to determine if the work being performed justified the salary an employee was receiving. If an employee's performance was less than ideal, a pay cut would follow. However, if his performance was better than expected, a pay raise was in order. This system was cut-and-dried and failed to take into account the developmental possibilities of an employee. Referring to the origin of the performance appraisal process, it was believed that an adjustment in pay should be the sole impetus for an employee to either improve or continue to perform well. Sometimes this basic system succeeded in getting the intended results, but more often than not it failed.

As a nurse-manager, you know this methodology has little to do with recruiting and retaining competent staff, especially professional staff, in today's health care setting. Most professionals want to work in an environment that satisfies them on personal, professional, and educational levels, above and beyond the monetary factors, with morale and self-esteem being key issues.

Measuring performance

Robert Mager, the famous educator, stated: "We teach and train because we hope that through our instruction students will some how be different than they were before the instruction. We provide a learning experience with the intent that each student will be a modified person in knowledge, in attitude, in belief and in skill." The process of measuring employee performance should have the same intent. It should be a learning experience, for the employer and manager that improves the areas of performance listed by Mager. Measuring performance has moved beyond the original intent established by Frederick Taylor and Henry Ford. It should be a continuous process that helps an employee grow in his job. (See *Understanding the performance appraisal process.*)

Because the performance appraisal process touches the heart of employment — that is, an employee's job responsibilities, abilities, and money — few other issues in management stir as much controversy as this process. Ideally the performance appraisal process allows management to specify exactly what an employee

Understanding the performance appraisal process

The *performance appraisal process* may be defined as a structured formal interaction between an employee and a manager, in which the employee's work performance is examined and discussed, with a goal of identifying weaknesses and strengths as well as identifying opportunities for improvement and skills development. The interview may be conducted annually, semiannually, or at another set period, depending on the organization.

From the employee viewpoint, the purpose of performance appraisal is fourfold:

➤ Tell me what you want me to do.
➤ Tell me how well I've done it.
➤ Help me improve my performance.
➤ Reward me for doing well.

In most health care facilities, the results of such performance appraisals are used to determine which employees deserve pay increases, bonuses, or promotions. Alternatively, such results are also used to identify a marginal employee who may need additional training, counseling, or in some cases, demotion or dismissal.

Many different techniques can be used during the performance appraisal process. Below are some examples.

Type	Characteristics
Rating scale	Employees are rated on a scale, usually from 1 to 10, on behavior and job skills, such as timeliness, accuracy, teamwork, and quantity of work accomplished.
Management by objectives	Objectives are set, plans determined, performance reviewed, and rewards given.
Forced choice	The evaluator chooses among descriptions of employee behavior — scored according to a key.
Simple ranking	Raters rank the their subordinates from best to worst on their perceived performances.
Critical incidents	Raters identify critical positive and negative employee performance. (*Note:* Behaviorally anchored rating scales can be derived from these.)
Essay	Performances are described in essays.

is expected to do and then set relevant goals and solicit employee feedback related to his meeting of such goals. Because this process is never totally objective and infallible, the measurement system should be job-specific, directly relevant to the job, practical in its application, and fair and useful in its outcome. The employee who is being evaluated should always have a say in the process and an opportunity to disagree if necessary. The process should be ongoing during the course of employment so when the time comes for a formal performance appraisal, nothing discussed is a surprise to the employee.

Process failure

The performance appraisal process can fail for a number of reasons, but inevitably falls back on the manager's ability to communicate expectations and give relevant feedback to an employee. Some of the more common reasons include:

> ➤ The manager conducting the performance appraisal has limited contact with the employee and thus doesn't really know how he performs.
> ➤ The manager isn't skilled in giving timely feedback or in dealing with an employee who doesn't take negative feedback well.
> ➤ The manager views the performance appraisal process as one more annual task that has to be done and checked off the list.
> ➤ The manager separates the objective performance appraisal process from the more subjective coaching process, failing to see that the two are inextricably linked.
> ➤ The manager is new and fears she doesn't know the employee or the job well enough to defend her observations—precisely why it's vital that the performance appraisal be based on written standards that are directly related to the critical job elements.

Again, the employee should know in advance what's expected, when the performance appraisal will occur, and what the outcomes could be for good or poor results. Managers should be thoroughly trained and familiar with the performance appraisal process their facility uses and should apply the elements individually. Successful appraisal requires an investment of the manager's time. The process should go on day-to-day, in addition to the annual or semiannual formal session. To make the process meaningful for the employee and manager, certain steps need to be taken before the actual performance appraisal session.

Before meeting with the employee

An employee should be given an opportunity to complete a self-evaluation using the same tool and criteria the manager uses. This process should allow the employee the opportunity to state the areas he thinks he has done well in as well as the areas he knows he needs additional work and assistance. This exercise sets

QUESTIONS & ANSWERS

Improving the outcome

Question: *What should I do as a manager if the performance appraisal has some negative components?*

Answer: The manager isn't there to pass judgment on an employee, but rather to find ways to help the employee improve, add skills, and move ahead with personal or career goals. Be aware, however, that if the employee isn't meeting the goals and expectations of the job, it's your job as manager to specifically discuss this with him. In most cases, an employee knows when he isn't doing what he's supposed to and is waiting for you to tell him.

If such a situation occurs, be prepared to ask the employee how he intends to correct his behavior or what steps or actions he intends to take to improve his skills. Set a time frame for this action, and schedule another meeting date to discuss the outcome. Ask the employee if he needs additional training or retraining. Finally, together develop short- and long-term career goals that will benefit the employee and the company.[5]

the framework for the actual performance appraisal because now the manager knows how the employee thinks he's functioning in his job.

The entire process should be approached from the perspective that the manager is there to learn from and assist the employee in reaching his full potential. As such, the manager must review the entire period that the performance appraisal covers, not just the most recent period. So how do you prepare for the interview? Review any notes, letters of thank you or complaint, projects completed, and anything else that has occurred with this employee since his last appraisal. With this information in hand and with the employee's self-evaluation, you should be able to remain objective as you work through the performance appraisal process.

The next step

The next step might be a little different than what's commonly done, but allow the employee to take the lead in the performance appraisal interview. Let him tell you how he thinks the job has gone since his last evaluation. Ask him what he has learned from any situations that could be perceived as less than desirable. Ask him what he needs from you or the company to be successful or to continue to grow in his job. Does he want to continue in this role, or is he interested in pursuing opportunities in other areas? (See *Improving the outcome.*)

Self-evaluation

The self-review performance appraisal model is based on the idea that an employee is most familiar with his own work. How he thinks he's doing his job is essential to the appraisal process. An employee rates himself on a number of criteria on a formal survey form that includes a section for self-improvement suggestions the employee feels are needed. He's given an opportunity to clarify his goals and state his areas of weakness as a focus for improvement during the next review period. In most cases, the self-review is done as part of the entire review process, usually in advance of the formal manager-and-employee interview.

Having an employee use the self-evaluation performance appraisal model can be an enlightening experience for the manager. In most cases, the employee scores himself lower than what the manager would score. Every once in a while, however, you'll have a poorly performing employee score himself highly. You can prepare for this by doing your homework before the formal review. When there's a wide discrepancy in scoring results, be prepared with objective data and questions to ascertain why the employee thinks he's doing a good job when the data proves otherwise. Perhaps he doesn't fully understand the job requirements or his role in the continuum of care where he works. It's also possible he may never have been given feedback on his performance and may truly think he's meeting all requirements. This is a good time to begin the redirection of this behavior and reestablish goals to get him on track.

The self-evaluation tool must be carefully selected and must correlate to the questions and criteria on the formal review tool. Both the tools and the process itself need to be carefully and thoroughly reviewed with each new employee at the time of hire as well as immediately before the actual review. Let the employee know the information you're looking for and how you'll use it. Allow time for him to ask questions so he can go into this process being comfortable with its level of fairness and applicability to the job.

A self-evaluation should be completed and turned in several weeks before the formal evaluation interview so you have time to compare notes and proceed with a meaningful and fair appraisal.

Be sure to reference the self-evaluation during the interview to acknowledge the importance of the employee's feedback. It's a good idea to have a copy of it with you in case you or the employee needs to refer to it during the interview.

Peer review

Peer review is a process through which team members give one another formal feedback on their performance. It usually replaces the traditional performance appraisal process in team-based organizations.

Peer review isn't a common way of measuring performance in a significant way. That is, it isn't used in most cases, and when it is, it may affect the employee's monetary compensation. Generally, it's more prevalent in organizations with a culture of openness, teamwork, and cooperation — for example, in nonprofit organizations.

In organizations that traditionally conduct business in a team model, the traditional performance appraisal process (where managers sit down one-on-one with an employee to rate and discuss his performance) doesn't always provide the employee with a solid understanding of how he's doing. This model provides feedback only from the manager and not from other team members — and team feedback is critical to the success of the performance appraisal, especially if the manager is new to the job and still getting to know the employee.

In a peer review model, an employee is evaluated by the people with whom he works and whom he has to back up and support on a daily basis. Also, the traditional performance appraisal process reinforces a hierarchical, paternalistic culture that's in opposition to the team-staffing model. It's vital that an employee not only be competent and skilled in his job but also perform as a cooperative team member, in order to provide the best service to the patient.

Laying the groundwork

For the peer review process to be effective, certain groundwork must be laid. The peer groups need extensive training so the

MANAGER'S TIP

Preparing for peer review

One of the best ways to prepare staff to participate in peer review is to allow them maximum input in establishing the ground rules for the process. They need to know the philosophy behind the system and the rationale for why it has been selected. They need assurance that their input will be considered and that they won't be held responsible for counseling peer team members who don't meet performance standards. This preparation is, and will always remain, part of the manager's or supervisor's job description.

Another area that tends to meet staff resistance is data collection for the aggregation of performance appraisal scores. Team members tend to not want to participate in this process because it takes them away from the job at hand, which is patient care.

Once the decision has been made to use the peer review model as a part of the overall performance appraisal process and the tools have been developed, the process must be piloted. Staff should be encouraged to provide feedback on the system itself. Training and support should be available. Pilot programs are important for any new system, because they provide the opportunity to iron out the bugs, without letting the program lose credibility among other workers.

process is valuable to them and not a means to reward friends or hurt foes. There must be an objective approach to the measurements being selected.

Most facilities that use the peer review process use the results for personal improvement issues and not pay increases or disciplinary actions. They typically use a combination of models in order to give thorough, accurate feedback to the employee being appraised. Facilities need to be aware that use of peer review or the 360-degree evaluation is a major cultural change for most people — and can be a threatening experience for the poor performer or insecure team member. It usually takes a lot of time, practice, and discussion to get the buy-in required to make peer review successful. (See *Preparing for peer review.*)

Implementing peer review

Peer reviews that are carefully thought out and fairly implemented can have a high level of worker acceptance and involvement. By helping peers understand each others' work and by airing grievances in a nonthreatening manner, peer reviews may also help people get along better and thus improve overall organizational performance. It can also help alleviate frustration in the workplace and minimize the role of workplace politics. It's also recommended that this not be the only method of performance appraisal used. It should never be used by management to shift their responsibility for evaluating and fostering the professional growth of an employee onto the employees themselves.

Additionally, somewhat apart from the performance appraisal process, it isn't uncommon in the health care environment for professionals to conduct a peer review of other professionals when an untoward incident has occurred. It's expected that in most cases such a review will occur; however, some nurses are offended by the idea of being judged in such a review process. The peer review process should include a committee consisting of staff and supervisory members who have a knowledgeable and nonbiased view of the incident.

The critical role of peer review in patient care is widely accepted in the health care profession. A major component of the peer review process is the peer evaluation of clinical judgment using written documentation, established clinical guidelines, and patient care protocols. Moreover, the process evaluates technical skills, appropriateness of the care, and the outcome of the care rendered.

The 360-degree evaluation

One of the best methods of performance appraisal combines several tools and is known as the 360-degree evaluation. This process solicits performance feedback from:

➤ self
➤ coworkers (peer review)
➤ supervisors and managers
➤ patients.

This method covers the gamut of job responsibilities, including "customer" service, with the "customer" (patient) being involved in the appraisal process. It also allows the manager to maintain control over such issues as merit and other pay increases that are based on behavior other than what the peer group sees.

Although costly in resources, the 360-degree feedback has been found to be the most comprehensive type of appraisal. The model includes self-assessment, peer review, customer review, and management review, with feedback being sought from everyone. It gives people a chance to learn how others see them, to see their skills and style, and to improve communications with others. Because this process solicits input from so many sources, the employee tends to receive a more honest, thorough evaluation of job performance. Also, because the input comes from many different sources — and because different people observe different things — the employee's behavior and work performance tend to improve at an accelerated rate.

Again, the process requires extensive preparation and training of all involved for it to be successful. All relevant employees need to be involved in the process because if they help build it, then they have ownership and buy-in to the process, and then it will work.

Components of performance appraisal

The performance appraisal process gives an employee recognition for his work efforts. Great power rests in such recognition and, in fact, it's well known that human beings prefer even negative recognition to no recognition at all!

Turnover, tardiness, and absenteeism might be reduced if more attention were paid to employee performance on a daily basis. People need to know that someone does care and does pay attention to what they do, or don't do. If it does nothing else, the time and effort spent in developing, implementing, and using a performance appraisal process shows an employee that the facility is interested in his job performance and professional growth. This gives him a sense of worth and value. In a general sense, the data collected from the individual appraisals should be used to monitor the effectiveness of the recruitment and retention activities of the facility. This method is effective for determining what the facility does well and what it needs to improve on as it relates to employee retention, education, and training.

The performance appraisal process typically consists of four inter-related steps.

Step 1: Clear expectations

The first step occurs well before an evaluation is ever done. A new employee must be told and must understand exactly what the job expectations are, how performance will be measured, who will "judge" the work, and how often. He needs to know what will be done to assist him if he isn't meeting expectations as well as opportunities for advancement if he meets and exceeds expectations.

Step 2: Regular feedback

An employee should also be aware that the performance appraisal process is just that, a process and not a once-a-year drill. Ongoing assessment of performance and the progress in meeting job expectations is vital. It isn't good management style to wait until an evaluation to tell an employee that he's consistently failing to meet expectations. Instead, tell him all along how he's doing, whether it's positive feedback or constructive criticism. Remember that every new job has a learning curve, even if the curve is getting used to the new facility, rather than new skills or competencies. Allow for this and mentor the new employee, as needed. The same holds true for a seasoned employee who's promoted into a new role, who may also need additional attention during this time.

Step 3: Documented progress

Thorough documentation of the employee's performance using the facility's policies, procedures, and forms is the next step. If the facility uses a self-appraisal, peer review, or 360-degree process, make sure the employee clearly understands how he's to be rated, before the actual meeting.

Step 4: Future direction

Finally, set up a time to conduct the performance appraisal interview with the employee. Allow adequate time, and have all documents ready. Make sure you have coverage for phone calls or other managerial duties so your time with the employee is uninterrupted. Be prepared to end the review with a discussion of a job-related development plan that's tailored to that employee. To-gether determine the areas where additional effort is needed as well as practical ways for the employee to make that happen within his job.

A matter of trust

Even though a manager is responsible for nurturing the professional growth of an employee, the employee is an adult who's responsible for his behavior and choice to be or not be compliant and professional in his job. Remember: One poor appraisal doesn't reflect badly on you as a manager. If an employee typically does a wonderful job and is willing to learn and change as the environment changes, then you're doing your job as a manager and leader. Never ignore poor performance or try to make someone look better than he is because you fear the situation may cause discord among your staff and may come back to haunt you.

You'll undoubtedly encounter times when your job isn't to foster the professional growth of an employee in his current job, but rather to help him find another job in which he'll have a better chance for success. On the other hand, if no employee ever meets your expectations, then you need to go to your supervisor for guidance because the problem may be that you have unrealistic expectations.

Preparation is key

The performance appraisal process should never be done on the fly. It's a vital part of the success of your employees, your facility, and yourself—and it requires preparation. Know the requirements of each position you supervise. Know who does what job and how well they do it. If you're directly responsible for multiple shifts, make sure you have a presence during the various work hours in order to be fair in your staff evaluation. Most employees want and need feedback more frequently than once per year, which is why it's important to have frequent, meaningful contact with each of your employees.

Extending the appraisal's use

The performance appraisal process can be used for many purposes other than the annual scheduled review. Based on the intent, the components reviewed or process followed might be different in various situations. Sometimes this process is used to determine who's promoted, separated, or transferred to another area. The process can be used if management wants to know how an employee views them. Sometimes the process can be used as part of a learning needs assessment or to evaluate the success of certain education and training programs. Finally, as related to budgets and finance issues, this process can be used to determine merit increases, promotions, and future budget and scheduling needs.

Expectations of the manager

Managers undoubtedly carry with them certain expectations about the performance appraisal process. Remember that the manager:

- ➤ translates the facility's mission, vision, and goals into individual job objectives
- ➤ communicates the expectations about employee performance
- ➤ provides frequent and meaningful feedback to the employee about job performance against management's objectives
- ➤ coaches the employee on how to achieve job objectives
- ➤ identifies the employee's strengths and weaknesses and determines which development activities might help him better use his kills to improve performance.

JCAHO standards

In the leadership chapter of the Comprehensive Accreditation Manual for Hospitals, the Joint Commission on Accreditation of Healthcare Organizations (JCAHO) states, "leaders regularly assess the success [of] hospital activities in achieving the hospital's mission. They support and participate in leadership training in the principles and methods of continuous quality measurement, assessment and improvement. They also promote staff self-development of the knowledge and skills required to maintain and enhance individual competence." To take this further into specific components of the performance appraisal process, the human resources section of the same manual states, "the goal of the management of the Human Resource function is to identify and provide the right number of *competent* staff to meet the needs of patients served by the facility. *Ongoing, periodic competence assess-*

ment evaluates staff members' continuing abilities to perform throughout their association with the hospital." The leaders create a culture that fosters staff self-development and continued learning. Staff members are encouraged to provide feedback about the work environment to the leaders.

Competence-based appraisal involves managers defining required elements of competence for each specific job and then comparing the employee's ability against these elements. In addition to these specific job requirements, a facility may also have a set of general, or core, competencies that are also measured with the performance appraisal. These core elements could encompass criteria, such as timeliness, attendance, customer satisfaction, and general mandatory training requirements, including infection control or body mechanics and safety.

Keep it simple

The most important point to stress as you review the components of the performance appraisal process is to keep it simple. Nothing is worse than a cumbersome process that forces managers to place employees into forced rankings. State the job requirements; the employee is either meeting them or isn't. If not, he should already be aware of this.

Based on the results, tell the employee what he needs to do. If he's exceeding the job requirements, what would he like to do next to challenge his skills? Are there any special projects he can work on? If he isn't meeting the requirements, what does he need to do to meet the standards? What's the time frame? What does *he* think needs to be done? (See *Basic manager responsibilities*.)

The importance of documentation

Documentation is a vital component of the nursing process that by extension is also an important component in the performance appraisal. The manager is required to document carefully and accurately. It's essential to thoroughly document good and bad issues in the employee's personnel file because doing so can help protect you and your facility if an employee is terminated.

Appraisals should be prepared regularly, accurately, and carefully. Never be afraid to state what you know when an employee consistently fails to meet the job requirements, and always document your discussions with the employee and your observations.

Basic manager responsibilities

Every manager has basic responsibilities in the performance review process. These include:
➤ Clarify job description and employee responsibilities related to the job.
➤ Clarify employee interests and needs.
➤ Identify and list specific development areas in which the employee needs to concentrate.
➤ Review performance objectives and standards.
➤ Review and discuss the employee's progress toward set objectives through ongoing feedback-established review periods.
➤ Give the employee answers to the following questions:
–What am I expected to do?
–How well am I doing?
–What are my strengths and weaknesses?
–How can I do a better job?
–How can I contribute more?

If you allow poor performance to slide without communicating it to the employee or putting it in writing until the day you terminate the employee for not meeting the job requirements, both you and your facility may be faced with a wrongful discharge lawsuit — and no documentation to show a history of poor performance.

Termination issues

Unfortunately, employee termination is an all-too-common part of a manager's professional life. Nearly every manager has had an employee who just wouldn't comply with or abide by the rules and regulations his position required. Oftentimes, the experience is traumatic, especially if it's the first time the manager has had to terminate an employee. (See *Falsifying care,* page 398.)

Some terminations can be avoided by counseling and coaching a new employee or an employee in a new position. A good manager takes the time to nurture the professional growth of an employee and never assumes that an employee understands something just because he nods his head in agreement. A good employee is an expensive commodity that shouldn't be wasted and, thus, personnel issues should take a big block of a manager's time. A manager's job is to remove as many speed bumps from

CASE IN POINT

Falsifying care

As a manager, I simply couldn't believe that a registered nurse would deliberately falsify care and actually lie about performing the care. I couldn't fathom how she could do this and risk the patient's health and well-being as well as her own license.

At the time this situation occurred, I was a new manager for a home health agency. Sometimes in home health care, as in any health care arena that cares for geriatric patients, patients tend to mix up their days and their nurses and not remember when the nurse was last there. I always took the individual patient and the nurse or other employee into consideration whenever a patient called to say that "their nurse hadn't been there."

This particular patient, however, was aware of her surroundings and care needs. When the first call came, I asked the nurse, and she assured me that she had been there. The patient must be confused. This was a good nurse that had never given me any reason to doubt her word. A few days later, when she was scheduled to see the same patient, another call came. I asked the nurse again, and again she assured me that it had to be an error, but that she would stop by the patient's house just to make it right.

At this point it was just too coincidental. The patient never called for anyone else, just this particular nurse. I reviewed the record and everything was documented appropriately. I decided to make the next visit myself without letting the other nurse know. I performed the patient's care and changed the dressing on her hip. Once the dressing change was completed, I put my initials and the date directly on the new dressing, and then scheduled this nurse for the next day and myself for the day after. Sure enough, when I returned the patient still had the same dressing in place that I had applied 2 days before, even though there was a clinical note stating otherwise.

When I finally determined that the nurse had falsified the visits and the documents, I notified the state board of nursing and made sure any visits she claimed to have done that didn't match what the patient said were removed from billing.

Although this experience was many years ago, I still remember it as a learning experience, reminding me that there are people out there who will falsify care and, also, preparing me to effectively deal with it.

the employee's path as possible. The biggest part of that job is telling people directly what you need, when you need it, why you need it, and what happens if they don't produce.

The manager's job begins with recruitment of qualified employees for the job, not just "warm bodies." Once an employee has been hired, most organizations have a 3- to 6-month trial period to determine if the right person was selected for the position and if the job is what the person expected it to be. In most states, employment relationships are considered to be *at will* and

Grounds for termination

To set the ground rules for employment with your organization, the new employee should be given a list of behaviors or actions that could result in immediate termination, to help dispel confusion up front. Some of the more common actions that result in immediate termination include:

➤ falsification of records or information
➤ theft of company or coworker property
➤ habitual tardiness or excessive absences (excused or unexcused)
➤ failure to report absences
➤ leaving job without manager permission or knowledge
➤ negligence or neglect of duty
➤ breach of confidentiality related to a patient, another employee, or the organization
➤ disrespect or unprofessional conduct
➤ dishonesty related to stealing, revealing trade or company secrets, punching another employee's timecard, or other such behavior
➤ insubordination or flagrant disobedience to organizational rules and regulations
➤ exceeding the authority of the job
➤ willful refusal to follow the directions of a supervisor, unless doing so is directly in opposition to what the employee knows or feels to be illegal or unethical
➤ assault, sexual harassment, abuse of others, unprovoked attack, or threat of harm against others
➤ use of or possession of drugs or alcohol while on company premises or on the job
➤ possession of weapons or firearms on company property
➤ intentional and willful negligence in performing duties or willfully hindering or preventing others from performing their duties.

terminable anytime by the company or the employee. Even though this is the case, employers must make sure they've covered all legal and ethical bases when terminating an employee. Some cases will inevitably go to court—and the facility may lose if all bases haven't been covered. Such cases could involve discrimination protection, false representations of the job requirements, or whistle-blowing. At the time of hire, the organizational policies and procedures related to employment should be carefully reviewed with the new employee, and the employee should sign such a statement. The employee should be given a company handbook or written employment agreement that covers all such requirements, and he should also be told that either party may terminate the employment agreement anytime, with or without cause and with or without notice. (See *Grounds for termination.*)

If you have an employee who consistently performs poorly or who "pushes the behavior envelope," know your company's progressive discipline guidelines and follow them to the letter. As

Preparing to respond

If you find that you must terminate an employee, be familiar and ready to respond to the following questions:

➤ Does your organization have a clearly written rule against the behavior for which the employee was terminated?

➤ Is the rule reasonable and related to the lawful, orderly, efficient, and safe operation of your organization?

➤ Was the employee given adequate time to learn the organization's rules, and was this documented?

➤ Have these rules, specifically the one that resulted in the employee's termination, been evenly enforced with all staff?

➤ Was the employee given a chance to respond, and was a fair investigation conducted of the offense that resulted in termination?

➤ How was guilt determined?

➤ Was the termination fairly based on the nature of the offense and on the employee's employment record?

discussed in the last section, some managers are reluctant to follow progressive discipline when dealing with inadequate performance or consistent behavior problems with an employee. As a manager, you have a duty to be even-handed in the application of all work rules. Employers must meet with employees early, discuss their performance problems frankly, and set written goals or objectives, which are acknowledged and signed by both. Doing so will help defend against termination litigation. (See *Preparing to respond.*)

Timing is everything

Termination is never easy for either party. Once the decision has been made and approved by management, the manager and a human resource (HR) representative will need to determine how and when the termination will occur.

Almost without exception, all terminations should be discussed in person with the employee, the manager, and an HR or other leadership representative. The meeting should be brief and to the point and should give the terminated employee immediate direction on how to proceed from the facility and when.

There's no best way to break such news to an employee, and each case needs to be handled on an individual basis. Some employees are terminated because of poor performance or actions

that result in immediate termination, whereas others are terminated because of downsizing or restructuring. How the terminated employee is approached and by whom can affect the risk of
that person seeking legal intervention for wrongful discharge.
The employee should be told specifically why he's being terminated, with some states requiring that these reasons be put in
writing and given to the employee.

Avoiding confrontation

Do your best to avoid confrontations with the terminated employee. If, however, you happen to get into one and the employee
won't back down, call security. It's also always best to have a third
party present while the termination meeting is taking place, simply as an observer for the benefit and protection of the facility.
Also, be prepared to give the employee any information he'll
need related to benefits.

Except in unusual cases of theft and bodily threats, avoid requiring the terminated person to clean out his belongings in
front of others. Rather, give him the option to come back after
hours to collect his things accompanied by a security representative. Even though the employee is being terminated, he still deserves to be treated with dignity and not unduly embarrassed.

Stopping the rumor monger

Finally, the termination of an employee can cause rumors and
trepidation among the other staff members. Be careful in what
you say and how much you reveal. In most cases, the other employees don't need to know this information. Always be cognizant that terminated employees might still have friends on the
job who will come back and tell them what they've heard about
the termination, so don't give them grounds for a lawsuit.

Points to remember

The following points summarize the importance of performance
appraisal in nursing management:

➤ The best performance review lets a manager and an employee *communicate* — share ideas, opinions, and information with the ultimate goal of higher performance and success. The well-orchestrated performance appraisal helps foster the professional growth of an employee and improves the facility's performance.

➤ The performance appraisal process is an ongoing process that prevents the employee from being surprised by anything that's said when the formal interview occurs.

➤ Progressive discipline should be instituted with the goal of turning a poor performer around. If this doesn't work, then termination may be the best solution.

➤ JCAHO standards require health care facilities to define their mission and purpose, define the qualifications of employees to meet that mission, recruit and retain competent staff and, finally, assess and improve the ongoing competency of the staff — the performance appraisal process.

References

1. Williams, A. *Pushing Up People.* Doraville, Ga.: Parklake Publishers, 1984.
2. Waddell, W. *Sales Coaching Playbook.* Coppell, Tex.: Winspirations, 1999.
3. "A Science Odyssey, People and Discoveries," PBS Online. WGBH Boston, 1997. *www.pbs.org/wgbh/aso/.*
4. Dwayne Simpson, D., and Benjamin, L.T., Jr. "In Memory, Founder and Formal Direction of IBR, Saul B. Sells," *American Psychologist* 43(12):1088, December 1988.
5. Lloyd, J. "Federal Human Resources Week," Online. LRP Publications, 1999. *www.lrpdartnell.com.*

Selected readings

Martin, V. "Assessing Staff Performance in a Rapidly Changing Service," *Journal of Nursing Management* 10(2):30-33, March 2002.
Meretoja, R., et al. "Indicators for Competent Nursing Practice," *Journal of Nursing Management* 10(2):95-103, March 2002.
Milio, N. "A New Leadership Role for Nursing in a Globalized World," *Topics in Advanced Practice Nursing eJournal* 2(1), 2002.

PART FIVE

Information technology skills

CHAPTER 18

Computers in nursing

George Harbeson, RN, MSN

> "The future masters of technology will have to be lighthearted and intelligent. The machine easily masters the grim and the dumb." — Marshall McLuhan, 1969

Throughout the country, nurses are at the leading edge of health care information technology (IT): They're writing software to better track wound management, heading the implementation of major information system projects, working with leading physiological monitoring companies, and researching how to better train the next generation of nurses. A nurse in California has developed a software application that will be used on handheld computers for home health nurses, allowing them to document patient assessment and care and record supplies, all on an unobtrusive handheld instrument. Similar technology is being used by the military for front-line medics, allowing them to do their triage, bring up treatment algorithms, and keep track of supplies in a similar fashion. Each soldier carries a chip, in place of the older dog tags, which contains his personal identification and medical history. The information on the chip is updated anytime he receives medical treatment.

While continuing to lag behind the rest of the civilized world in information technology, health care is catching up with a vengeance, blasting ahead with just about every kind of application that can be written to automate every conceivable thought, piece of data, schedule, or roster. Much of this activity has been driven by nonclinical forces, such as reimbursement issues, governmental regulatory bodies, and credentialing agencies. IT has also become a mainstay of clinical practices and research at all levels, from the office visit to the Human Genome Project. What's more, the last 10 years or so have seen tremendous change in health care, and these changes have helped bring about its ever-increasing reliance on computers.

So what does all of this mean to the nurse-manager? A nurse-manager is bombarded daily with information — including patient reports, administration memos, and staff productivity, quality assurance, and product information. Therefore, nurse-managers need to be proficient at information technology in order to better manage their time and attentions. They must continually evaluate finances, staffing schedules, staff education, evaluations, and patient care issues. Being knowledgeable about the information technology available and the resources to support it are essential to the success of any nurse-manager.

What's nursing informatics?

Nursing has always involved collecting, managing, processing, transforming, and communicating information. It wasn't until the late 1960s, however, that nurses started using electronic tools to assist with these activities. Mayers'[1] described efforts at El Camino Hospital in Mountain View, California, to automate nursing documentation within the Technicon Hospital Information System (now TDS Healthcare Systems Corporation). During the same period, Cornell and Brush[2] and Wesseling[3] described different approaches to the nursing care plan, and Beggs and colleagues[4] reported on a system for online computer scheduling of patient care activities in a rehabilitation center.

A nursing specialty called *informatics* has emerged within the last 20 years to fill a void between the clinician at the bedside and information technology. The field is expanding with the growth of technology and the realization of the impact that technology can have on patient care and nursing science.

Informatics is the union of technology and information — and nursing informatics adds the critically important feature of nursing science. Blum[5] described the framework of nursing informatics by defining the central concepts of *data, information,* and *knowledge.* He defined *data* as discrete entities that are described objectively without interpretation; *information* as data that are interpreted, organized, or structured; and *knowledge* as information that has been synthesized so that interrelationships are identified and formalized. The management and processing components may be considered the functional components of informatics.

The informatics theory proposes that computerized data collection and recall, knowledge base access, and a properly structured information format promotes better clinical documentation; this has been proven true in clinical practices by both nursing staff and physicians. A well-thought-out, well-implemented electronic medical record (EMR) allows professional providers latitude to document their clinical practice in an intelligent manner consistent with their practice, while prompting them through the structure of screens and forms to do a more complete job than if they had been using either a printed form or writing freehand on a blank sheet.

The *science* of informatics is seen in everything from planning a database to building a screen for data display to investigating the latest radio frequency wireless system. The *art* of informatics, on the other hand, carries the ability to accurately interpret the documentation needs of the clinician and translate these needs into a computer system for storage and retrieval. Such a system shouldn't add to the clinician's charting time and must yield a finished document that's complete, easy to read, clinically sound, and recoverable at another time and in another setting with adequately secure access measures. The information must also be available to other providers who benefit from an easily accessible document that also serves as a multidisciplinary medical record. In addition, the data should be available for trending, research, productivity, resource management, and billing. (See *The Health Insurance Portability Accounting Act of 1996.*)

The greatest challenge to implementing a computerized system for those who have been solely charting on paper is the old question, "Will it save me time?" The answer: "If it's good, then it will." Will this time savings be at the moment of the initial charting or when doing an admission assessment? No, it probably won't. Will it save time when the physician sees the patient for the next visit and the patient's history, allergy information, immunization record, and current and past medication lists are readily accessible? Will it save charting time when the nurse does

The Health Insurance Portability Accounting Act of 1996

The Health Insurance Portability Accounting Act of 1996 is a broad-ranging set of federal statutes that started out as a way to codify patient billing information, doing away with the scores of existing billing codes and languages to provide faster reimbursement from third-party payers — thus benefiting the patient. It became evident at the beginning of this project that although information would be standardized for more rapid processing, unauthorized parties would have many more avenues to access a patient's clinical information.

As efforts to standardize data continue, strict guidelines must be written for handling of all patient information to restrict unauthorized access. Health care facilities throughout the United States are now in the process of evaluating software systems that involve patient identification. After these statutes are enforced in April 2003, each system will need to pass a strict set of security standards before health care providers can use it. Noncompliance could bring criminal charges and substantial fines for the provider as well as the facility.

a shift assessment and information from earlier assessments comes forward? Yes to both.

The nurse as IT specialist

A nurse-manager should have not only knowledge and skills of current computer technology but also excellent organizational skills and the ability to present technological information to clinicians in an informative, nondemeaning way. The manager should bring, at a minimum, an ability to create simple spreadsheets, use a database and word processor, and use electronic mail. (See *Informatics specialty skills,* page 408.)

Keeping up with current nursing theory and being able to speak with some knowledge about the issues of end-user clinicians (those nurses on your staff) is key for all nurse-managers. Much of what managers do in the unit involves assessing current clinical processes. Although automation may be necessary, successful managers help prioritize projects. Working to bring fellow care providers online is an art that comes with experience. You'll find some staff nurses eager to jump into online charting, and others who'll need some prodding.

The growing host of health care applications, from old staffing software written in DOS to a home health system that uses the latest handheld technology, demands a specialized clinician who

Informatics specialty skills

Mills and colleagues[6] recommend the following knowledge and skills for nurses specializing in informatics:
➤ an understanding of nursing, information science, and systems theory in clinical and management decision making
➤ proficiency in organizational and group dynamics
➤ a comprehensive understanding of the interrelationship between people, organizations, information technology, nursing, and health care delivery
➤ the ability to identify the properties, structure, use, and flow of clinical and management information from the patient to the health care provider
➤ the ability to assess real and potential problems related to communication, accessibility, availability, and use of information for decision making
➤ skill in creatively determining alternative methods of information handling and system design options
➤ the ability to evaluate cost risks in relation to benefits or effectiveness
➤ skill in orchestrating change.

can successfully help improve the state of information management in the unit, office, clinic, or laboratory. (See *You can do it.*)

As you explore the intricacies of designing, implementing, and supporting clinical systems, it may appear that there are more pitfalls than successes. If that were true, the field of nursing informatics wouldn't be growing as it is. All the effort of a large implementation project are forgotten when you walk onto your unit and see your staff using the system, benefiting from the enhancements it brings to clinical practice, and loving it!"

What's an HIS?

As a nurse-manager, you'll need to know about your current hospital information system (HIS). The term *HIS* means different things to different people in different facilities, and it's rare to find a facility that has a completely integrated HIS. More likely, even if the facility had an integrated system 10 years ago, it has probably suffered many traumas. The admissions piece may still work pretty well, the outpatient scheduling portion can last a bit longer (with an upgrade), and the old medical records module has some life, but the laboratory system must be replaced, and how are you going to incorporate rules-driven physician order entry (OE) with that antique OE piece?

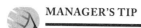

You can do it

Don't allow a shaky background in PC skills to deter you from volunteering to be part of a clinical software implementation. Enthusiasm and the ability to listen to the needs of end-users will carry you a long way. Show your staff that you're willing to pave the way to new technology without fear — it may help decrease their fear of change. After all, you can always sneak out for evening classes at your local college for that class in "MS Project."

Technology and end-user sophistication drive the development of newer systems. What happens? A "system" of worthy components is put together, but it certainly can't be called completely "integrated." With such a hybrid system, the interfacing becomes the focal point to the detriment of developing new features for enhanced functionality. Although not the desired outcome, it certainly is more the norm. Because the components of an integrated HIS have different life spans, it's important to focus on the central function of this system — the data repository. A well-built, sturdy, clinical data repository allows for modification and enhancement over time.

The store-bought system

Unless your facility is a large medical center with considerable IT resources, the days of the successful homegrown clinical information system seem about gone. The need for systems integration for billing compliance, governmental auditing, research, clinical documentation, sharing of secured databases, and Internet integration within the system, all point toward the new generation of HIS vendors. These vendors are developing the software as entrepreneurs, with integration of systems as a chief feature of their product. Much of the implementation of a new system will probably include wrestling with the interfacing or coping with data transfers from older systems that were developed without an eye toward standardized protocols, such as Health Level 7. (See *Explaining Health Level 7,* page 410.)

Explaining Health Level 7

Health Level 7 (HL7) is an organization founded in 1987 to develop standards for electronic interchange of clinical, financial, and administrative information among independent health care–oriented computer systems. Accredited by the American National Standards Institute, it continues to be developed by volunteers committed to improving communication in the health care field using computer technology.

Obtaining an HIS

If you're to be involved in the installation of a new HIS, just remember there aren't any "one size fits all" systems. The purchase and installation of a system is often a long and sometimes painful process. Becoming a member of the HIS search team can be a beneficial experience, but you'll likely find yourself at odds with other departments who are looking at the automation of clinical services with more of a focus on capital budget constraints, connectivity, and interfacing capabilities. There must be a lot of room for compromise in this process.

The list of vendors who build and support clinical information systems has shrunk considerably over the past 5 years. The problems in the technology fields and general economy have caused the downfall of many smaller software vendors who failed to get the numbers of needed installations to make them big-time players in the volatile HIS market. Those that remain are larger, well-established software vendors whose products may not be as great a fit for your facility. A software vendor who has a good product but a limited base of installations will likely be more attentive to your unique needs and more willing to work within your budget. Weighed against these positives are the potential pitfalls of the product, which probably still needs a lot of tuning, and the possibility of dwindling vendor resources. Your best bet is to spend time looking at the product demonstrations and presentations of the newer, smaller vendors as well as the older, larger systems. (See *Expanding your knowledge*.)

If your administration has decided to buy a new integrated HIS, you can expect implementation to take several years. Hopefully, your facility has a nurse informaticist who has been included in the vendor selection process. The process of vendor demonstrations, site visits to other installations, and drafting of the Request for Proposal (RFP) will give the informatics specialist a

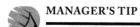

MANAGER'S TIP

Expanding your knowledge

As a nurse-manager involved in the purchasing of a new software product, you should try to attend one of the large national health information conferences. If it's in the budget, have another staff member go with you — one who might be interested and become involved in the implementation of a new system. These conferences are truly impressive in the number and types of vendors showing their wares. And, while you're there, consider attending a seminar session or two — for example, by the American Medical Informatics Association, the Healthcare Information and Management Systems Society, or the American Nursing Informatics Association. You may walk away with some valuable, cutting-edge information.

chance to uncover potential problems. If your facility doesn't have an informaticist on staff, spend as much time as possible at other installations, and make contacts with the informatics staff at those facilities. A call to another facility that's implementing such a system can help solve or avoid potential problems.

Vendor selection

After the initial contact with a software vendor is made and both parties express interest, the vendor will make a presentation at your location. The audience is usually the administration, key medical staff, and heads of the clinical departments that will be involved in the project. The presentation will include a demonstration of the requested system.

Next, make a site visit to another facility that's using the system. Try to find a site that's similar to yours, such as a pediatrics-only facility, a teaching facility, or a smaller community hospital. Your implementation team should arrange the visit, not the vendor. If possible, ask for a demonstration of the system in use for the facility's patients. Schedule some time at the end of the site visit to talk about the experience and issues that the facility had with the vendor; however, don't include the vendor's representatives. To optimize the site visit, have an agenda of processes you want to see the system accomplish and a thorough set of questions to ask the users. This is the time to ask the users about the vendor's support record — a crucial factor.

What's an RFP?

The RFP is a document written with input from clinicians, information systems, and administration. It's a request from your facility to the software vendor for a bid. The RFP must be carefully written and include as detailed a description as possible of what the facility wants. Areas covered in the RFP include hardware platforms, documentation, operating systems, and connectivity to other applications. Technical and software support items are included. In many such documents and ensuing negotiations, provisions are made for disposition of the software in the eventuality that the company goes out of business. The accounting office and chief financial officer will want detailed information on payment conditions for the purchase as well as future support.

The nurse-manager and the nurse informaticist should be actively involved in the drafting the clinical specifications of this document. The nurse informaticist acts as the resource for the administrators, medical staff, nursing staff, and other end users.

What's a CPOE?

Currently, there's a nationwide focus on medication errors. In 1999, the Institute of Medicine published a report, "To Err is Human," which presented astonishing statistics about the numbers of preventable medication errors and their impact on human lives and the cost of health care. This report has been the impetus for legislation aimed at reducing such errors. Many of these changes will become law and will be implemented by clinical informatics. Computerized physician order entry (CPOE) will become the standard. This mandate alone will drive many facilities to completely revamp their HIS, with many having no recourse other than to purchase new systems; many will have to install new order entry systems at the least.

The new order entry systems being built today are rules-based, one of the keys to CPOE being a deterrent to medication errors. Elaborate dictionaries of "rules" must be compiled. The permutations of each rule are tremendous. The new rules-based systems will have to be closely linked by interface to the pharmacy, admissions, medical records, nursing, and laboratory systems. If a physician wants to order a medication for an inpatient, that order would rapidly search the databases of the clinical system, the patient's laboratory results, diagnosis, demographics (to ensure the correct patient), pharmacy dosage, and interactions database; then, by following the rules, the transaction would — or wouldn't — be allowed. Depending on the variance of the rules, a warning might appear on the screen or the transaction might not be allowed due to alerts built into the system.

By eliminating verbal, telephone, faxed, and handwritten orders, this ordering process can eliminate misunderstood verbal orders and misinterpreted written orders. Both of these factors are cited as leading causes of medication errors. With the rules-based feature in place, orders that might otherwise have been administered or carried out due to a lack of access to all pertinent clinical data can be intercepted and corrected.

For this piece of the HIS, many applications will likely be sold with rules-based CPOE already in place. The individual facility's implementation team will still have a tremendous chore coordinating these clinical decisions with current facility and practice policy. Because it's unlikely that any vendor will have a package that will solve all ordering issues at any single facility, this feature will require diligent research and cooperation between departments.

Interfaces

Interface refers to the special programming that translates data from one application so that it can be used in another application; this is a *one-way interface*. A *two-way interface* also translates data from the second application so it can move back to the first.

For any modern facility, regardless of size, no completely integrated system will take care of all computer needs. As mentioned previously, certain stand-alone systems may be left in place, with the plan for integration into the new HIS. For the informatics specialist, the ability to easily interface smaller specialty applications to your HIS will be the icing on the cake, if this indeed is a feature of your new system. However, don't count on it, because interfacing rarely comes easily or inexpensively.

When selecting a vendor, be aware of interface capabilities and established history of your new vendor's product. Also, make sure you've inventoried all in-house systems in your facility and know which are going to stay, and for how long. It's best to prioritize these potential interfaces from the standpoint of criticality.

As part of the selection process, ask the HIS vendor where they've installed interfaces to the systems on your list. Contact the facilities that have the interfaces in place, and find out how difficult the interface was to install and support. The most common response from software vendors when asked about a potential interface is the standard, "No problem!" Your RFP should contain information about the cost of existing interfaces and interfaces that will need to be written.

Putting it all together

After the RFP has been written and sent to the vendor (or possibly several vendors), the contact between vendors and the facility will become a bit more formal. The software vendor will carefully read the document and prepare a bid that will have answers and information for all issues in the RFP. During contract negotiations, all items in the RFP will be addressed and the cost for the software and support will be agreed upon. At facilities with smaller information technology departments, this contract commonly includes connectivity and hardware as well. The HIS is one of the most costly purchases most facilities make. And, with all concerned parties having a good idea of the life of computer technology, it's usually a tense period.

Take advantage of contract negotiation time to develop an implementation plan and start assembling a good implementation team. This will be an important factor to the success of a new computer system on your unit.

During this hectic time, there will be many meetings with internal facility shareholders as well as with vendors. The eager sales representatives will be replaced with project engineers, account executives, implementation consultants, and trainers from the home office.

Hardware

Hardware is the equipment required to run and operate the software program. It includes mainframe computers, servers, personal computers (PCs), handheld devices, monitors, printers, and bar code scanners. Presuming that your new HIS will be of the client/server type of installation, you'll need to decide where the PC workstations are going for use by physicians, nurses, and ancillary personnel. The number of workstations to be used with the system is a large issue. For every documentation location, the cost of a new networked PC must be added.

HIS architecture

A significant part of the installation process of a new system is interaction with the technology side of the project. You must develop a relationship with your facility's information technology department as well as become proficient with the technical specifications and requirements of your new system. If you're in the early stages on such a project, learn about the current HIS computer architecture.

Until recently, there was more of a variety of system types for data management. Many facilities relied on large in-house "main frame" computers attached to "dumb terminals." What this means is that the entire application ran from, and data were stored in, a main computer. Benefits of this type of system included less-expensive workstations and a networking system that was easier to support. Drawbacks included capital costs, especially for system-stressing upgrades and new technologies, such as more graphics, color, and Internet connectivity. Mainframe systems remain popular for high-volume, high-speed computing of data that are more narrowly defined than for health care.

Vendor support

Another popular configuration of mainframe computers was to have the mainframe with applications and databases housed and supported by the vendor. The system was shared by customers who avoided the large expense of buying and supporting the mainframe computers. This worked well for many smaller to medium-sized facilities. Although not as popular today, a variation of this idea is thriving on the Internet where applications run on larger servers to be accessed by PCs from homes, clinics, and offices. These shared systems (called application service providers [ASPs]) are in use by several clinical system vendors. The good and bad side of these is who controls and maintains the application and servers. Internet security is a concern.

Client/server hardware

Most vendors steer toward the client/server hardware. In this setup, much of the application resides on a workstation, which is usually a standard PC. Databases, large reports, and large dictionaries (such as the master patient index) reside on larger servers, which are usually housed in the information technology department. Having the application on the individual workstation makes the input-output process much quicker for the end user.

Implementing a new HIS

Nursing informatics is a key resource in the implementation process. The nurse informatics specialist will likely be working on the clinical applications end of the project but will necessarily be concerned with technology issues, project staffing, and project integration.

Your involvement in the new system is important. Your vendor will supply early training to you and provide materials outlining the implementation project from the standpoint of the software application. You'll need to coordinate this information with your own implementation plan that accurately addresses internal issues, such as prioritization of potential users. Those clinical areas that show a strong eager staff and management will serve as models for subsequent areas. It's never wise to begin in areas that aren't in the least similar to others. Recruiting and training implementation team members from the clinical staff is critical to success. End-user training for implementation and ongoing support must be assessed and resources allocated. Hardware and connectivity needs throughout the facility must be cataloged.

Documentation issues

Ideally, the new HIS will produce a paperless record, and staff will gather data in the the patient's presence. This raises numerous questions. How and on what equipment will this best be done? Will clinicians use a PC in a patient room? What security issues arise with a network PC in a patient room? Many HIS project mangers and informaticists shy away from in-room workstations.

The obvious alternative is PC workstations outside the room. Having them in a public area is also a big security risk. Having them behind nurse's stations and in secluded charting areas places them too far from the patient. What happens with this scenario is return to a paper form for data collection or, at least, written observations on a blank paper pad to be transcribed into the system later. No one wants to duplicate documentation. This dual system creates *longer* documentation time, greatly increases staff dissatisfaction, and is probably as guilty as any other HIS issue of causing the project to fail.

This critical issue must be addressed by the entire project early on, to help head off some crippling problems. If standard PC workstations are going to be the terminals for the system, it would be worthwhile to have some trial runs with the use of PC's on carts with network jacks in the patient's rooms as well as in clinical work areas.

Terminal placement

Performing an examination on a patient, documenting a nursing assessment, or capturing a respiratory therapy treatment online is tricky when done on a terminal in the patient's room. Most likely the information will be entered only once, which is the goal. However, the difficulty comes from the awkward placement of an imposing piece of computer equipment while this is being done. Having the screen and keyboard between the patient and clinician allows the caregiver to face the patient, but places the computer so that the back of the monitor faces the patient.

An alternative is a charting desk, which places the monitor against a wall and perhaps the clinician's back to the patient. Some angles may not seem to be too antagonizing for patient and clinician, but all in all, the PC workstation in the patient room on a cart is less than optimal. If alternatives are lacking because of hardware budget issues, the moveable workstation that can be positioned for each patient encounter may be the best solution.

Alternative systems

A laptop computer is the least obtrusive option but brings up the questions of cost and fragility. (See *The best approach,* page 418.) Even better than laptops are smaller, more portable, handheld devices, such as notebook computers or personal digital assistants. If you're considering one of these systems, obviously, it will

The best approach

Question: *How do I decide which computer is best for the unit — and where is the best place to put it?*

Answer: Without a doubt the way to proceed, if at all possible, is with a newer technology approach. A laptop computer is less obtrusive when in the lap of an interviewer than the much larger PC. However, laptops raise flags for administrators about theft, cost, and fragility. Despite these issues, they've proven to be successful. A bare-bones laptop without multimedia devices can be reasonably priced. Although not perfect, they're preferable to PCs when used in patient care areas.

If possible, set up a "lab" for your clinical system implementation. You may have a typical patient room that can stay empty for a month or so, or maybe you have a skills laboratory already set up by your clinical educators. Placement of workstations, data ports, and printers in patient care areas is unfortunately treated as an afterthought to purchasing a large expensive system. Time spent trying out different workstation placements, doing mock examinations and documentation, and retrieving printed material can highlight some potential workflow nightmares. Do this exercise before decisions are made on computer furniture purchases and placement. It will be time well spent.

need to be compatible with the main database. Handheld systems will need to be constantly "docked" so that data can be sent to the main database and new information from the database can be transferred into the handheld device. This can generate staff dissatisfaction and additional technical issues.

Handheld devices might be able to handle enough information to complete data intake, but accessing database information, such as laboratory results and order entry, would require accessing the servers. Interest in these small computers is growing, and they would lend themselves to patient-caregiver interactions very well. There are already many applications for the clinical use of handheld devices.

At this time, the ultimate hardware configuration for those clinical areas where a PC workstation is too cumbersome may just be the portable workbook or handheld device that's linked to the application server real-time via radio frequency. The equipment keeps getting better, and this technology is now much more able to handle the demands of a large HIS clinical documentation system.

Getting the team together

An implementation team of clinicians is critically important to the success of the project. They'll bring their issues and concerns and be a valuable sounding board for ongoing evaluation of the project from the end-user perspective. As a manager, you're part of the team because of your unique perspective and buy-in. As you recruit staff members, be sure to include members from every shift. Choose those staff members who show an interest in the upcoming automation of their clinical processes and documentation. To keep them at their most productive, have regularly scheduled, well-organized meetings. Create forms (computer templates) for meeting agenda and minutes, and use them. Plan your project meetings, and publish the draft plan early on in the process. Give your implementation teams a synopsis of the project meeting agenda items and time line. If they're more knowledgeable of the time line, they'll be better prepared to provide needed input and complete their implementation projects when you need them. Having a set meeting time is important because it will help set a routine for the implementation. In your meetings, take time to listen to concerns from the potential end-users. By keeping an open ear to the staff (the end-users), you'll not only avoid big problems but also get their critical support.

The specialness of the specialist

The nurse informatics specialist will most likely be involved in developing the end-user product as well as in organizing the implementation. Implementing a product for staff and physician documentation, or departmental implementation, requires building dictionaries of users, access levels, titles, locations, medications, diagnosis codes, allergies, laboratory tests, imaging tests, and on and on. Some of these compilations might be facilitated with data transfers from existing systems, such as a stand-alone pharmacy system, but many will be built by hand. You can't do this without well-coordinated help from the different departments in your facility.

Many of these lists and dictionaries are contingent on others being in place, so having these milestones on your project plan is important. There will be many critical deadlines for your team members to build these dictionaries or collect the required data.

Building a form

Screens or on-line forms are the tools that end-users will be using — and such tools will save them a second or two, which can add up to a lot of time by the end of the day. This example will give you a better idea:

Say that you want to order a prothrombin time (PT) to be done on a patient. The laboratory will want to know if the patient takes an anticoagulant. Is this information critical? If it is, you'll need to somehow make this a "required" field, or flag it some way. You must build a query asking the question, "Does the patient take an anticoagulant?" A "yes" and a "no" answer are available. If the clinician answers "yes," then a list of current anticoagulants will appear and allow for a single response or the ability to choose more than one medication. You'd probably make this response a "multiple choice."

In the end, you've written a short dictionary of anticoagulants, and it's stored in your "dictionary of dictionaries." Down the line, you may build a more complicated form for a clinical assessment, and in the history section you may again want to ask the questions used on the order entry PT form. When the laboratory order form was built, you made the two queries "recallable." When these queries appear on the same patient's assessment history, the data will be automatically entered by the system.

Although by definition the nursing informatics specialist deals with end-user patient care and documentation issues, much time is spent in upper-level implementation meetings coordinating other branches of the HIS, such as pharmacy, admission department, laboratory, billing department, and medical records.

BE A BUILDER You'll probably build online forms with your new system. All software applications must be modifiable to handle your facility's unique information needs and use their existing data. For instance, for the order entry portion of your system, you'll probably need an order "form" for the clinicians to complete when ordering. The software vendor will provide tools and instructions for building this form; most likely you and your team will construct the final form. (See *Building a form*.)

Forms must be built for ordering diagnostic tests; making changes in a patient's admission, transfer, or discharge status (ADT); and doing clinical assessments and documentation. The information specialist will likely work with the vendor to build templates for the presentation of unit rosters and staffing patterns. All of these templates must contribute data to a repository from which the nurse informaticist can build ad hoc and scheduled reports of patient census, staff productivity, quality assur-

COPING WITH CHANGE

Getting help!

Developing new forms means changing the way things were done in the past, which is sometimes a difficult thing to do. However, you aren't suffering alone! Other facilities are undoubtedly going through the same laborious process. Contact them. Join user groups, and share your forms. It's much easier to modify a complicated clinical intake form for your facility's unique needs than to build one from scratch. What's more, taking such a shortcut can help make dealing with the change a little easier.

ance, supplies control, and so on— information vital to run a unit efficiently. (See *Getting help!*)

One goal should be to create and operate a successful emergency medical record (EMR). One of the cornerstones of success is the ability to easily and quickly share clinical data among all health care providers. Whether the EMR is an inpatient chart or an ambulatory clinic visit document, the system should be built so that the data collected and recorded are stored in such a manner as to provide an accurate clinical picture of the patient's condition and treatment.

Much of this data must be available for recall on subsequent assessments or clinic visits. This recall is a key satisfier for the end user. Not only is it a timesaver, it also can be formatted to provide trend analysis or simple comparison.

The system must be available to multiple providers from different disciplines simultaneously for it to be most effective. No longer is the physical location of the medical record a key to patient care. Health care is delivered by specialists and subspecialists who should be able to access the record anytime.

Security issues

Patient confidentiality and system security are important concerns— as important as ease of use and accessibility to patient data. Current legislation and federal statutes are mandating tighter control for all clinical systems that contain patient information. Improper access to this information is major concern. Discussions on data security must be an important part of your discussions with software vendors. If your facility is building its

Security issues

For the informatics nurse, all components of a system's security are important. The Joint Commission on Accreditation of Healthcare Organizations has brought attention to some of these issues; others concern keeping up with facility, professional, and governmental mandates. Here are some features that will be found on all hospital information systems on the market today, with some confidentiality issues that reside outside of the system:
➤ thorough documentation of confidentiality training during the application for access and initial training period. A duplicate copy must be filed with the information technology department and in the user's human resource record.
➤ a working policy and procedure for getting new users into the system with appropriate access and removing them as soon as they leave your facility.
➤ facility and departmental policies and procedures covering system access and security issues as related to patient confidentiality and facility business. The policies should contain a section outlining strict disciplinary standards for noncompliance.

Before purchasing any clinical system, the information technology security supervisor, facility privacy officer, or informaticist with knowledge of these issues must be assured by the vendor that the system will meet the security needs of the facility.

own home-grown system, these new mandates will present a significant challenge. (See *Security issues*.)

The clinical information system must provide features written into the application to satisfy current and forecasted needs. The following features are a minimum requirement:

➤ The system must have scalable access levels to limit access to patient data to providers who need the information for patient care. For example, admissions personnel need access to all patients in the facility, but certainly not to their clinical data.

➤ Access should be limited to patients under the care of that provider. You may consider restricting access to location of care or unit. This needs to be a flexible operation because of the workflow and the provider's need for patient information. For example, nursery staff would need to be able to access information about a postpartum patient, whereas intensive care staff would need to be able to closely monitor the care of an emergency department cardiac patient before transport to the intensive care unit.

➤ All users must have a distinctly identifiable access code. They must have an encrypted password, which must be changed after a set period by forcing a new password to be entered.

➤ An automatic timeout feature should close the chart and entire application after a set period of inactivity.

➤ The system must be able to tightly restrict certain documents. This additional level of access control must be available to allow access only by the primary care provider and the system security officer. This feature is for subpoenaed documents and those records protected by statute, such as employee charts.

➤ A second tier of user authentication must be available for transcription electronic signatures. A personal identification number is usually sufficient.

➤ All access to any record must be easily tracked by audit trail. This audit should show not only who had access to a patient's record but also how long it was open. Access reports must be available both from an individual known user and from a patient's record.

Additional security and privacy concerns must be addressed in the actual implementation of the system. Much thought must go into the placement of end-user workstations and how they can best serve the staff, yet remain secure from any kind of public viewing. Unless the staff is using portable devices, it will be difficult to position workstations in a completely secure area. Additional emphasis must be placed on the user logging off when leaving a station. The ability to easily "bookmark" a desired file and to log off are features that would be of great advantage, although they're missing on most systems. The timeout feature is a critical part of the resolution of this issue.

What's an NIS?

An NIS is a clinical system that all patient care providers who care for the patient and contribute to the patient's record use, including those in nursing, social work, case management, child life therapy, wound and ostomy care, education, respiratory care, physical therapy, occupational therapy, speech therapy, and nutrition, among others. The most important function of a clinical information system is the building of a true multidisciplinary patient record. To see a chronological cross section of multidepartmental charting is much more worthwhile to all health care providers than separate sections for each discipline. Realistically, this can only be done through an NIS. The NIS must be completely integrated into the existing HIS or developed and implemented as part of a new HIS. Most NIS implementations are best formulated after several pieces of the HIS are in place. These include medical records, ADTs, diagnostic order entries, and, preferably, pharmacy records.

Perhaps no system can impact patient care as much as a clinical documentation system for use by all facility caregivers. Unfortunately, because of both internal and external factors, many nursing information systems (NIS) haven't gone well, even though there are nursing and clinical documentation systems on the market that do work well. Invariably the systems that are the most successful also seem to be the most labor-intensive to build and implement inside the facility.

Implementation plan

The keys to a successful implementation are a good product that's easily modified for your processes, complete and unwavering support from administration, and staff buy-in. Selling a nursing documentation system to the administration might be a bit easier if it can produce positive changes in patient care and satisfaction, show an ability to capture charges in a better way, and be able to facilitate reporting to regulatory agencies (minimum data set reports for skilled nursing facilities).

Resistance to a computerized system may be high among staff and managers. Facilities with an acute staffing shortage or high turnover rate may be reluctant to embrace a new system, which will obviously require a significant investment of resources for the short term and additional resources for continued support. The preimplementation period is critical to becoming intimate with the benefits of the new system and developing a thorough assessment of the needs of the clinicians and the current and future issues that may act as deterrents to the project. (See *Convincing the troops.*)

Documentation tools

An NIS should have, as a minimum, easy-to-use documentation tools to both help plan and record patient care. The clinician should be able to quickly bring up a unit census. A method for patient assignments should also be a feature. Computerized forms for completing an assessment at admission, discharge, and

COPING WITH CHANGE

Convincing the troops

The nurse-manager of the emergency department mentioned to her staff during a meeting that there was a new documentation system "in the works." The response was a lot of groaning and eye rolling. The nurses said that they didn't have time to learn a new system — they felt like they had just learned the old system — and maybe it was better to leave well enough alone.

Realizing that the success of the new system depended on staff cooperation and satisfaction, the nurse-manager arranged for the chief nursing officer and nursing informatics specialist to come and speak to the staff about the new system. They came supplied with schedules for training and an explanation of the system. They related how the new system would actually save the staff time when documenting patient care. The new system would allow more time at the bedside and less time with the pen.

Once the staff had all of their concerns addressed and questions answered, there was a cautious excitement for the new system. Many staff members volunteered for the implementation team.

during each shift must be offered. These assessments must be built to the practice standards of each facility as well as promote the development of an automatic care plan that represents the current clinical standards of care. The care plan must be a dynamic tool that can change as the acuity and needs of the patient change. Measurable goals must automatically be presented to the clinician. An easy way to document clinician interventions must be a part of any NIS. Narrative notes must be available as needed and present themselves in both a departmentally exclusive and multidisciplinary format. Values that are collected as part of the assessment or interventions must be plotted on a graph or chart to identify trends.

All interventions should have acuity values attached to them; these values can be used to create accurate patient and unit acuity reports that are valuable to supervisory staff. This same feature could also be linked to the billing system, allowing for real-time billing for such ancillary personnel as respiratory therapy. As therapists document patient care, each intervention triggers a charge in billing. Ancillary departments traditionally have therapists working from a patient roster and "worksheet," checking off their charges at shift end. These departments can expect to see at least a 50% increase in revenues starting with the day of "going live" as a result of billing being generated from intervention documentation.

An interface to the HIS is absolutely mandatory, allowing for diagnostic and procedural orders to be added to the care plan with the automatic building of the plan. This methodology works with and without clinical pathways.

Computerized care plans

The quality of the computer-generated care plan is key to NIS success. The days of looking at the admitting diagnosis and digging into the care plan drawer to pull out the folder with the care plan nearest the needs for the patient are over. Today's care plan must be driven by real-time factors, including the care standards of your organization (for example, patient-family teaching record will be done), unit level (for example, vital signs every 15 minutes × 4 then every 30 minutes, and so on), and the assessments documented on the patient. The care plan should reflect facility-wide nursing goals and interventions, unit-specific goals and interventions, and the goals and interventions produced by the computer after analyzing the input data from the assessments. The care plan should be unique to each patient. Data items from assessments must be linked to both nursing diagnosis and interventions with appropriate outcomes. This must be an ever-changing process because the care plan is constantly updated as new data are entered into the NIS after the patient is reassessed.

For the informatics nurse, this entails significant networking with unit staff and eventual dictionary building. Along with more than a thousand interventions, a dictionary must be built of measurable goals, expected outcomes, links to order entry, and acuity values for the interventions. Remember that as units and clinical missions change, so do the types of care plans and acuity.

Access to online nursing resources

The most popular form of accessing clinical data banks comes with the ability to toggle from the clinical system to an online nurse data "dot com". If Internet connectivity isn't an option, there are clinical data vendors whose products can be piggy-backed on your system. The MICROMEDIX system offers a variety of clinical data from medication databases to poison control, diagnostic information, and patient-teaching aids. Having these resources readily available within the information system has proven to be a positive feature for users.

The audit trail

A key feature to look for on any clinical system is the audit trail of intervention documentation, with the ability for the nurse to easily make corrections. There are two kinds of errors: Documenting on the wrong patient and putting incorrect data on the record of the right patient. Correcting both errors must be well documented in the system and fast. Both types of changes must have an audit trail showing the original entries; however, the data from the incorrect patient must be erased — "hidden" — from flowsheets and reports and only the corrected entry left showing.

This system must also allow "back timing." Every intervention must record two times, the actual time the intervention was done, and the automatic time stamp showing when it was put into the document.

Time versus benefits

Although implementation can take six months to 1 year or more, the right HIS can produce positive results for patient care improvement, staff satisfaction, and an accurate clinical record. The nurse-manager's ability to monitor the occurrence and documentation of such interventions as restraints makes a profound difference in the way the intervention is used, assessed, and documented. Being able to read clear, precise nursing and other clinician notes is an immediate benefit.

Having nursing documentation available for recall and editing lends to a multitude of reporting possibilities. Staff productivity can better be gauged. Evaluations, with all chart auditing done from the manager's desk computer, become a breeze. And tracking and trending clinical processes is easier.

Having respiratory, case management, social work, and other ancillary clinicians write notes in the same system and having these notes appear chronologically allows clinicians to read other provider's notes and provide better care for the patient.

Managing the nursing student

Much has been said about security, but it's worth mentioning here how critically important it is to keep on top of the access of active users and deletion of those who have left. This includes nursing students, who will be doing a nursing program clinical rotation through your facility. However, few facilities make arrangements for nursing students to use their clinical systems.

This exclusion is bothersome for several reasons. Nursing students should be exposed to computerized documentation and electronic medical records well before they're taught to log on during orientation at their first job. Regardless of the makeup of the program—LPN, ADN RN, or BSN RN—all students should get more of an introduction to informatics than they currently do. Some of the most prestigious baccalaureate nursing programs send their graduates into the workforce with minimal knowledge and experience in informatics. (See *A bold step.*)

Another goal in allowing nursing students to chart online is to benefit the staff. If the facility is doing online documentation and the students can't chart on the NIS, problems arise. Although the students may be doing a series of vital signs, they won't have access or training to enter them into the patient's EMR. The data will be given to a staff nurse who will face the dilemma of entering vital signs taken by someone else. Most student nurses do a wonderful job of documentation with some mentoring from their instructors and the facility nursing staff. Their input into the patient's record should be valued and encouraged.

Obviously, the biggest drawbacks to allowing nursing students online are access, security, and training. Nursing students probably won't be doing many of the functions you would need to teach regular full-time nursing staff, so the training should take little time. And, fortunately, the size of the rotation group is limited by the number of students an instructor supervises. One possibility is to have the students complete the regular system security access form, where they're clearly identified as student nurses from "XYZ Nursing Program, ABC College." The system would allow these users to be grouped together in the user dictionary by folder so it would be relatively easy to delete them from the system at the end of their rotation. The students may also be given a limited set of online documentation privileges in the system, with the signature credentials of "SN" for student

MANAGER'S TIP

A bold step

More facility programs would be wise to follow the lead of the ADN RN program at Lee College in Baytown, Texas. This school has taken the bold step to partner with a nearby facility and have the facility's clinical system's training version available at a series of workstations in their skills laboratory. These students are getting valuable experience building care plans, writing critical pathways, and practicing soon-to-be-needed management skills — all online. In addition, because the nursing students become familiar and comfortable with the facility's system, it may also serve as a recruitment technique.

nurse. They could also have their own "Student Nurse Note" type built and assigned and be permitted to do limited assessment on certain units, document the interventions they made, and write student nurse notes, which will ultimately become part of the permanent patient chart.

Students from health care programs are much easier to teach how to effectively use online clinical systems than established clinicians. Students of this generation have had more exposure to computer systems than the older nurses with 20 years' experience at the same facility. After all, nursing school libraries are using online cataloging, and Internet accessible databases are substituting for many texts.

All-important training

One of the most neglected parts of a clinical implementation is that of application training for end users. It always seems to be an underestimated issue. When the implementation of the system is nearly done and all users are online, the project is over in the eyes of many administrators and managers. However, depending on the size of the facility and total number of users, you'll need at least one full-time educator. This person must be knowledgeable about the system, preferably having been a member of the implementation team from the start of the project.

Part of the work of the educator will be training new hires. The educator will need appropriate classes and training to meet the needs of the different levels of users. Another duty will be getting access forms completed and submitting them to whoever places new users on the system. The educator will need to be included in all meetings that concern real and potential changes to the system because these changes will impact the curriculum.

The amount of time spent on training new hires, in-house transfers to new positions, nursing and other caregiver students, rotating residents, and medical students, among others, will be a real problem for the implementation team. The role of the informatics nurse will swing from an activist role to a support role. As the clinicians thrive on your system, they'll develop ideas for enhancements, note errors that they've discovered, and staff workflow issues that need to be changed. All these issues will need to be addressed. Any changes will need to be continually disseminated to the other users and become part of all future training.

The training schedule

All nursing information systems will have a training, development, or test system as part of the installation before the system goes "live." The test system will be as identical to the live system as possible. These systems are used for training new users as well as for doing a lot of the screen and form building already described. They shouldn't contain real patient names. Your responsibility as a manager is to make sure that all staff members attend the required sessions, even if it results in short staffing.

Points to remember

The following points summarize the role of computer technology in nursing:

➤ Computer technology is a growing presence in health care. The nurse-manager needs to embrace the resources provided by this technology to improve time and information management.
➤ Computerized data collection, data recall, and knowledge base access promote clinical documentation.
➤ Implementation of a new or revised computer system can create challenges for the managers and staff, but is critically important to the success of any computer system.

➤ An NIS improves communication among members of the multidisciplinary team by providing documentation tools that can be readily available for recall.

References

1. Mayers, M.G. *A Systematic Approach to the Nursing Care Plan,* 3rd ed. New York: Appleton-Century-Crofts, 1983.
2. Cornell, S.A., and Brush, F. "Systems Approach to Nursing Care Plans," *AJN* 71(7):1376-378, July 1971.
3. Wesseling, E. "Automating the Nursing History and Care Plan," *Journal of Nursing Administration* 2(3):34-38, May-June 1972.
4. Beggs, S., et al. "Evaluation of a System for Online Computer Scheduling of Patient Care Activities," *Computers & Biomedical Research* 4(6):634-54, December 1971.
5. Blum, B.L., ed. *Clinical Information Systems.* New York: Springer, 1986.
6. Mills, M., et al. *Information Management in Nursing and Health Care.* Springhouse, Pa.: Springhouse Corp., 1996.

Selected readings

Azzarello, J. "Nursing Informatics: Could This New Specialty be for You?" *Home Healthcare Nurse* 17(10):634-41, October 1999. Ball, M.J., et al. *Nursing Informatics: Where Caring and Technology Meet,* 3rd ed. New York: Springer-Verlag, 2000.

Graves, J.R., and Corcoran, S. "The Study of Nursing Informatics," *Image — The Journal of Nursing Scholarship* 21(4):227-31, Winter 1989.

Hannah, K., et al. *Introduction to Nursing Informatics,* 2nd ed. New York: Springer-Verlag, 1999.

Hebda, T., et al. *Handbook of Informatics for Nurses and Healthcare Professionals,* 2nd ed. Upper Saddle River, N.J.: Prentice Hall, 2001.

Kreider, N., and Haselton, B. for the Midwest Alliance for Nursing Informatics. *The Systems Challenge: Getting the Clinical Information Support You Need to Improve Patient Care.* Chicago: American Hospital Publishing Inc., 1997Lorenzi, N.M., and Riley, R. *Organizational Aspects of Health Informatics: Managing Technological Change.* New York: Springer-Verlag, 1995.

Romano, C., and Heller, B. "Nursing Informatics: A Model Curriculum for an Emerging Role," *Nurse Educator* 15(2):16-19, March-April 1990.

Saba, V.K., and McCormick, K.A. *Essentials of Computers for Nurses: Informatics for the New Millennium,* 3rd ed. New York: McGraw-Hill Book Co., 2001.

Veronesi, J.F. "Ethical Issues in Computerized Medical Records," *Critical Care Nursing Quarterly* 22(3):75-80, November 1999.

CHAPTER 19

Managing the data

Martha Morris, RN, BSN, BC

> "An individual without information cannot take responsibility; an individual who is given information cannot help but take responsibility."
> — Jan Carlzon

Now that you're familiar with the role of computers in the nursing field, you need to become more aware of the data that are floating around. How are the data handled? What do they mean? Is there a regulating force that controls the right to privacy? Computer technology continues to rapidly expand and, as a manager, it's your responsibility to know about data management. This is somewhat of a technical chapter — so put on your cyber cap!

Information manager

Nurse-managers are in a position that requires them to gather, process, and use data. They're called upon to manage changing facility- and unit-based missions, to be flexible and timely in goal setting, and to acquire knowledge, skill, and ability in managing data. That's why it's crucial that today's managers be organizers, administrators, communicators, and analyzers of data. (See *Duty calls*.) Success at managing the mounds of information that a nurse-manager deals with helps deal with the stress of time constraints, staff demands, and administrative duties.

Duty calls

Nurse managers are commonly called upon to wear many hats. This chart depicts the various informatics duties that they may be called upon to perform.

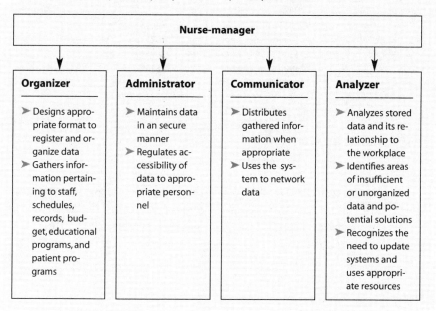

Nurse-manager			
Organizer	**Administrator**	**Communicator**	**Analyzer**
➤ Designs appropriate format to register and organize data ➤ Gathers information pertaining to staff, schedules, records, budget, educational programs, and patient programs	➤ Maintains data in an secure manner ➤ Regulates accessibility of data to appropriate personnel	➤ Distributes gathered information when appropriate ➤ Uses the system to network data	➤ Analyzes stored data and its relationship to the workplace ➤ Identifies areas of insufficient or unorganized data and potential solutions ➤ Recognizes the need to update systems and uses appropriate resources

Information anxiety

When there's inability to access or control information, information anxiety may result. Described by Wurman,[1] information anxiety results from a gap in the information that we understand and the information that we think we should understand. The factors that contribute to information anxiety include:

➤ inability to access needed information because of the inability to work the system appropriately or because it's controlled by others

➤ complexity of data presentation that makes it difficult to understand

➤ need for technical assistance in order to access or manipulate data.

Telltale signs

Wurman[1] identifies these signs and symptoms as possible indicators of information anxiety:

➤ feeling unable to keep up with work-related events occurring around you, while giving time and attention to unrelated events
➤ feeling guilty about being unable to follow a new procedure, keep up with periodicals and journals, or explain something that you thought you understood
➤ communicating understanding or knowledge of a new product or procedure when that understanding or knowledge doesn't exist
➤ avoiding learning about new equipment or procedures for fear that you'll be unable to understand what's being taught or reacting emotionally when such a situation occurs
➤ feeling that you aren't as smart as other managers
➤ being afraid to say "I don't know" and being afraid of relaying wrong information.

Information anxiety can decrease with improved understanding and successful data management. Enlisting the assistance of an informatics nurse can prove beneficial. (For signs of information anxiety, see *Telltale signs.*)

Data management

Data is information that's processed in a way that increases the knowledge of the person who uses it. Data consists of facts, text, graphs, images, sounds, or video that have meaning for the user. As a nurse, you collect data; as a nurse-manager, you organize and manage different forms of data from various sources. In the past, data such as common medications were commonly stored on index cards. Now with the proliferation of new drugs, the best place to store drug information is on a computer. The place on the computer where you can store, manipulate, and retrieve data is a *database.* (See *Functions of a database.*)

Everyone in the facility uses a database to manage information — single users, work groups of 2 to 25 people, departments of 2 to 100 people, as well as the facility as a whole. The most common desktop database applications include:

➤ Microsoft Access
➤ Filemaker Pro
➤ Paradox

Functions of a database

Database applications perform four basic functions:
➤ adding new data
➤ reading current data
➤ updating or modifying data
➤ deleting data.

➤ Lotus Approach
➤ FoxPro.

Using Microsoft Access

The most common database program is probably Microsoft Access. This program is user-friendly and ideal for managing the type of information that nurse leaders are required to manage. What's more, it has the same look and feel as other applications in Microsoft Office, so learning the program is that much easier. You can even create a shortcut to it on your computer desktop, enabling you to go directly to the program quickly and easily as soon as you sit down at your computer. It comes with the necessary help information, complete with Wizards to troubleshoot the more complex tasks. What's more, a sample database called Northwind comes with the software.

Each Access database contains related tables where data is stored. This "relationship" among tables enables you to update information in one table while the program automatically updates it in the others. For example, you can enter employee information in one table and employee work hours in another; if an employee changes her phone number, you need change it in only one table and it will automatically be changed in all of that employee's record. Each employee's characteristic is an *attribute*, each data column is a *field*, and each row is a *record*. (See *Looking at Microsoft Access*, page 436.)

Finding data

You can view stored data in forms, reports, or queries. Microsoft Access *forms* are used for adding new data and editing and looking at an existing record. The Report Wizard in Access is used to build *reports* to print out or to view information formatted and

Looking at Microsoft Access

Here's an example of a table you can create using Microsoft Access.

Employee ID	Employee number	First name	Middle name	Last name	Title	Home phone
1	123456	Judith	J.	Test	RN	(616) 999-8888
2	345678	Mary	K.	Simply	RN	(616) 999-2222
3	678901	Pete	W.	View	RN	(616) 999-3232

organized to your specifications. Examples of reports include employee lists and unit supply usage reports.

A *query*, which can be thought of as a question, finds the information you need without your having to wade through multiple records. You can create a query by using the Query Wizard, going through the process in steps and selecting the tables and fields that you want. The Wizard can also help you build more elaborate forms and reports, which you can enhance with clip art from the Web or Microsoft's Clip gallery.

What's an SQL server?

Microsoft Access is used as a front-end development tool and is attached at the back end to an SQL server. (SQL, or structured query language, is a database programming language used to create, modify, control, and retrieve data from a database.) The SQL server enables work groups, departments, and single users within the facility to share data, offering those facilities that have the server an advantage over those that have single stand-alone databases.

Relational databases

Microsoft Access is a relational database, the most common type of database. Information within this database is organized in tables with rows and columns. The data may then be manipulated using SQL language. Programs are also available that don't need to use SQL language. Relational databases constitute second-generation database management; with earlier systems from the 1970s, data access was difficult because programmers had to work with one record at a time, and the systems lacked a theoretical foundation.

In a relational database, queries and reports can be done using Crystal Report Writer. These reports can be distributed to management using intranet-ready software called Seagate Info. With this software, your information technology (I.T.) programmer can produce Crystal reports, analysis, and information delivery from databases. Seagate Info software can be purchased from: *www.crystaldecisions.net/products/crystalreports.*

In the 1990s, third-generation data management systems were developed to handle images, audio, video, and geographic data. Object-relational database systems are hybrids that can handle both objects and data.

Understanding standards

The Joint Commission on Accreditation of Healthcare Organizations (JCAHO) has established standards for managing information. For accreditation to be obtained, your facility must follow the reporting requirements set concerning all areas relating to the care of individuals and management of the health care facility. As a manger, you're responsible for becoming familiar with the latest revisions of JCAHO and establishing the appropriate information system to adequately maintain and report required information.

Language standards: Dealing with nursing data

Two key things need to be established in order to computerize nursing data: clarification of what constitutes nursing data and standardized nursing language. To facilitate the process, organizations such as the American Organization of Nurse Executives (AONE) and JCAHO have developed *minimum data sets* and *standardized terminology sets.* Although the definition of *data* could encompass both things, the two are different, despite the fact that they share the same purpose, which is to assist nurses in making decisions about health care.

Nursing Minimum Data Sets (NMDS) help to clarify what constitutes nursing data. These sets of information have clear definitions for each category of nursing information, although they don't define the data that's used in each category. For example,

The role of the NIDSEC

The Nursing Information and Data Set Evaluation Center (NIDSEC) has developed standards to evaluate four dimensions of nursing data sets and the systems that contain them.[2]

➤ Nomenclature (the terms used) American Nursing Association–Recognized Classification Systems:

–North American Nursing Diagnosis Association (NANDA)

–Nursing Interventions Classification System (NIC)

–Nursing Outcomes Classification System (NOC)

–Nursing Management Minimum Data Set (NMMDS)

–Home Health Care Classifications

–Omaha System

–Patient Care Data Set

–PeriOperative Nursing Data Set

–Systematized Nomenclature of Medicine Reference Technology

–Nursing Minimum Data Set (NMDS)

–International Classification for Nursing

–ABC Codes by Alternative Link Practice (ICNPR)

➤ Clinical Content (the "linkages" among terms)

➤ Clinical Data Repository (how the data are stored and made accessible for retrieval)

➤ General System Characteristics (such as performance and attention to security and confidentiality)

although NMDS defines *nursing diagnosis,* it doesn't list the individual nursing diagnoses. For this, a standardized nursing language is used—in the case of nursing diagnoses, that means the taxonomy codes established by the North American Nursing Diagnosis Association. For nurse-managers, AONE developed the Nursing Management Minimum Data Set (NMMDS), which helps nurse-managers make more informed decisions about nursing environment, nurse resources, and financial resources, thus leading to better unit management.

Nursing language classification sets help to standardize nursing language, thus improving communication about patient care and helping to maintain JCAHO's nursing documentation standards. These sets were developed to document nursing care in the areas of acute care, ambulatory care, and home care.

Following JCAHO standards, the American Nurses Association (ANA) established the Nursing Information and Data Set Evaluation Center (NIDSEC). The function of the NIDSEC is to review, evaluate, and recognize information systems that support documentation of nursing care. The ANA recognizes 12 established sets of nursing language. (See *The role of the NIDSEC*.)

Security standards: Getting "hip" with HIPAA

Security concerning data collection, storage, and accessibility is a key concern and a primary responsibility for nurse-managers. That includes learning about federal standards that affect these issues and monitoring complaints where appropriate. If your facility has an informatics nurse on staff, enlist her help in communicating and maintaining appropriate standards.

The Health Insurance Portability and Accountability Act (HIPAA) became a federal law on August 21, 1996. This law deals with issues involving health insurance, health care fraud and abuse, implementation of health information standards, and security of patient's health information. An outgrowth of HIPAA is the Fraud and Abuse Control System, which gives the Department of Health and Human Services (HHS) and the Department of Justice more power to go after suspected facilities.

HIPAA rules established accountability for a patient's medical record. The maximum penalty for the misuse of unique health identifiers and individual health information is $250,000 and up to 10 years' imprisonment.

New rights for patients

The HIPAA Privacy Rule became effective April 14, 2001, and health plans and providers must comply with these regulations by April 14, 2003. Smaller health plans have until 2004 to comply, and the Health and Human Service's Office for Civil Rights (OCR) will enforce this ruling. OCR has a Web site for detailed information including frequently asked questions at *www.hhs. gov/ocr/hipaa/*. For the first time in history, the federal government is protecting the privacy of health information, giving patients new rights on how health information is used. What does that specifically mean for patients? They'll be given clear written explanations on how health providers use and keep their health information. They'll be able to obtain a history of any health information that was disclosed for new treatment purposes as well as to whom it was disclosed and when. They'll have the right to see, get copies, and make amendments to their own medical record. The privacy rule covers records and individually identifiable health information that's in written, oral, or electronic form. State rulings that give patients higher levels of privacy and confidentiality (for example, mental health patients) will remain in effect.

Covered entities

Covered entities include health plans, health care clearinghouses, and health care providers (hospitals, other facilities, and private practices) that electronically transmit any health information for billing, transfer of funds, and other financial and administrative transactions. Covered entities and their contracted business associates must comply with the standards, requirements, and implementation specifications of the HIPAA privacy rule. A business associate may be another covered entity. A business associate isn't a member of a covered entity's workforce and performs a function that involves patient-unique identifiable health information.

Compliance

Facilities must designate a privacy official, who will be responsible for HIPAA privacy compliance, and they must train all employees in the new privacy standards. Nursing and ancillary departments will be involved in writing new policies and procedures and reviewing present policies for gaps in compliance. Facilities must also establish a patient grievance process in writing and then implement it so that patients have a way to file complaints or inquires about the privacy of their medical record.

Authorization is a customized document that's detailed and specific. It's required for psychotherapy notes and the release of psychotherapy notes, regardless of reason. Authorization is also needed for research.

Modifications to the legislation

HHS was given permission by Congress to modify the privacy rules. Changes are being proposed so that personal health information may be used for first-time referrals to hospitals and specialists, allowing surgery, procedures, and appointments to be scheduled without having to wait for written consent. Pharmacists encounter the same problem, prohibiting them from filling prescriptions that are phoned in for new patients, unless the rule changed.

More changes on the way

The Security and Electronic Signature standard was proposed in August of 1998 and, as of this writing, is awaiting a final ruling. This standard will heavily involve information technology and upgrading systems, documenting systems, backup plans, and policies and procedures. All users of information within the health system — including nurses, those in ancillary departments, those in risk management, physicians, and security personnel — will also be required to comply with the new standards. To plan, organize, implement, and maintain the security of patient records, facilities will need to assign or hire someone for the job of data security officer.

The proposed Security rule is made up of administrative procedures, physical safeguards, and technical security services to guard data integrity, confidentiality, availability, and technical security mechanisms, to protect against unauthorized access to data transmitted over the network. The Electronic Signature proposal rule requires a digital signature, which is encrypted and ensures that the person's signature wasn't tampered with after it was applied. (See *Complying with HIPAA security rules,* pages 442 to 444.)

Standard codes and formats

Standard codes provide a universal language for health care information — and they help ensure HIPAA compliance. The standard codes for diseases, impairments, and injuries are the *International Classification of Diseases,* 9th revision (ICD-9-CM), volumes 1 and 2; for inpatient procedures, volume 3 of ICD-9-CM is used. For outpatient procedures, Health Care Financing Administration (HCFA) Common Procedure Coding System (HCPCS) and *Current Procedural Terminology,* 4th edition (CPT-4) are used. Others include National Drug Codes (NDC) for drugs and HCPCS for medical supplies and devices.

HIPAA also mandates specific formats for health claims, payment and remittance, coordination of benefits, health claim status, enrollment, disenrollment, eligibility, premium payments, referral certification, and authorization. These standards are available free at *www.wpc-edi.com* and can be downloaded at no charge. You must completely document your transaction stan-

(Text continues on page 445.)

Complying with HIPAA security rules

Under the Health Insurance Portability and Accountability Act (HIPAA) of 1996, policies and procedures that health care facilities must establish to safeguard the security of patient records include the following.

Administrative procedures
➤ Evaluate and certify your facility's computer system and network.
➤ Certify that appropriate security has been implemented. Either your facility or an accrediting agency can do this.
➤ Have a formal mechanism for processing health records that includes having a policy and procedure for how your facility receives, manipulates, stores, disseminates, transmits, and disposes of health information in place.
➤ Review system activity through internal audits, such as logins, file access, and security incidents.
➤ If you or a third party use multiple two parties at the same level, make sure you have a chain-of-trust agreement and maintain the same level of security.

Planning for emergencies
➤ Create a contingency plan for system emergencies.
➤ Perform an application and data criticality analysis. You must know what applications and data are critical to patient care and to the facility's business, and they must be functional 24 hours a day, 7 days a week.
➤ Have a data backup plan that includes how you obtain and make copies of applications and users' computer systems.
➤ Have a disaster recovery plan.
➤ Have an emergency operation plan, including a plan for manually processing data. If the system is critical, you need to have equipment available that can be substituted in an emergency, plus alternative power sources to keep your critical systems functioning.
➤ Write and maintain procedures for testing and revising contingency plans.

Restricting access
➤ Put into place policies and procedures for facility-wide information access control, including access authorization, access establishment, and access modification.
➤ Make these policies and procedures uniform across all types and kinds of media, including electronic, paper, and fax.
➤ Ensure that they cover:
– accessing health information by the user's role or job description
– who will authorize user sign-on and who's accountable
– special authorization for sensitive health data
– how you'll monitor user access to health data
– how clinicians will access data remotely
– what you'll do about user noncompliance
– how you'll modify or terminate an employee's access.

Complying with HIPAA security rules *(continued)*

Training users
➤ Set up security awareness training for all personnel, including management.
➤ Educate employees with periodic security reminders.
➤ Require user education in password management and virus protection.

Safeguarding password access
➤ Don't allow temporary or shared passwords. *Note:* Alphanumeric passwords are the most secure, but they're difficult for users to remember.
➤ Make sure users know how to change their passwords.
➤ Having password assistance available for critical systems 24 hours a day, 7 days a week.

Ensuring personnel security
➤ Have only authorized, knowledgeable personnel supervise those who perform technical systems maintenance activities.
➤ Keep records of who authorized access and when.
➤ Ensure that operating and maintenance personnel have proper access.
➤ Observe personnel security policy and procedures.
➤ Make sure system users and technical maintenance personnel are trained in system security.

Managing system configuration
➤ Keep system documentation on file.
➤ Make sure hardware and software installation and maintenance have been reviewed and security features tested.
➤ Inventory your computer assets.
➤ Test your security.
➤ Install virus-scanning software and fixes on computers and servers, and check the system regularly for viruses.

Handling incidents
➤ Establish security incident procedures that contain reporting and response procedures.
➤ Set up a security management process to address security issues.
➤ Do a system risk analysis.

Handling terminations
➤ Institute termination procedures for when employees depart. These must include:
– changing user combination locks
– removing users from access lists
– removing user accounts from the system
– mandating the return of keys, tokens, or cards that allow access.

Physical safeguards
➤ Assign security responsibility to a specific person or organization, who'll be responsible for:

(continued)

Complying with HIPAA security rules *(continued)*

- – management and supervision of the use of security measures
- – protection of data
- – the conduct of personnel in relation to the protection of data.
- ➤ Establish policies and procedures governing how hardware and software, including tapes and diskettes, are received and removed from a facility.
- ➤ Have a facility security plan that controls physical access to your facility, including procedures for:
- – control of equipment in and out of your site
- – verifying access authorizations prior to physical access
- – maintaining maintenance records
- – visitor sign-in and escorts
- – testing and revising your access plan.
- ➤ Set up policies and procedures for workstation use and instruction for how to keep patient data secure.
- ➤ Secure workstation locations to minimize unauthorized access to patient data.
- ➤ Do security awareness training.

Technical security services

- ➤ Institute access control.
- ➤ Implement a procedure for emergency access and at least one of the following:
- – context-based access.
- – encryption.
- – role-based access.
- – user-based access.
- ➤ Institute audit controls through mechanisms to record and examine system activity (audit logs).
- ➤ Institute data authentication controls, requiring each organization to provide validation that their data hasn't been altered or destroyed in an unauthorized way. This could be ensured by the use of check sum, double keying, and message authentication code or by digital signature.
- ➤ Institute entity authentication controls, including:
- – automatic logoff and unique user identification
- – one of the following: unique passwords, personal identification numbers (PINs), telephone call-back procedure, token system, or biometric access that could include finger scan, retina or iris scan, speech recognition, face recognition, hand geometry, or signature verification.
- ➤ Ensure that communication networks have integrity controls and message authentication as well as one of the following:
- – access controls.
- – alarm.
- – audit trail.
- – encryption.
- – entity authorization.
- – event reporting.

dards, and this documentation must include your implementation guide, a data dictionary, and data conditions.

HIPAA standards for unique identifiers for providers of health care, employers, health plans, and patients will reduce confusion, cost, and error. The proposed standards for the health care provider are the National Provider Identifier (NPI), which HCFA will issue and maintain. The Employer Identification Number (EIN) is the existing Internal Revenue Service number. The Health Plan Identifier is the payer I.D., and the individual identifier is still on hold.

You need to begin assessing your computer system's patient medical record numbers. Have your information technology department review its system to see if duplicate records for the same person or more than one patient assigned the same medical record number is a problem. Ask if you have a Master Patient Index and if your medical record numbers have been cleaned up so that each patient identifier is unique. Your facility may need to consult and purchase new hardware and software to accomplish this major task.

Although HIPAA standards are extensive and somewhat confusing, the nurse-manager is responsible for maintaining some of those standards. The facility should have systems and personnel in place to maintain and check the security of data. The nurse-manager should also be aware of the extent and importance of these systems, as well as who is responsible for them.

Making the connection

A network is a system made up of computer hardware and software. A network provides computers the ability to interconnect, work together, and transport communications from one computer to another. It gives computers the ability to share hardware: printers, servers, and modems. Networked computers can also share software applications, files, and databases. For this reason, networks have advanced security features.

Two types of networks are available: peer-to-peer and client/server. In your home or office, setting up peer-to-peer networking is easier and more economical. In a large facility, client/server networks are built to handle the large amount of data being transported. You might even work with both systems in the same setting.

Servers are dedicated computers in a network shared by users. They have both hardware and software components. Servers are used for applications, communications, directories, faxes, Internet and intranet access, e-mail, databases, and video, proxy, print, terminal, and remote access.

Larger, more powerful, and more stable application servers linked to the network are mainframes, AS 400s, and reduced instruction set computers (RISCs). Facilities store, centralize, and secure servers in environmentally controlled rooms called *data centers*.

Fat client network computers

One type of client on a network is the personal computer (PC) workstation. Powerful personal computers are needed for *fat client networks*. Fat clients store the data on the server, but the application is manipulated on the PC workstation. These workstations can be purchased with different operating systems. Smaller, much older applications use DOS, Windows 3.1, or OS2 operating systems, although Windows 3.1 and OS2 are now outdated and lack support. Most computers purchased today have Windows 2000 preloaded. If you want to convert to Windows NT (new technology) or backload to a previous version of Windows, that's an additional charge. The cost of licensing the software operation system is also included in the charge of the computer.

The operation you purchase depends on the software applications you want or need to run on your computer. Linux is a free version of UNIX operating system that runs on various hardware platforms. Software and technical support and training can be obtained from vendors for a fee. Large and small facilities are exploring the transition to Linux operating system for their servers and computers because of the reduced licensing cost.

Thin client network computers

Computers that do very little processing are termed *thin client network computers*. Similar to "dumb terminals," they're computer devices without hard drives or floppy disks. Thin clients can't function on their own; they download applications from the network server and obtain all data from that server. All application changes are then stored back to the server, with the network using the server to manipulate the data.

The use of thin clients is growing. Many computer applications using Internet and intranet browsers don't require a personal computer. With thin client network computers, cost and maintenance can be controlled. Because everything is maintained at the server side, software doesn't need to be installed and upgraded at each client. Also, because thin clients occupy small areas, they are ideal for areas with limited space.

To support Windows applications, additional software from Citrix or terminal services must be purchased to run on the thin computer's Windows NT or 2000 server. These software and licensing costs are additional.

To connect a thin computer to the network, you'll need to purchase a network interface card (NIC) for your computer. Mobile laptop computers come with PCMCIA card slots, which enable you to add a NIC or a wireless LAN PC card. The 3Com wireless cards now have an XJACK antenna that extends for wireless reception while in use and retracts for safety and convenience when not in use.

The NIC card is then attached to a cable with a connector for Ethernet and Type 3 Token Ring networks, which has been mistaken for the four-wire or six-wire connection that's commonly used for a phone or modem connection; Type 1 connectors are used only for Token Ring networks. To prevent confusion for computer users, contractors installing the computer cables can make the computer connection in the wall a different color so that users always plug in to the correct site.

Going wireless

Use of wireless networks in the health care industry is growing. One such network uses Citrix clients and 3Com for the access points, with Ethernet wireless cards, and works well. (Visit *www.3com.com/index2.html.*) However, implementing a wireless network requires specialized support and knowledge — and patience. Mobile computer hardware, including personal digital assistants (PDAs), are an alternative. Physicians today are using PDAs for tracking patient data and referencing clinical information. Nurses are beginning to use them too, as more programs are being developed for the practicing nurse.

Other mobile hardware

A mobile hardware device currently being used is the Tremont, which is especially useful in the operating room. This computer has a large monitor screen, rugged cabinets, and can be washed down, keyboard covers and all. It costs more, but it's durable. It also has a 12-hour battery so that it doesn't always need to be connected to an electrical outlet. The Tremont system is also used in dialysis.

Both the Tremont system and laptops affixed to a pole (also called "computers on a stick" — for example, a laptop PC roll stand with sliding tray, with a laptop security cable to lock the laptop down) are used in critical care areas. Poles are ideal for use with a computer system because they can be used to mount patient monitoring equipment, video displays, information systems hardware, and other equipment that requires adjustable positioning, accessibility, and security.

Other useful ideas include assigning one mobile computer to each critical-care patient room, with a few Ethernet cables and electrical cables placed in the hallways so that if the room is too full, the workstation can be transferred to the hall. This option is also less disturbing to the patient, especially at night. Although these "computers on a stick" are replacing the bedside fixed computers, laptop computers have only a 2-hour battery, and staff must keep that in mind when using them. Also, surge protectors can be placed in the baskets along with a long Ethernet cable so they can be moved around a patient's room.

Connecting with e-mail

Electronic mail (e-mail), which involves sending a message to a recipient over the network, is a speedy and efficient way to communicate within an organization. In today's technological world, many people are already familiar with e-mail and how it works. Everyone given access can send and receive immediate messages.

E-mail programs

Netscape Messenger, Outlook Express, Lotus Notes, and Eudora Light are all e-mail programs. These programs can be used through an Internet browser linked to your intranet, enabling managers and staff to access and send e-mail from any computer on the network, 24 hours a day, 7 days a week. The disadvantage of older Web-based products is that they lack the full functionality of newer Web-based and single-access e-mail programs, which allow users to format text (including changing text color), add images, schedule appointments, and manage messages, calendars, and links to other Internet addresses (called uniform resource locators [URLs]). Users also have the capability of downloading and uploading messages and appointments to a PDA or pocket computer. The latest e-mails allow wireless mobile access, so users on the go are always connected. Managers who want the ability to use networked computers to access and respond to e-mail from anywhere in the organization and to have their own personalized e-mail configured for their office need both single access and Web access for their e-mail.

E-mail programs require a server, networked computers, and user training. Therefore, your facility would need to have on staff an information technology department server specialist to manage the server, a network specialist to manage the network, a personal computer specialist to do upkeep on the computers, and computer system trainers. User training can be done using either e-learning modules for experienced Web users or as classroom hands-on training for new users.

Facility administration and management can also access their e-mail from home via a modem. If you have Windows NT server for network dial-in capabilities, someone in your information technology department can set up remote access service (RAS) on your laptop. Some companies also set up remote dial-in access via the Internet, which enables users to communicate with their staff, peers, and boss anyplace, anytime.

E-mail has numerous positive aspects, the major ones being immediacy, convenience, and ability to reach numerous people at one time. Other aspects associated with e-mail use that should be considered include:

➤ *Appropriate use.* Some users may use e-mail to transmit inappropriate messages or even threats. A user's guide on e-mail etiquette, called *netiquette,* is a good tool to promote proper communication. Books on e-mail etiquette are available in stores.

➤ *Virus attack.* A virus can cause extensive damage to your entire network. To prevent such damage, the information technology department, which is responsible for system reliability and security, may install and maintain virus-checking software on the e-mail system and on user's computers.

➤ *Misinterpreted message.* E-mail is a delayed conversation, and such delays can cause a message to be misinterpreted. If you need an immediate response to a question or immediate feedback from a comment, a real-time conversation by phone or in person is your best bet. For this reason and others, e-mail shouldn't be your sole means of communication.

➤ *Depersonalization.* Some users may use e-mail to avoid social contact. From a manager's standpoint, this could be detrimental to developing a strong working relationship with your staff. Therefore, try to maintain a healthy mix of personal interaction and electronic communication. (See *Sending the wrong message.*)

Other e-mail uses

Databases within the e-mail system are made up of user names and e-mail accounts. Within Lotus Notes, software databases can be built by programmers to automate workflow, track, broadcast, reference, and enable user discussions. Lotus Notes is more than an e-mail provider, it's also a business tool. By following the

MANAGER'S TIP

Sending the wrong message

The manager of a busy trauma unit frequently used e-mail to inform her employees about hospital events as well as upcoming changes that affected the unit. In fact, she replaced staff meetings with these messages. She felt that this was the best way to get information to her staff, especially those who worked on the night shift, whom she didn't see very often. She felt that she was being very informative, as well as saving time for the staff by not pulling them away from their busy day.

The Director of Critical Care received several complaints about this particular manager's e-mails. Staff members saw them as a method of avoiding personal contact. They felt there was no opportunity to ask questions or relay ideas and opinions and didn't believe that sending an e-mail would relay their ideas with the same feeling. The director met with the manager and communicated these concerns. The manager immediately scheduled a staff meeting to apologize for using this method of communication and to allow open discussion of feelings and concerns about e-mail.

E-mail should be used as a supplemental tool to relay information. Although it's a convenient communication method, each person views it differently. Some people hate e-mail. Others don't have time to access it; if it's the main method of communicating information, they could feel that they're left "out of the loop." Although you should acknowledge e-mail that you receive from your staff, avoid using it as the sole method of communication. Speaking to your staff personally can establish a much stronger relationship than the technological touch.

workflow of a document such as an incident report, you can expedite and track the process. For a medication error, the nurse completes the document online and then it's routed to nursing management, who can send requests for feedback from other departments, such as pharmacy, and then to its final resting place in risk management. You can track where a process began, stopped, or slowed down and how long it took to get to its destination. Using this process can be an effective timesaver for a demanding schedule.

Intranet (not Internet)

Do you want to increase productivity, save the cost of manually copying and distributing paper, and increase communication? Then the intranet is your answer. The intranet uses the same protocols as the Internet, but resides on the facility's network. It's used within your facility and is protected from the Internet by "firewalls." Firewalls are a method of keeping out the public and trespassers and consist of hardware and software.

Windows computers are preloaded with an Internet browser, such as Netscape Navigator and Microsoft Internet Explorer, which can be used for your intranet

Building an intranet

To build your own intranet, you'll need to consult someone who is knowledgeable in that area, if your facility doesn't already have someone on staff in I.T. Start with a simple a home page. Remember: A page that's simple is also quick to load, whereas a fancy page with a lot of graphics takes more time and computer power, which doesn't translate into time savings for your employees.

Web pages can be built using Front Page, Dream Weaver, or other Web site–building software. If you want a robust Web site, you'll need to purchase a server and server licenses. For ease of maintenance, link your intranet to a database instead of a lot of pages. Simply keep in mind that this option requires purchasing an additional database server and licenses, and database expertise. You'll also need to look into your facility's policies for support on these items.

The main intranet site must contain a primary search for quick access to information — just like the Yahoo and Google search engines on the Internet. This can be a real time-saver if your facility has all your policies and procedures online. Which books and information does your unit purchase and distribute? If these were distributed electronically, would it reduce labor and distribution costs? JCAHO manuals are now intranet-ready, and facility policies and procedures can be organized, centrally stored, and managed using document management software.

Net-It-Central is an example of document management software by Informative Graphics that may be useful for your facility. The information technology department manages the server hardware and software: Department personnel configures the user's site on the server and then sets up a network drive on the user's computer and maps it to Net-It-Central. The department content experts prepare the documents that they want to have displayed on the intranet. Then a secretary or support staff member copies the documents to be published from the hard drive and pastes the documents to the system on the network drive.

Documents to be published can be in a variety of forms: Word, WordPerfect, Acrobat, Excel, Power Point, Visio, or Project. The sites can be password protected and configured on the server to look for and post updates every 10 minutes if needed. Therefore, if a new procedure is written and approved and needs to be replaced, it can be done in minutes. The system even flags document updates so users know what's has been newly added or updated. Each document site is then linked to the intranet, and the site is live.

Intranet and ancillary departments

Think about ancillary departments. What databases have they built to distribute manuals that could also be displayed via the Web? How about radiology procedures preps and information about laboratory tests? For example, users could easily search and find which colored-top tube and how many milliliters of blood are needed for a laboratory draw. Drug companies sell intranet-ready software. Rather than hunting for the drug manuals, it can be as quick as a search on the drug database via the intranet. Many clinical systems on the market today either have a Web browser front end or can be converted. View laboratory, transcription, computerized patient record, and radiology results linked to your intranet home page. Employee job postings, e-mail, whiteboards, phone and pager directories, newsletters, surveys, department Web pages, and Internet links can also be both viewable and interactive on the intranet.

The library offers clinicians a wealth of information. With just a few clicks of the mouse, these resources can be found on your Web site. Also, many journals and manuals are intranet-ready. Users can search one resource or all resources in the software package. What's more, your facility can save money by purchasing the intranet version of the resource as opposed to buying multiple copies for every unit in the facility.

Intranet and education

The Intranet can also be used for E-learning, or electronic learning. The market has many prebuilt programs for meeting corporate compliance. Microsoft and other vendors have built within the software packages the ability to be Web enabled. Do your nursing educators have presentations that could be loaded on an educational page for clinicians to view and learn from? Let your creativity flow.

In the field of information technology, all projects have a life cycle, called the *Information Systems Cycle*. The first phase of the cycle is project analysis; the second phase, design; the third phase, development; and the final phase is implementation, which includes ongoing evaluation.

Start with a meeting, and "mix well." Calculate your return on investment. A quick way to calculate this is to calculate the cost you spend now to copy, print, update, and then distribute the unit's many policies, procedures, and newsletters. Also, calculate if you distribute information to other areas of your facility and to employees, physicians, and facility affiliations within your network. Compare that cost against the cost of implementing a documentation management system. Heat things up by determining who will manage the project and obtain capital monies. When things cool down, plan how you'll implement, evaluate, and maintain your intranet site. Top this off with a hearty congratulation to all when the job is done.

Points to remember

The following points summarize the importance of data management:

➤ Successful data management helps deal with the stress of time constraints, staff demands, and administrative duties.
➤ Standards for managing information are in place to adequately maintain and report required information.
➤ Nursing language classification sets help to standardize nursing language, thus improving communication about nursing care as well as maintaining established nursing documentation standards.
➤ Nurse-managers have the responsibility of being knowledgeable on security issues regarding data collection, storage, and accessibility.
➤ E-mail is a communication tool that can be used by nurse-managers to reach numerous staff members as well as other administrators in an immediate and convenient fashion.

References

1. Wurman, R.S. Information Anxiety. New York: Doubleday, 1989.
2. Nursing Information and Data Set Evaluation Center. *www.nursingworld.org/nidsec/class1st.htm.*

Selected readings

Anderson, T. "Curing Privacy Problems: HIPAA/Healthcare," *Journal of Healthcare Protocol Management* 18(1):97-107, Winter 2002.

Bleich, M., and Bratton, M. *Information Management and Computers.* Baltimore: Williams & Wilkins, 1990.

Brown, R. "An Overview of the Federal Legislation and the Accompanying Rules Developed by the Department of Health and Human Services." [White paper] 2002.

Delaney, C., and Huber, D. "A Nursing Management Minimum Data Set (NMMDS): A Report of an Invitational Conference." Chicago: American Organization of Nurse Executives, 1996.

Dennis, J.C. *Privacy and Confidentiality of Health Information.* New York: Jossey-Bass, 2000.

Freedman, A. *Computer Desktop Encyclopedia,* 9th ed. New York: Osborne/McGraw-Hill Book Co., 2001.

Frye, C. *Microsoft Access Version 2002 Plain and Simple.* Redmond, Wash.: Microsoft Press, 2001. *www.dabases.about.com/library/weekly/aa120300b.htm*

Gillespie, G. "Defining the Roles of HIPAA Officers," *Health Data Management* 10(3):52, March 2002.

Levine, J.R, et al. *The Internet for Dummies,* 8th ed. New York: Hungry Minds, 2002.

McFadden, F., et al. *Modern Database Management,* 5th ed. Reading, Mass.: Addison-Wesley, 1998.

Paul, L. "Leading the Way to HIPAA Security Requirements." July 1999. *www.healthcare-informatics.com/issues/1999/07_99/expo.htm.* Available through Healthcare Informatics Online: *www.healthcare-informatics.com.*

Richards, C., et al. *Using Lotus Notes 4.5.* Indianapolis: Que Corp., 1997.

U.S. Public Law 104-191, Health Insurance Portability and Accountability Act of 1996.

Wagner, B., and Negus, C. *The Complete Idiot's Guide to Networking,* 2nd ed. Indianapolis: Que Corp., 1999.

Young, K. *Informatics for Healthcare Professionals.* Philadelphia: F.A. Davis Co., 2000.

CHAPTER 20

Meeting information challenges

George Harbeson, RN, MSN

> "Never before has so much technology and information been available to mankind. Never before has mankind been so utterly confused. It's time for clarity." — KPMG advertisement

As health care delivery systems become more complex, nurses are relying more on information technology (I.T.) to carry out their primary mission — patient care. Long-standing issues facing nurses will be magnified in the coming years, and nurses will undoubtedly face even more challenges. The nursing shortage, inadequate staffing, shorter patient stays, and patients with more complex problems are immediate issues that can directly benefit from technology. Increased scrutiny by regulatory and accrediting agencies and the resulting need for more complete, more accurate, and more timely reporting demand the use of computerized data collection and processing.

Today's effective manager will look to technology for more effective ways to automate many of the time- and effort-consuming duties that keep nurse-managers from supervising nurses.

Identifying a need for I.T.

Nursing practice continues to mature alongside the field of I.T. Data collection has always been a primary responsibility of nursing care, with nurses using the actual data to enhance their knowledge. Whether in the context of a nursing assessment, a history, or a simple set of vital signs, patient data helps guide the care plan for each patient and serves as the basis for clinical decision making.

However, now more than ever, patient data must be standardized for ready access and interpretation by other caregivers, quality outcomes managers, and third-party payers. Today's more-streamlined health care systems are demanding standardization of clinical languages and outcomes predictions that require a dramatic increase on reliance of I.T.

Standardization of staff documentation

As health care facilities turn to computerized data management systems for their business transaction needs, they're typically confronted with inadequate, sloppy, illegible, and late patient clinical data that doesn't meet the new reporting and billing needs. This fact alone has caused many facilities to computerize their health care providers' records.

Nursing documentation that remains paperbound will undoubtedly become a bottleneck for smooth billing, materials management, and quality outcomes monitoring after these departments have become automated. The nurse-manager will spend an increasing amount of time doing time-consuming chart audits to supply the information needed. No matter whether the clinical documentation application or the patient billing record comes first, implementation of one will soon drive implementation of the other.

The Health Information Portability and Accounting Act of 1996 (HIPAA) mandates standardization of health care payer information for business transactions between a health care provider and payer. This standardization will cut the time and cost of these transactions, benefiting the facility as well as the patient. It will, however, require much tighter parameters on clinical documentation. Even for those facilities whose documentation is primarily paperbound, the adaptation of the HIPAA standards will surely drive the move toward charting standardization.

Quality of documentation

As staff documentation becomes standardized, a manager will be able to recount the horror stories that come out of chart audits. Nurses who are under stress will tend to revert to "blind charting." Nursing assessments will be written more from rote than from actual subjective and objective data. Nursing notes will sound the same from patient to patient. Then there's the case of the missing information: "Did anyone actually see this patient during this shift?"

The nursing clinical record has suffered because it's perceived (especially by physicians) as an afterthought to patient care. At most facilities that rely on manual charting, nursing documentation is more of a testimony to how industrious staff nurses are for that shift. Staff nurses still view charting as a record of what they did for 8 to 12 hours. No wonder the nurse documentation section of a patient's chart is the least accessed by other provider staff. Physicians rarely look at anything other than vital signs in the nursing section — that is, unless a problem arises, in which case they may look at narrative notes. This situation perpetuates dissatisfaction among nurses in their jobs because they feel that others don't appreciate their work.

Standardizing documentation, however, will quickly and clearly elevate the caliber of documentation in the health care setting. The new computerized patient medical record will be easier to access, read, and evaluate because it will appear in the same format from patient to patient and from unit to unit. This in turn will subtly raise nursing department standards of documentation. (See *Appreciating quality.*)

As a nurse-manager, you need to promote a standard for clinical charting, and this is easily done with a clinical system, with input data helping to create a computerized medical record. Through the use of formatted screens and templates, charting is more meaningful for patient outcomes and less centered on the clinician.

Today's complex patients demand a multidisciplinary approach to their care, which can only happen when information and knowledge is freely shared and easily accessible Although a change to computerized charting can present some challenges, it's important to realize that computerized charting is a direct means to raising standards. After successful implementation in

MANAGER'S TIP

Appreciating quality

If nurses felt that more care providers accessed their documentation, the quality of the charting would undoubtedly improve. Charted information would be more accurate and more pertinent, thus directly impacting patient care.

As a nurse-manager, you must not only be an advocate for quality documentation but also stress to other disciplines the value of nursing documentation. While attending grand rounds, formulate a plan that will look at the nursing notes on the topic patient. Develop short multidisciplinary meetings that focus on patient documentation and the impact it plays in every discipline's care of the patient. Use information technology whenever possible to demonstrate the role it plays in storing and obtaining patient data. Your involvement could greatly impact the quality of documentation.

some nursing units, implementation in ancillary support departments most closely tied to nursing will naturally follow. The case management, food and nutrition, and social services departments are natural candidates for coming up on the electronic record. Their needs are fairly straightforward and directly linked to the nursing interventions.

Decision support

The body of medical and nursing literature is doubling every 19 years. For example, information on acquired immunodeficiency syndrome care increases twofold every 2 years. Today's patient is more complicated and more likely to have come in contact with medical equipment and procedures that have been around only for the past 10 years.

The nurse can no longer rely on standardized nursing care plans from the drawer in the nurse's station. The care plans must be customized for each patient, according to his unique diagnosis, problems, and expected outcomes. In even the most prestigious nursing schools, a nurse is taught only a fraction of the knowledge and skills she'll need to have at hand in the workplace. Information retrieval will be the most important component of the curriculum. A nurse must be a decision maker and can no longer be content with the task-oriented practices so prevalent in health care settings today.

Evidence-based practice

Evidence-based practice is a growing topic in health care. A nurse wants to know what's going to be clinically effective in her practice. However, journals may contain suspect information, and textbooks are too time-consuming to be readily used. Although literature searches have always been available, they've historically been too cumbersome to work in the clinical setting and, thus, were left in academic settings. The solution? Hardware and software development in recent years has brought the entire body of nursing knowledge to the patient's bedside. Practice guidelines can be readily accessed to support a nurse in her critical thinking. These guidelines can also support the delivery of complex patient care and serve as an indispensable part of care planning and unit and department policy making.

The modern nurse-manager should seek out these resources, evaluate them, and lobby to make the appropriate ones available to her staff. Even if implementation requires a great deal of staff input as to the content and eventual use of the information, it's likely to be worthwhile. The validation and implementation effort, in itself, will be a wonderful learning exercise.

Medication administration

Drug dispensing by a nurse and drug ordering by a physician are two activities being scrutinized now more than ever. A nurse must have quick and easy access to drug information, including adverse effects and interactions. Instant access to diagnostic test results must be available to staff as part of this process. With new drugs being approved every day and new indications and warnings being issued, a set of drug cards or a drug handbook is no longer adequate. Even the most scholarly nurse can't be expected to keep up with all critical interactions among a patient's medications. To ensure that drug information is current and complete and to enable a nurse to make the critical clinical decisions she must make, sophisticated data management tools — specifically computerization of clinical data — is necessary.

Drug information support must be closely linked digitally to the patient clinical database as well as to the order-entry and laboratory systems. With all of this information linked, the nurse is not only able to gather accurate drug information from an up-to-date drug literature source but can also relate the information to the patient's real-time diagnosis, condition, and other medications.

Accessing clinical data

Today's nurse-manager is being asked to do more detailed and focused monitoring of clinical documentation than ever before. Much of this is because case management is more important. The manager needs to have ready access to accurate data about patient census, potential admissions and discharges, and patient outcomes. As resources are being managed on a tighter time and dollar budget, the manager can't afford to have beds remain unoccupied or patients who can be moved to a less-acute setting remain in a unit bed while the intensive care unit (ICU) is waiting for a room to empty. More complex procedures are being performed in the ambulatory areas, and still many other procedures require in-patient care, are complex, yet have shorter stays. Being able to instantly access clinical data as well as accurate bed resource information is a key to patient care and business survival.

Relying on documentation

With managers needing so much information at their fingertips, relying on documentation that comes in as many formats as there are staff nurses simply won't work anymore. Speedy access to a patient's chart, unit census, acuity levels, and facility bed resources requires a standardization of clinical documentation. Online clinical charting is the only answer.

Another issue facing the manager is patient care reimbursement. Governmental payers and health insurance companies are demanding better and more standardized documentation when they call for chart auditing. They're setting standards for the content and quality of the patient's record. Diagnosis must be accurately coded, physician documentation must be present and legally signed, and nursing and ancillary interventions must be accessible and pertinent to the patient's coded diagnosis. Documentation on a clinical information system will help organize the various chart components as well as drive more accurate and pertinent charting by all providers.

Standardization in charting protocols is also beneficial to the nurse-manager who is juggling staff from unit to unit. Float pool nurses can adapt more quickly and effectively on a new unit that's using standardized charting tools.

Nursing quality management

Quality management, outcomes monitoring, and utilization review are among the several patient documentation audits with which the nurse-manager is charged. Whether the manager is a supervisor for a single unit or a director with several areas to manage, access to the information needed for these audits is commonly difficult to find and time-consuming to obtain. The nursing areas on a paper document must requisition charts from medical records, and lengthy chart audits must be conducted.

Data input and collated into an automated computerized medical record can be used to run audits and build pertinent reports. Reports can be keyed to a focus quality indicator, such as I.V. patency or restraint assessment, or they can monitor the interventions of a single staff caregiver. This information can be accessed from the manager's office without a desk full of patients' records, which saves the time of medical records personnel.

Many nurse-managers are required to monitor utilization review. Whether they're case managers or unit managers with the case management task, a great deal of time must be spent reviewing the charts.

Minimum data sets (MDS) of patient demographics, assessments, care plans, and records of interventions are now a routine yet resource-intensive requirement for federal and state reimbursement for hospitals. Ultimately the responsibility of collecting and transmitting this information falls to the unit manager. To have the ability to quickly access patient records in order to track a particular nursing procedure and to monitor the times the procedure was performed, by which nurse, and how often can be a wonderful tool for monitoring the quality of patient care in a nursing department.

A nurse-manager who's expected to be a key figure in quality outcomes monitoring must have a process in place to easily identify, quantify, and evaluate clinical data that staff nurses input. This involves a great deal of chart auditing and searching for missing records that need auditing. The actual chart audit can be time-consuming because it involves reviewing notes taken manually and reviewing quality indicators — that is, data that must be transferred to a report.

I.T. and nursing operations

Information technology can help with all of the administrative chores that nurse-managers face.

Time and attendance

What nurse-manager likes to do payroll? How much time and energy is wasted verifying clock-ins and sorting out staffers who forgot to clock out or who contend that they worked a shift that doesn't show on the time roster? To find the staffing sheets, call charge nurses, or track down the shift supervisor takes the manager away from more important tasks. A computerized time clock system that's linked to the unit staff and scheduling application can save a nurse-manager valuable time and energy. Quick access to time sheets from the manager's workstation saves time and resources when the manager needs to monitor a nurse's tardiness, excessive time past shift change, or absence record.

Staffing and scheduling

Automated scheduling gives back to a nurse-manager better use of her time, easier accommodation of a nurse's preferred work schedule, and improved availability of data to staff units according to need. Good staffing through a well-constructed staffing software program can reduce costly overtime and enhance care. Several good staffing tools are available in the health care automation marketplace. Building scheduling matrices and automating a unit's scheduling leads to great staff satisfaction—an important factor in these days of widespread nursing shortages and use of agency staff.

A good integrated hospital information system (HIS) will have a module dedicated to unit staffing as part of the system. Implementation of these applications is fairly straightforward, with a modest amount of dictionary building. The nurse-manager is typically expected to build templates for the staffing matrices and maintain updated unit staff rosters. All systems require credentials, "home" shift, and facility level job title. These job titles must be consistent across the facility for float pool staff. Many systems are sophisticated enough to allow for modifiers to be attached to individual staffers, such as scalable preferences, holiday time off-record, and unique skills or training, such as cross-training to other units.

For the unit manager and nursing directors, the reporting capabilities of all currently available staffing systems will offer a new tool to help with budgeting and work flow analysis. Control of unnecessary overtime is much simpler when the individual staff member's schedule and times are easily analyzed across different time periods. Auditing the on-duty times of agency nurses for comparison to the billing invoices from these agencies can help identify variances.

The nurse-manager must also build templates for the staffing matrix. Most staffing systems allow for a range of matrices, which can be called up to allow for dramatic census changes or special circumstances, such as changing the patient acuity level for ICU overflow, disasters, and so on.

Although most nursing departments prefer to staff on a strict acuity basis, the reality is most are usually staffed based on the number of occupied beds. A quality scheduling system should accommodate each as well as a combination. The software should be able to facilitate the rotation of qualified nurses to different areas where they're proficient and comfortable. This system promotes more efficient and capable nurses and can help head off nursing burnout from being on the same unit too long.

So how does an automated staffing system work? The shift supervisor inputs census data, and the system presents a screen or report plugging the nursing unit staff into the appropriate role assignments for both licensed and unlicensed personnel. The system should be able to factor in previous role assignments for each staffer and, by looking at this recent history and analyzing the job titles, present an automated staffing report that's fair and clinically sound. A nurse is generally more satisfied with staffing assignments after implementation of an automated staffing system, perhaps because she perceives the system as being nonbiased in its assignments.

The integration of scheduling programs to the facility's payroll and human resources system can go a long way toward freeing the nurse-manager from having to figure the payroll out biweekly. What's more, the new generation of schedulers can finely tune shifts to reflect historic peak and quiet times in such areas as the emergency department (ED). (See *Overcoming staffing challenges.*)

Overcoming staffing challenges

Staffing remains a challenge for nurse-managers and for the nurse administrator. It's a never ending balancing act between adequate staffing for good patient care and the bottom line. Today, administrators are further challenged with a nursing shortage and the need to budget for increased agency and contract staff and increase resources for nurse recruitment and retention. Many new software applications are available to help harried nursing departments with these issues.

Strict control of agency expenses demands maximum efficiency with use of hospital staff. Use of a good scheduling system provides the administrator with reporting capabilities to see the big picture. These questions should be asked:
➤ Which units are losing nurses?
➤ Which units are using an unusually high amount of overtime?
➤ Is the nursing float pool operating as it was designed to operate?
➤ Are all float pool nurses going to the same areas day after day?

An automated staffing system can accurately track agency use. Where agency staff is being used the most and why is valuable information. A simple spreadsheet should be built to track agency nurses by agencies and by individual names. Tracking performance by agency might show a trend to overall quality from one agency to another — something that's hard to do when looking only at the supervisor's report after a shift ends. Tracking temporary agency nurses by performance on different units also highlights those nurses your hospital might want to offer full-time or longer contracts to.

The nursing shortage and trend toward higher salaries and sign-on bonuses is going to move the pool of nurses around more than ever before. Nursing turnover is going to increase at a time when administrators are longing for a core staff of loyal, satisfied professionals. More licensed nurses are going to be interviewing with nursing departments. In response, the savvy nurse-manager and nurse administrator will have quick and easy access to state boards so they can do online checks for license status and disciplinary problems. This access should be used for querying those other states where the prospective nurse has been licensed. Simple investigating up front can avoid trouble down the line.

Acuity systems

Most new staffing and scheduling applications have an acuity system, which should be implemented and used. When done accurately and honestly, this system can produce a staffing schedule that will ensure better patient care and prevent overstaffing over the long haul. By using the system across all nursing units, communication between units improves; by using the input fields of cross-training, it will be easier to control the number of nurses who are canceled at the last moment because of low census and fill those staffing shortages on other units, whether caused by unexpected rises in census or staff call-ins.

The acuity module in the staffing and scheduling application should be invisible. The acuity scoring and resultant patient, unit, and facility acuity level scores should be built for the documentation module. The acuity score levels should be driven by the care plans for each patient. Nursing acuity can be scored in various units, but the units are driven by the time required for a given nursing intervention.

No one in the facility other than the nurse-managers and staff nurses can build these acuity score dictionaries. After all, they're the end users of the system who really know the time and energy required for each nursing action and assessment. This building will require some unit level time studies and chart audits. The actual identification of intervention will probably already have happened during the building of the documentation piece. Every intervention will need to be assigned an acuity unit value and a minimum staff skill level that can perform it.

The system should allow for scalability with regard to acuity units attached to nursing interventions and extensive tweaking after going live. The nurse-managers will be able to compare unit acuity levels to census numbers and adjust acuity units early on. For an acuity-driven staffing system to work, staff must believe in it, yet they will do so only when they feel that the acuity levels that the system is reporting are in line with the amount of nursing effort expended to provide good care. The implementation process shouldn't be painful, but it must be viewed as an import step toward full acceptance.

The acuity scoring system will probably be tied to the staffing and scheduling piece, and if the unit is to be staffed by acuity levels, this operation will be automatic and won't require the input of census numbers. However, care must be taken when setting up this system to factor in leeway for scheduled and unscheduled admissions during the shift.

Acuity level reports are useful to facility administration and all departments impacted by patient needs. Long-term acuity forecasting can be done and, over time, a better picture of seasonal trends can be seen. Although bed census will always be a critical indicator for health care facilities, acuity level is sure to become a significant factor in performance improvement management.

Staff nurse evaluations

Most nurse-managers loathe staff nurse evaluations. No matter how well intentioned, you never seem to be able to space them out over a reasonable period, and they inevitably end up stacking up as the deadline looms. Doing a quality evaluation takes time and effort. Unfortunately, much of the work put into doing these reports comes from gathering the needed information. Chart audits need to be done, and time and attendance sheets must be reviewed. What's more, midyear evaluations and last year's evaluations must be tracked down.

The ability to run reports from the manager's workstation is a big benefit of nursing department automation. Having information management tools accessible from a single physical source can greatly speed up the evaluation process. Instead of ferreting out staffing sheets to find out which patients a particular nurse cared for so that medical records can be requisitioned or how many times this nurse called in sick, standard reports can be called up and the information displayed on the monitor. Patients' computerized medical records can then be accessed on the same screen and a charting audit can be done. This type of data access and management is an absolute necessity for today's managers who don't have the time to chase down information.

E-mail

E-mail is no stranger to nurses today. Most nurses use e-mail from their home computers, and most nurse-managers use e-mail at their facilities as the official medium of intra-staff communication, for all but the highest level of subject.

A lot of facilities on different I.T. platforms have discovered the benefits of e-mail access for all employees. It offers a fast, convenient method of rapidly getting the word out to the entire body of personnel or to a targeted subset of employees.

The facility e-mail system should be easy for all staff members to use. Managers should be able to build "sets" of their own personnel so they can easily get a message out to their unit. Perhaps they would want to break this set down further for licensed nurses, nursing aides, and clerical staff. Having staff e-mail address sets for each shift could come in handy if a memo is meant for the night shift only. What's more, having these subsets available can save time and energy.

Nursing personnel can benefit greatly by learning how to build personal folders to better organize their e-mail messages. Some systems even have the ability to send messages or files to folders that staff can access but that are "read only" — that is, they contain information that can't be edited or deleted, except by designated users. Examples of "read only" files include staff schedules or unit policies.

Policies and procedures

Computers are useful not only for educational materials but also for official communications. Facility, nursing service, and unit policies and procedures are always problematic: The sheer volume typically deters staff nurses from accessing them as often as they should. By putting policies and procedures on the facility's computer network, access can be extremely easy with the help of some keywords and a search engine. Even without this level of technology, simply being able to log on and review your facility's policies and procedures can be an improvement over the paper system. What's more, with the wider access that comes with computerization of such information, you should notice fewer incidents caused by a staff nurse's lack of knowledge of official policy.

I.T. and teaching

Information technology also offers help with documenting patient teaching and staff education needs.

Documenting patient and family teaching

Patients are leaving the hospital sooner—and staff nurses, specialty nurses, and ancillary support personnel are faced with the task of teaching these patients what they need to know before they go home. Whether the teaching is in response to orders given by the physician or a need perceived by the nurse clinician, the teaching must be properly documented, with the same diligence as any other diagnostic or care order.

Although certain mandated data fields must be documented on any teaching record, even the best-drafted paper form will still fall short of providing an accurate assessment of learning needs, subject matter, and postteaching assessment. To fulfill current requirements, the new teaching record must adequately assess the learning status of the student. The record must document learning barriers and physical and mental limitations, including the need for interpreters, signing, large print, and so on. Both ability and motivation should be recorded. The best methods for learning must also be part of the assessment. Remediation for each barrier must be listed.

The teaching subject and presentation method must be documented as well as a quantifiable assessment of the effectiveness of the session. A score below complete and verifiable learning must be accompanied with a follow-up education strategy.

This type of data collection lends itself to online documentation. Data collection fields are easily tailored to the standards of each facility and to the requirements of accrediting agencies. For example, a data field where the discipline of the clinician doing the teaching (such as nursing, physical therapy, nutrition, or social work) can be added. Most documentation systems have the intervention of patient and family teaching structured to be reportable. These reports should present a multidisciplinary approach to the teaching needed for good outcomes for most patients. The teaching record should be a prominent piece of the patient's electronic medical record.

The intervention of patient and family teaching must be a standard part of the care plan for all patients.

Handling patient-teaching aids

Flyers, pamphlets, and fact sheets have always been a part of patient teaching, but now they must be thoroughly documented and meet certain standards. The manager needing to monitor patient teaching must be able to document their validity and applicability to the patient.

An information management system is a wonderful tool to print out information for the patient. Today's system allows the nurse-manager to build a unit-standard patient-teaching aid (PTA) library, with PTAs that are always ready for printing. No longer will the file drawer be stuffed with poor quality copies of patient-teaching materials. No longer will the needed PTA go missing because a staffer gave out the last copy. In addition, many systems include a virtual copy of the PTA produced as part of the electronic medical record.

Many facilities purchase software packages of PTAs, which can then be uploaded into the data management system. These packages can be entire information libraries, covering disease processes, surgical procedures, medications, minor procedures, and health maintenance subjects. Because these PTAs are in the form of instructions to the patient, the appropriate medical-legal committee in the facility must approve them. These purchased PTAs are commonly available in different languages.

Most computerized publication libraries support varied levels of graphics. Before purchasing such a library, it's a good idea to inquire about customization of the PTAs, which should have the ability to be edited. After all, not all information applies or is appropriate in every case. What's more, the PTAs should look professional and should be tailored to the patient, with his name included in the header area. The PTAs should also print clear accurate follow-up instructions for patient and family questions.

Most systems that support these computerized libraries allow for new PTAs to be built from scratch. Simply keep in mind that staff members need to adhere to copyright laws when building their PTA files. For those PTAs created using a word processor, most applications support cut-and-paste techniques for creating a new PTA format.

Enhancing staff education

The average nurse-manager is probably familiar with computerized education tools as any other nursing operation software. The nurse in even the most technologically backward facility has embraced the many avenues available on computers for professional education.

Nursing schools today make great use of e-mail systems, computerized reference materials, teaching materials, and testing. As a result, today's nurse graduate is entering the clinical setting with a more sophisticated computer background. The modern nurse-manager should be able to use this resource to raise the standards of staff education. Whether an education program is unit based or produced by the facility's education department, computerization allows more flexible presentation methods as well as more innovative programs.

More facilities are using client-server hardware technology as a platform for their clinical systems, which usually places a personal computer (PC) workstation within easy reach of all clinicians on every shift. The possibilities for nurse education are endless. If the facility has built an intranet system, it can allow secure placement of training programs to be uploaded and accessed by staff during slow hours or during off-shift times.

All accredited facilities have minimum standards for in-service education. There are mandatory courses on safety, patient rights, and ethics, and then there are programs unique to the nursing department. Attendance at these sessions must be documented, and records kept at the department level as well as in the personnel folder of the nurse. This leads to a filing nightmare for understaffed education departments and for the unit nurse-manager. Software applications that serve as the educational medium and that can be used for record keeping and reporting of the employee's entire in-service education record are now coming to the rescue.

Tests and simulations

These new systems are easy to upload with formatted educational courses that can be presented to a group or to an individual sitting at a workstation. For many clinical-based programs, there may be a pretest, an educational offering, and a posttest. The time online, program title and details, and test scores are added to the application database. Educational programs that aren't uploaded into the facility's network can be presented and attendance and testing scores input manually by the nurse-manager or education department. These systems can be queried by the manager to see at a glance who has attended mandatory in-services as well as who has taken online courses for professional advancement. The quantity and subjects available for computerized presentation are staggering, and the quality of the new breed of programs makes these offerings more interesting and relevant to the staff nurses.

Computers are also widely used for programs that have clinical simulations. Learning heart sounds and 12-lead electrocardiograms is easier with today's interactive programs, and a multimedia presentation for practicing for advanced cardiac life support certification can prove realistic and effective. Nursing schools are using software that presents a virtual hospital unit for nursing management training. The possibilities are endless.

The Internet as teacher

The Internet, or World Wide Web, has come to the forefront as one of the greatest teaching tools ever. It's beneficial to the nurse-manager and staff, and it has numerous applications. Promoting computer skills at the facility or at various nursing department levels can show a great return when the facility is moving toward greater automation. Nurses with computers at home have access to more professional knowledge through the Internet and, thus, may be faster to get on board when you start to discuss an electronic health record.

Various web-based applications are available to help nursing units operate. Many computerized nursing operation applications described here can be accessed from the Internet. Use of application shared provider (ASP) software is a viable alternative to purchasing expensive hardware and software for smaller facilities. In the case of ASP programs, the program and databases are usually maintained by the software vendor, and the clinician customer pays a subscription fee to tap into this system, with only high-speed Internet capabilities and locally networked PC workstations as hardware requirements.

In addition to an enormous savings in capital expenses when compared to a hospital-based system, the software, databases, and servers are maintained and supported by the vendor. However, it's more difficult to get the software vendor to customize the system for your facility's unique needs, so there's a tradeoff. What you see is what you get.

For nursing personnel, the Internet offers access to clinical knowledge bases, online professional journals, information on conferences and seminars, and opportunities for web-based continuing education. However, strict policies should be firmly in place before giving a staff nurse access to the Internet. Your information services department security personnel should be able to help set up some screening protocols on the facility's firewall to prevent staff from misusing or abusing their Internet privileges.

I.T. and physical operations

Information technology offers solutions for physical plant management.

Forms and printing control

A clinical information system reduces the need for forms. Most notable in its absence is the unit nursing assessment documentation forms. These charting tools tend to take on a life of their own and grow in size rather dramatically. Nursing documentation forms rarely get simpler. The revision of an assessment and care documentation form presents a large project to the unit staff. Necessary edits are commonly put off because of the high cost of printing, and an eye must be keep toward the forms inventory. This warehouse inventory typically drives form development.

Regardless of the model and vendor of a modern documentation application, a great deal of time goes into developing the actual documentation tools. Although form building can become a lengthy process, subsequent editions, tweaks, and major and minor edits can be done quickly and easily.

The building of the documentation tools falls to the unit manager, providing a good opportunity for you to make those changes you've wanted to make for the last few years. The overall magnitude of the changeover from paper forms to online forms requires input from staff members, which in turn drives ownership by the unit staff of the new product.

Those involved on the project team will undoubtedly want to make changes. It's important for the nurse-manager to keep the staff nurses involved in the development, implementation, and phases of the project after it's instituted. The end user clinicians must always feel that the system is theirs and that they have a strong voice in making changes as needed.

Materials management

With the move toward a leaner, more streamlined health care delivery system go many of the luxuries that are commonly taken for granted. Even large university medical centers are doing more outsourcing of many support functions, such as medical supplies and food management. Facility administrators have finally discovered what the automobile industry has known for decades: Keeping a large stock of parts on hand is inefficient. In every facility, an entire department and bureaucracy was needed to warehouse, inventory, and distribute these items. Many supplies have short shelf lives and consequently were wasted due to expiration dates. More facilities are looking to reliable outside suppliers who can supply clinical needs quickly. Where at one time a year's worth of a certain item was available, now perhaps only several days' supply is on hand.

Outsourcing may be great for the facility's bottom line, but what about your unit nurses having the right supply and the proper quantity of that supply required to care for their patients? Automation of supplies at the nursing level usually means using one of the new generation of "vending machine" type devices. These devices should be set up to relieve nurses from having to document the use of disposable, chargeable supplies for the sake of resupply and patient billing. Nurses should be documenting supplies only within the context of patient care.

Medications management

With the spotlight on reducing medication errors, computerized order entry isn't only going to make the nurse-manager's life easier, it's probably going to be mandated—and fairly soon. Several states are already requiring physician-entered computerized ordering of medication. The need for purchase and implementation of order entry automation will be the catalyst for bringing the integrated hospital computer system to many facilities that resisted these large changes until now. (See *An important letter.*)

Order tracking and order status monitoring will be a benefit for the nurse-manager as well as for staff nurses. So much of the manager's time is spent fielding questions from a physician over the phone about a particular medication order when the chart can't be found to check allergies or laboratory results, which would impact the administration of a particular medication.

How many patients have been adversely affected by a wrong medication that was given by a nurse who misread a physician's handwriting, didn't adequately review recent laboratory values, or missed the handwritten notation lost in the chart, about a newly

An important letter

The following note was sent from the Healthcare Information and Management Society's *E-News* to subscriber's to the *Health Information Management Newsletter* on April 25, 2002:

"Medical errors impact more Americans than previously reported. An estimated 22.8 million people — one in five Americans — report that they or a family member experienced a medical mistake. According to a new study from the Commonwealth Fund, an estimated 8.1 million households have experienced an error that caused a serious problem. The report, based on a national survey of nearly 7,000 adults, points to serious problems of communication between patients and doctors as well as a widespread failure to monitor chronic medical conditions such as heart disease, breast cancer, and diabetes.

The survey indicates that medical and prescription drug errors are far more common than previously believed. Karen Davis, president of the Commonwealth Fund, said the 1999 Institute of Medicine report on medical errors, which caused a stir at the time, may have revealed just the tip of the iceberg. She advised that computerized reminder systems and drug cross-checks could help ensure better care — as well as prevent errors. But, she said, most hospitals haven't invested in the information technology that could help.

discovered drug allergy. Although automating order entry won't completely eliminate errors, adverse events should drop dramatically when ready access to a computerized medical record and physician's orders are available.

As facilities look for new ways to reduce errors and control waste, they're now purchasing and installing pharmacy-based robotic systems that are interfaced to the nursing unit's order entry system. The electronic medication order is verified and the system automatically fills a container with a short-term supply of the needed medication and delivers it to the nursing station. The medications are usually packaged in single doses. The shorter time and the reduced supply, such as only a day's worth, works well with the faster turnover of today's patient census. If the medication isn't canceled, the system will repeat the supply the next day, without any additional human intervention.

The system also cuts down the numbers of "leftovers," which invariably end up in medication rooms after a patient is discharged. The nursing unit is credited for lowering wasted medication charges, and the patient's itemized statement doesn't contain medications that were charged for and not administered. These systems have shown to reduce errors that had originated in the pharmacy. However, even with this new technology the administering nurse remains the ultimate safeguard against medication errors.

Bed management

One key to patient satisfaction is prompt and efficient admissions, discharges, and transfers (ADT) operations. As facilities continue to be at full in-patient capacity, a major effort for the nurse-manager is to promptly execute ADT. A common scenario has a physician telling a patient and his family that the patient has improved and will be immediately transferred to a step-down unit. Hours go by and a series of process malfunctions keep the patient in ICU and the family stewing in the ICU waiting room. The physician wrote the transfer order, but the medical-surgical bed that the charge nurse thought was assigned to the patient was pre-empted by another patient coming in as a direct admission. Of course, an expert admissions department, good communications, and good policies may have prevented this, but the scenario would occur less frequently with an automated admissions system.

The nurse-manager who works with a bed tracking system can immediately access bed availability, status of readiness of the bed for a new patient, and scheduled direct admissions. Many things can change by midshift from the report given by the off-going charge nurse 4 hours earlier. Having immediate information on ADT needs and resources will head off many patient flow snags.

All nurses working on a unit should be able to transfer and discharge patients. Manual systems that rely on telephone calls to and from admissions personnel and bed controls generally will break down on a regular basis. A patient who's discharged home usually wants to get up, get dressed, get discharged by the nursing staff and leave! Nurses often tell a patient he's going home, and then the patient and family wait hours for paperwork to be generated from the admissions department. Two bad things happen: First and most important, the patient is no longer impressed with the skill and efficiency of the hospital; and, second, a patient might be lying on an uncomfortable stretcher in the ED waiting for the same bed. A well-constructed, automated ADT system keeps an information link up between nurses and admission staff. (See *Changing the system.*)

COPING WITH CHANGE

Changing the system

The emergency department (ED) of a busy city hospital faced the daily challenge of finding beds for those patients requiring admission. One day there would be a shortage of critical care beds, the next it would be medical-surgical beds that were in need. The ED staff felt that they were continually playing "phone tag" with the admissions office and the floors themselves, because there would be changes or delays continually throughout the day on the status of these beds.

The manager of the ED recognized the need to change the system to one that's more efficient — not only to improve patient satisfaction, but also to relieve staff of an unnecessary stress. She investigated and proposed a computer system specific for tracking bed availability and status. However, she was surprised at the negative response from the staff when she related the news of this system. They communicated that they felt that the system would take too much time and they didn't want another thing added to their workload.

Implementation of change always meets with some resistance. However, there are some actions that the manager could have taken to promote a smooth implementation of this system. First, the manager should have had staff "buy in" of the idea as well as participation in the selection process. Although they might not have had any "official" say as to what system was chosen — they would have felt that they were recognized as part of a team, and since the system would impact them, they would have had the opportunity to voice concerns at an early stage. Second, the staff members should have had the opportunity to volunteer to become the "super users" of the system — that is — appointed staff members would learn the system well and be the designated teacher and trouble shooter during the implementation period. These super users help generate enthusiasm and decrease anxiety about change in the system. They help to get a new system "up and running".

The manager of this particular ED was quick to recognize the fear of change in her staff. She took on the role as super user in this situation and arranged her time so that she participated in the initiation of the new system. She spent time with each staff member to answer their questions and review the process as many times as was needed to make them comfortable and proficient with using the system. Although this implementation may have taken longer, the staff came to realize that they were spending less time on acquiring beds as well as being less frustrated over the whole procedure of admitting patients.

Census management is a direct product of the ADT system. Nurse-managers covering several units or the entire house can immediately locate a patient, track unit patient flow, and manage bed assignments when the facility is near capacity and the ED is stacked up. Shift supervisors will also benefit from this real-time information.

ED tracking

The perpetual dilemma of too many patients for too few rooms and too few emergency staffers isn't going away anytime soon. However, computerized ED resources and a patient tracking system can eliminate part of the problem. Through the use of this system, the departments stressed resources can be used more efficiently. The tracking system should be able to present a patient census of those patients in a department examination room as well as those patients who are in the waiting room. All patients triaged to the waiting room should be identified in the system and their chief complaint presented. The system should have the ability to "flag" or alert after a period of time if the triage nurse feels that the patient should be reassessed for some reason while they wait for an examination room to become available.

What the ED nurse-manager wants is to be able to control patient flow and room utilization. With a good ED system, the manager can track a patient's flow through the department and continuously monitor which resources are available or are about to become available. The ED manager is geared toward running the department when it's under the highest stress. Information management at this time is critical. A tracking system allows the clinical staff not only to monitor those patients who have made it to the "back" but also to have data access for those who are still in the waiting areas.

A system can be set to monitor all waiting patients with some immediate information such as age, sex, chief complaint, or acuity. Many systems have the ability to program "flags" or alerts. An asthmatic may not be acute enough to get into a crash room, but needs to have extra monitoring. A flag system can have the patient's name blink after 15 minutes as a signal for the triage and front desk personnel to do a quick status check out in the waiting area.

When the ED is completely packed with no chance of relief from a full ICU, the manager will need to be able to use every bed and stretcher space available. The system will likely have been set up with ghost locations, otherwise known as the "hallway spot #1," and so on. The patient will need to get into an examination room so he can be adequately cared for by the staff. A tracking system should be able to monitor orders management as well as resource and patient flow. A patient may need to go to imaging for a lengthy test, perhaps even for an emergency endoscopy. By monitoring orders management, the now-empty room could well be used for another patient who needs only a short procedure, such as having a fish hook removed under the examination room treatment light.

Most EDs are loss leaders and are commonly written off financially as a necessary evil that has to exist for public service or as an admission portal for private practice staff physicians. The technology savvy manager will explore ways to attach billable charges for care, equipment use, and supplies to point of care charge capture. A busy ED staff will relegate filling out charge forms to the last task done. Stickers will get lost, charge sheets won't be completed, and medications won't be properly counted. Although vital to the bottom line, it isn't usually looked upon as a priority of the clinical staff. If the nursing and medical staffs of the ED can capture accurate charges while they document their care — and this charge capture doesn't create another layer of paperwork — they'll happily get on board.

Operating room scheduling and documentation

Because of the unique business and operating styles in surgical departments, there seems to be a sort of disconnect with the clinical charting on the patient. The operating room and the surgical department have a large physician presence, and surgical documentation in the form of the surgical workup, operative report, and anesthesia record are critical pieces of the medical record. The different entities in the department — including surgeon and staff, nursing operating room staff, anesthesia, scheduling, and supplies — rarely document in a coordinated manner. Add to this preoperative nursing and postanesthesia care, and the documentation can become even more disjointed. (See *Meeting the need,* page 480.)

The heart of a surgery department is the scheduling system. Today's operating room and hospital surgeons must have a high level of cooperation and coordination. Most surgeons have specific days and rooms blocked out for them, but when cancellations or add-on cases come up, flexibility and rapid response can

QUESTIONS & ANSWERS

Meeting the need

Question: *How can I.T. benefit the operating room manager?*
Answer: The manager of any surgical department must spend a lot of time:
➤ auditing different charting documents
➤ managing staff and department resources
➤ coordinating cases
➤ managing sterile supplies.

All of these responsibilities cry out for an integrated and coordinated I.T. department system. Although the implementation for all but the simplest remains an enormous project, the operating department management system will probably produce the most dramatic results in improved department operations.

keep the surgeons happy and the rooms in full use, which is great for the budget.

There are several well-known, well-accepted surgery department software applications available that share a common architecture: they all center on the schedule. Implementing the scheduling module with its preferences, room management, and so on can be a long, arduous, heartbreaking project for the operating room manager and staff, but should show immediate positive returns when the system is turned on.

Along with patient, surgeon, and room scheduling, preference cards are another key piece of the operating room system and a time-consuming part of the implementation. The cards are actually online preferences built for each surgeon. Whereas these preferences were previously typed on index cards and stored in a box, they're now online for quick access. The preference cards are usually procedure-specific for an individual surgeon, with the desired equipment, sutures, gloves (type and size), patient positioning, and draping instructions.

The anesthesia record is a critical part of the operating room system and is possibly the most technologically challenging. A good anesthesia documentation system must be interfaced with the physiological monitoring system, bypass machine, and anesthesia machine. The raw data from these devices must fill in a meaningful flow sheet that will provide a good picture of the patient's condition. Systems will also prompt postprocedure narrative data and verification from the anesthesiologists.

The nursing staff running the preoperative or staging area in the surgical suite documents the patient's surgical record as well. Staff should have online preprocedure checklists, documentation for consents, and the ability to make clinical observations.

Postanesthesia, or recovery, units receive the anesthetized or sedated patient, and monitor recovery before sending him to a postsurgical unit. The operating room system should offer a customizable and scalable postanesthesia record with interfaced data input from physiological monitoring devices. The system should support plug-in interfaces to the I.V. pumps as well.

Surgery departments use various types of supplies — those that are reusable or disposable, those that require sterilization, and those that are implantable to name a few. In such a high-use environment, computerized supply management isn't an option. By piggybacking supply and equipment charges onto operating room procedure documentation, charge capture is much higher than doing manual reconciliation at the end of the day on paper.

ICU documentation

The ICU manager will certainly benefit from most of the computerized applications mentioned, but online clinical charting in the unit is a tough challenge. Many otherwise-successful software vendors haven't quite solved the ICU charting issues satisfactorily.

ICUs are labor intensive, and the patients require a high number of nursing interventions. They're also highly dependent on equipment and procedure. However, the documentation tools built for noncritical care units usually don't present the unique picture of monitoring and care required for good ICU charting. ICU nurses want to see a graphic representation of physiologic signs that can be easily compared to infusion of medications or other mitigating factors. The flowsheet approach to patient documentation is a cornerstone of ICU charting.

Documentation is done by the ICU nurse on a real-time basis and, except for a complex bedside procedure or a patient taking a turn for the worse, charting isn't as great a stressor for the ICU staff as it is for the medical-surgical staff. New clinical applications for the ICU interface the monitoring system to the documentation system. While nurses continue to do assessments, narrative charting, and notes, much of the data is automatically recorded. The ability to trend vasoactive medication drips' action on vitals signs and monitor I.V.s by rate and quantity takes a lot of burden off of the staff. Critical care units can benefit from automated supply and pharmacy dispensing systems.

Ideally, the integrated clinical documentation system will be sophisticated enough to bring forward pertinent ICU data to the assessment and charting record when the patient goes to a step-down unit.

Barriers to computerization

For a nurse-manager, the biggest barrier to going forward with I.T. is a reluctant administration. Although a lack of capital funding for I.T. projects and a lack of support for their implementation on nursing units may have been common 10 years ago, the pressures on administrators today — with increased demands from government regulatory agencies, accrediting bodies, and insurance companies for fast accurate reporting — all lead to the installation of information management systems.

Unfortunately, the clinical documentation piece of the larger integrated system may not get the immediate attention (and funding) that it deserves. Nurse-managers should meet with their nursing officers to present to administration a united, knowledgeable appeal for clinical systems implementation that focuses on patient care, staff satisfaction, and cost savings. The return on investment might be difficult to quantify, but it's significant. Survey other facilities about their experiences with computerized information management; ask if they've done cost savings studies of their own that can get you started.

Staff resistance to change

The clinical nurse-manager is the ultimate change agent when it comes to implementing a nursing documentation, scheduling, time and attendance, or other large-scale software system. She must be forward thinking, and as one of the strongest lobbyists for these technologies she must be focused on the task of running the unit more efficiently and safely, with better patient outcomes. After all it's typically the manager who introduces the implementation to the staff, so be sure to do your homework.

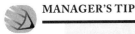

Selling technology

Many different strategies can be used to "sell" a new technology to a nursing unit staff. The manager should spend time with the implementation analysts or trainers to get a background in the features of the system. It's so much easier to allay the concerns of the staff if you can answer the questions they pose about the operation and implications of using the system. This point is probably the most crucial to winning over the staff to automation of some of their processes. The manager as a "super user" might spend time individually with apprehensive staffers to show some of the rudiments of the system and explain why the implementation is important for quality of care, resource management, or charge capture. Keep the lines of communiation open.

Usually, the project team installing a large system will ask the unit manager to recommend someone from the unit to be on the team. Choose a nurse who has the respect of the staff, is a critical thinker, and has shown interest in other unit and department projects. These implementation team members will probably be involved in building the clinical parts of the system, so select someone with a strong clinical background. She'll become an advocate for the system and a cheerleader for its acceptance by the staff.

Despite the benefits that automation offers, you'll inevitably have some staff nurses who resist the change. They may believe it to be a waste of time, too time-consuming, or not worth the trouble. They may be convinced that the new technology will degrade the standard of care on the unit. They may be afraid that they'll have so much difficulty learning the program that they won't be as well respected by their peers. Also, they may feel that their lack of language sophistication will be highlighted. The best strategy for handling such resistance is to spend time with these staff nurses to get to the root of why they're so resistant to the changes and reassure them with the benefits of automation.

Involve the staff nurses in the development and building of clinical input tools for their units. Their experience and expertise, especially on their own unit, will be invaluable. Best of all, these staff nurses will "buy in" to the system and become believers. (See *Selling technology.*)

Staffing instability

Before volunteering to be the next nursing unit to go forward with implementation of a departmental or facility-wide online documentation program, take a good look at the state of your unit's staff. If you have staffing shortages and the problem appears to be short-term, put off the implementation if possible. Moving from a paperbound system to an electronic-based system will put additional stress on your staff, which is already coping with float and agency nurses supplementing their numbers. With other pressing unit issues, it will be difficult to get the necessary buy-in and support for the project. What's more, implementation meetings can be difficult to organize in the face of unit vacancies, not to mention mobilizing staff resources to help build the nursing documentation tools.

Staff turnover

For optimal use of a sophisticated, integrated information system with clinical charting, a stable, well-trained staff of nurses must be in place. When this isn't the case, the nurse-manager and application educators must have a workable plan in place to get new staffers appropriate access and training as quickly as possible. No matter how thorough the training, there will still be a lot of catching up to do to reach the skill and efficiency on the system that only comes with experience. As part of the "new user" plan, postimplementation should have protocols for clinical setting mentoring and unit assignments. Hopefully, as nursing schools start to introduce more informatics into their curriculum, new graduates starting on your unit will learn the new system with a moderate amount of training and orientation.

Agency nurses' unfamiliarity

Probably the toughest issue for a nurse-manager on a unit that uses computerized documentation is continuing normal operations when short-term agency nurses are working on the unit. No matter how competent and professional these nurses are, they still need to be trained in how to use your unit's documentation system. If your facility is large or is affiliated with other facilities, lobby for creating an in-house staffing pool that can be trained on the system and given access as part of their orientation.

Need for adequate training and resources

For new technology to work effectively, the facility must provide the resources for training new staffers and retaining staff system upgrades. Staff shortages can stress the manager as well as the entire staff. Getting a new hire trained and familiar with the system as soon as possible requires coordination and cooperation with the trainers. They must have enough classes scheduled on the different applications not to impede the orientation process. If the unit educator carries out the training, you'll still need to develop a system to obtain appropriate access for new staff, usually through your I.T. security department.

Things break. Systems go down, and always at a bad time. Managers must have strict guidelines for reporting malfunctions, and for getting the word out to other caregivers. Use of PC workstation banner messaging, overhead paging, and beeper systems might be developed as part of systems downtime policy. Downtime policies aren't just a good idea; they're now a mandate of accreditation and regulatory agencies. The policies must be workable. Downtime procedures must be drilled on the unit and facility levels. There are different types and sources of failures, and the policies must cover them all. A downtime policy should plan for scheduled downtimes, such as system upgrades, and unscheduled downtimes such as system crashes. Both types of downtime should be broken down to cover brief outages and the major catastrophe. The recovery process will depend on the facility's status as to whether the electronic version or the paper printed out at discharge is the official chart.

Future trends for nursing use of I.T.

The shift toward knowledge-based practice that you see now will accelerate as the staff nurse gains more access to information. Use of evidence-based knowledge at the point of care will complement the trend toward more tailored outcomes oriented to planning and care. Structured data will provide better reporting and trending for health care research, financial information, performance improvement, and clinical operations.

The accessibility of the electronic medical record to all caregivers will foster a more holistic approach to patient care. The clinical chart will reflect a multidiscipline record. Information technology and health information management will become a prominent part of nursing school curriculum.

Hardware

Workstations will no longer exist in charting alcoves and at the nurse's station. They'll reside in the nurse's pocket. They'll be small and light, and they'll be easy to read and to enter data. They'll use biometrics to quickly log on a new user and to identify a patient, and they'll be cheap. Workstations that require a larger display will use touch-screen technology. All applications will be faster and more intuitive.

Accessing a patient's data will be as quick as using a swipe card to load demographics and health data in the ED. All physiologic monitoring will be wireless.

Medical and surgical technology development continues ahead at mach speed. Soon you'll have a noninvasive diagnostic chamber that will provide a complete scan and readout of a patient's condition, including hematology, chemistries, metabolic state, organ function, and so on.

Technologies soon to affect nurses include:

➤ wider use of telehealth, in underserved areas and education
➤ portable documentation devices, including handheld devices and mini-laptops
➤ wireless connectivity used inside and outside of health care facilities by nurses
➤ instant wireless links to orders management, laboratory results, and imaging reports
➤ handheld biosensor devices that take instant physiologic states and then transfer the data onto clinical documentation applications
➤ secure linkups between a patient's providers to integrate ambulatory and in-patient records
➤ greater use of "smart" identification tags available to seniors and children with demographic and health care information.

Points to remember

The following points summarize the importance of I.T. in nursing management:

➤ I.T. offers timesaving applications for staff management and communication, patient care, and documentation for accreditation.
➤ I.T can help increase job satisfaction and patient satisfaction by facilitating patient care and improving patient outcomes.
➤ Standardization of health care information is achieved through implementation of I.T. systems, which improves compliance with federal standards and accreditation agencies.
➤ Multidisciplinary care is more focused with proper use of I.T. because it offers easy communication between users.

Selected readings

Abbott, P., and Lee, S. "Informatics: A New Dimension in Nursing," *Imprint* 48(3):33, 51-52, April-May 2001.

Cherry, B. *Contemporary Nursing: Issues, Trends, and Management.* St. Louis: Mosby–Year Book, 2002.

Larrabee, J., et al. "Evaluation of Documentation Before and After Implementation of a Nursing Information System in an Acute Care Hospital," *CIN: Computers, Informatics, Nursing* 19(2):56, March-April 2001.

Parker, J., and Abbott, P. "The New Millennium Brings Nursing Informatics into the O.R.," *AORN Journal* 72(6):101-107, December 2000.

Rewick, D., and Caffey, E. "Nursing System Makes a Difference. Northwest IDS Reaps the Benefits of Using Automated Tools to Support Nursing," *Health Management Technology* 22(8):24-26, August 2001.

Staggers, N., et al. "Informatics Competencies for Nurses at Four Levels of Practice," *Journal of Nursing Education* 40(7):303-16, October 2001.

INDEX

Index